MW00844017

1. Acknowledge or another

2. GATHER How System should work (look like healthy) Universal design

3. SEE How it is

4. Evaluate the difference

5. Treat The MECHANISM FIRST, Then the STRAIN

7. Examine involuntary movement in non SD area. Compare c̄ SD area. Eval SD area after tx. IF involuntary movement similar function is restored. IF not - The base dysfunction has not been restored.

8. Evaluate Vitality. Do not go beyond the vitality level of the Pt. (quality of the vitality.

Life In Motion

Principle of PERMITED MOTION 226
Cranial Rhythm 10+4 /minute

RESPOND NOT REACT 319 + OTHERS
whiplash 319,
disipating TECHNIQUES 32#4
* clinical OBSERVATIONS 331-336 *
Sinus 348
MOTION OF FACIAL BONES 350

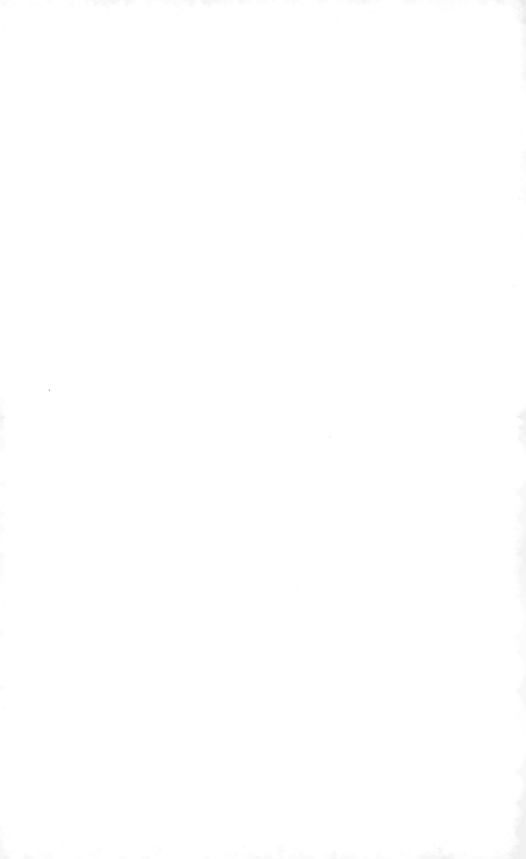

Life In Motion

The Osteopathic Vision
of Rollin E. Becker, D.O.

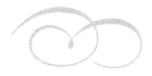

Edited by Rachel E. Brooks, M.D.

STILLNESS PRESS

Stillness Press, LLC
214 SE 14th Ave
Portland, Oregon 97214
phone/fax: 503.265.5002
www.stillnesspress.com

For ordering information see page 380.

Fifth Impression 2010: With Index added.

Edited by Rachel E. Brooks, M.D.
Book and cover design by Lubosh Cech
Cover: Close-up of a sculpture entitled "Dynamic Stillness." Photo by Duncan Soule.

Grateful acknowledgement is made to the American Academy of Osteopathy for permission to reprint, in edited form, articles that first appeared in the *Year Books* of the Academy of Applied Osteopathy. These articles include: "Force Factors With Body Physiology," "X...........Whiplash Injury," "Whiplash," and Parts I-IV of "Diagnostic Touch: Its Principles and Application."

(Previously published by Rudra Press, ISBN 0-915801-82-5)

ISBN 978-0-9675851-0-9

DEDICATED TO ARDATH BECKER

Contents

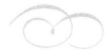

Chapter Seven: The Nature Of Trauma

Chapter Eight: Clinical Considerations

Foreword

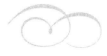

Rollin E. Becker, D.O., was among those students of William Garner Sutherland, D.O., D.Sc.(hon) who listened and thought about the meaning and the significance of what he learned. He was a physician who practiced osteopathy and also a teacher on Dr. Sutherland's associate faculty. It is fortunate that Dr. Becker wrote down something of what he learned from his study and also from his experience as an operator in the practice of osteopathy.

This collection of his writings reflects nearly 60 years of clinical experience. Even though the teaching of osteopathy is now over 100 years old, there is not a large body of literature developed from actual experience in osteopathic diagnosis and treatment of clinical problems. This book of Dr. Becker's work will make a significant contribution to that body of literature.

Dr. Becker told members of the classes of instruction provided by the Sutherland Cranial Teaching Foundation, Inc. that further learning would follow from their experience as operators in their own practices. This is true because no two patients are exactly alike when it comes to the diagnosis of problems in the body. There are many problems which the physician who practices osteopathy today meets in his patients' bodies that neither Dr. Still nor Dr. Sutherland ever saw. It is equally true that the osteopath today will probably not meet some of the problems Dr. Still found in his professional experience.

There is much information available today from the physical and biological sciences that aids in the diagnosis and understanding of how problems in body mechanics manifest in physiologic disturbances. Yet the simple mechanical principles of manual operations in the practice of osteopathy are just as sound today as when they were taught 100 years ago, and these simple principles carry within them the promise of something far-reaching. For as Dr. Sutherland said, "The possibilities in the Science of Osteopathy are as great as the magnitude of the Heavens."

It was with these "possibilities" in mind that Dr. Becker practiced osteopathy and learned from his patients' predicaments. And it was the exploration of these possibilities which gave him so much of value to say as a teacher.

–Anne L. Wales, D.O., D.Sc.(hon)

Preface

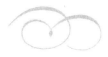

THIS PROJECT OF PUBLISHING the teachings of Rollin E. Becker, D.O., began in 1991 when I started to gather the available source materials. I had expected the quantity to be limited because Dr. Becker was known as a man of relatively few words in his conversations, and he was best known for emphasizing the same points over and over again. But, instead, my search was rewarded with a wealth and diversity of material. This current volume contains the written and verbal discussions he carried on in the public domain amongst his colleagues. A second volume will contain his more personal and private communications.

The material in this book spans a thirty-year period, from 1958 to 1988. It is derived from a variety of sources, which includes papers written for lectures to be presented and articles to be published, transcribed tape recordings of lectures given and conversations with his son (Donald Becker, M.D.), and outlines and notes jotted down for various uses. Given this variety of sources, it was not always possible to reference the quotations Dr. Becker used. In particular, the quotations he read in lectures often could not be fully credited.

Dr. Becker spoke and wrote in a free-ranging and idiosyncratic style. In the editing process, there has been an effort to keep the essence of that style, while at the same time improving the readability and accessibility of the information. Some of the repetition that existed has been edited out, but much remains. Whenever Dr. Becker wrote or spoke about any piece of a subject, he always was addressing the whole. In addition, the concepts he repeatedly emphasized bear repetition because they are only slowly grasped on an ever-deepening level. Also, the small but constant variations in his articulation of these ideas bring further understanding and insight. Dr. Becker often said this work cannot be taught, but it can be learned.

Dr. Becker always felt free to incorporate into his own communication the words of Drs. Andrew Taylor Still and William Garner Sutherland. In this text, the words of these two men often appear in formal quotations. However the informed reader will recognize other passing allusions to and use of Still's and Sutherland's words. The reader will also note that Dr. Becker's use of certain words is different at different times. In particular the meaning he implies by the terms "stillness," "potency," and "fulcrum" shows some subtle and not-so-subtle shifts over time and when used in different contexts.

Most of the pieces presented in this volume were edited to a moderate degree from their original form. This was done to improve readability and to remove extraneous or repetitive information. Careful attention was given to maintaining the meaning Dr. Becker intended. If ever there was any uncertainty as to what his meaning was, the ambiguity was left in place for the reader to ponder.

Only minor grammatical changes were made to the lecture, "Be Still and Know," because this piece, a special tribute to his teacher, Dr. Sutherland, had great personal meaning to Dr. Becker. On the other end of the spectrum, two sets of articles received extensive editing—they were rearranged and edited to about half their original length. The two sets are the series of "Diagnostic Touch" articles and the series on trauma, which includes "Force Factors With Body Physiology" and the articles on whiplash. Both sets of articles were originally published in the *Yearbook* of the Academy of Applied Osteopathy. They are reprinted here with permission from the American Academy of Osteopathy. A number of the items in this book were printed over the last six years in the newsletter of The Cranial Academy; most have been edited further since appearing there.

My thanks go to many people in connection with this project. No amount of appreciation can match the effort volunteered by Patricia Tarzian. She took this project to heart and contributed her considerable editorial skills to help this book achieve the level of quality a work of Dr. Becker's teachings deserves. Other people who gave support include Duncan Soule, M.D., Laura Washington, Julie Hankin, Harold Goodman, D.O., and the board of trustees of the Sutherland Cranial Teaching Foundation, Inc. I am also very grateful for the warm support for both me and this project that has come from the Becker family—his wife, Ardath, and his children, Don and Ginny.

Finally, I must express my gratitude to Dr. Rollin Becker himself. He touched and nourished a place deep inside me and gave me more than my life's work. He asked nothing in return except that I do the best I can with what was given. This book represents a part of that effort.

Introduction

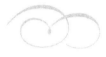

THROUGHOUT ITS HUNDRED YEARS of existence, the science and art of osteopathy has been passed on from hand to hand and heart to heart. Dr. Rollin E. Becker and his teachings represent a vital link in this continuity. He was both an inspired student and a compelling teacher.

Dr. Becker dedicated himself unendingly to being a student of osteopathy. After graduating from osteopathic college and practicing as he had been taught for some years, he found himself drawn to a more in-depth study of what Dr. Andrew Taylor Still, the founder of osteopathy, had to say. In Dr. Still's writings, he found a wealth of ideas for exploration as well as the specific guidance he needed to pursue his study.

Dr. Becker's endeavor to learn what Dr. Still had to teach was initially one of self-study. He shared his questions and ideas with colleagues, but ultimately the effort was carried out quietly in his office as he worked with his patients. After a few years of this type of study, he came to meet William G. Sutherland, D.O., the originator of the cranial concept in osteopathy. In the decade of their close association, Dr. Sutherland gave to Dr. Becker a method and forum for delving even deeper into his own studies and understanding.

The guidance of both Still and Sutherland led Dr. Becker to learn from the most authoritative source available—the living forces present within the living body. He became a ceaseless observer, continually seeking an answer to the question, What is *health* and what is the most efficient and effective way to help bring it about?

Osteopathy in Dr. Becker's hands focused on "Life in motion" and Stillness. He appreciated that everything alive is in motion–that Life itself manifests as motion. For him, one way of describing the state called health is the presence of totally free motion within a being on all levels. Helping patients to restore their health, then, requires that the restrictions to free motion be released.

While recognizing that life manifests as motion, he also understood that the power of life resides in Stillness. He recognized that there is a fundamental Potency or Power that exists within all things that are alive for as long as they are alive. All life springs forth from this power, and the nature of this power is stillness–a dynamic stillness full of potential and a stillness that one can learn to palpate as surely as one can palpate motion. These properties of life, motion, potency, and stillness are all available resources in the restoration of health.

Accepting this view of the nature of health leads to another key concept in Dr. Becker's practice and teaching. This is the understanding of the role of the physician. The physician no longer functions by deciding what the patient's problem is and then doing something to fix it. Dr. Becker always emphasized the view that the same stillness and life in motion exists within both the physician and the patient. Within the patient, these properties represent the self-correcting capacities that are continually in operation. And the physician, through his or her conscious awareness and hands-on contacts, is able to arouse these health mechanisms within the patient to a more effective level of functioning.

Dr. Becker lived the osteopathy that he taught–being both simple and profound. His understanding of health and healing was profound, as was his capacity to apply it for the benefit of his patients and students. Yet this great depth of understanding was always delivered in the simplest and most direct way possible. He met the needs of each person who came to him as best he could and strove to learn something more about life from each encounter.

Osteopathy and the Cranial Concept

The science of osteopathy was discovered in 1874 by Dr. Andrew Taylor Still, a medical physician ardently searching for a more effective system of healing. His intense study brought insights that led him to articulate a number of fundamental principles. He taught that the structure of the body and how it functions are inextricably linked and that each person contains within himself the resources necessary for health. He also maintained that the body is a unit of function—that body, mind, and spirit operate as a unified whole continually working to heal itself. Dr. Still conceived of all diseases and ailments as involving some impairment in the free flow of the material and energetic elements within the body, thereby impeding the self-correcting process within.

Based on an understanding of these principles, Dr. Still developed an approach which used the physician's knowledge, understanding, and hands as the primary tools in both diagnosis and treatment. The college he established taught the full array of medical and surgical knowledge, but Dr. Still's emphasis always remained on a thorough understanding of anatomy and physiology and the application of palpatory skills. Over time, various osteopathic manipulative approaches have been developed to apply these principles to the treatment of patients.

It was in 1892 that Dr. Still established the American School of Osteopathy in Kirksville, Missouri, and in the class of 1900 was a man named William Garner Sutherland. While a student at the college, Dr. Sutherland also had a flash of insight into the inherent mechanisms within the human body. He had the thought strike him that the bones of the living cranium maintain a movement throughout life which indicates the presence of a type of respiration. Through dedicated study, observation, and self-experimentation over a period of 40 years, Dr. Sutherland worked out the details of this respiratory mechanism. He then spent the last 15 years of his life teaching others this *cranial concept* and the practical application of it to patient care, which became known as *cranial osteopathy* or *osteopathy in the cranial field*. In all his teaching, Dr. Sutherland never failed to emphasize that the cranial concept was only an extension of, not apart from, Dr. Still's science of osteopathy.

Dr. Sutherland's discovery went far beyond the description of a mechanical system; he came to understand that the movement he observed is the basic life force in operation. It is a manifestation of life in motion—an outward sign of the fundamental self-regulating, self-healing mechanisms in the body.

Because of this mechanism's fundamental nature and its rhythmic quality, Dr. Sutherland termed it the *primary respiratory mechanism* (also called the *craniosacral mechanism*). He described five components of this mechanism that function as a unified whole. The five components are: 1) the fluctuation of the cerebrospinal fluid, with the potency of the tide; 2) the inherent motility of the central nervous system; 3) the mobility of the cranial and spinal dural membranes (reciprocal tension membrane); 4) the articular mobility of the cranial bones; and 5) the involuntary mobility of the sacrum between the ilia.

Having come to an understanding of the anatomy and physiology of this subtle but powerful mechanism, Dr. Sutherland was also able to establish treatment principles for working *with* this mechanism. He developed an approach, using hands-on manipulation, that was as subtle and powerful as the mechanism it was working with. Dr. Sutherland's approach to treatment can be summarized in his injunction, "Allow physiologic functioning within to manifest its own unerring potency, rather than apply blind force from without."

The understanding and approach taught by Dr. Sutherland was never limited to the cranial mechanism. This primary respiratory mechanism is represented in all of body physiology. Therefore, while it is uniquely suited to treat problems in the cranial field, it can potentially effect any situation arising from disease or trauma in the body.

Dr. Sutherland developed a course of instruction to teach physicians the necessary understanding and palpatory skills to begin to treat patients in this way. His dedicated students, including Dr. Rollin Becker, continued these courses, and in this way, Dr. Sutherland's work has been passed on.

Biographical Information

Rollin E. Becker (1910-1996) grew up in an osteopathic household. His father, Arthur D. Becker, D.O., was a prominent and respected osteopath, serving on the faculty with Dr. Andrew Taylor Still and later as dean of two osteopathic colleges. Rollin graduated from the American School of Osteopathy (later renamed the Kirksville College of Osteopathic Medicine) in 1934, and following a few years in Oklahoma, he moved to Michigan, where he practiced for thirteen years.

In 1944, after about a decade in Michigan, he met William Garner Sutherland, D.O. In 1948, he first served on the teaching faculty at one of Dr. Sutherland's courses. Dr. Becker moved to Texas in 1949, where he practiced until 1989. Throughout that time, he continued to serve Dr. Sutherland and his work. Dr. Becker was the president, from 1962 through 1979, of the Sutherland Cranial Teaching Foundation, an educational organization dedicated to perpetuating the teachings of W. G. Sutherland.

For more information on the Sutherland Cranial Teaching Foundation, Inc., see page 371.

To Study And Practice Osteopathy

A DEEP OCEAN OF STUDY

*This is an edited transcription of a lecture given in 1982
at a Sutherland Cranial Teaching Foundation basic course in
Alexandria, Virginia.*

THERE IS A TREMENDOUS transition that has to take place now, to bring
that which you have been using in your practice to that which you are
going to be exposed to during this week. As the faculty, our primary
job is to help you cross that bridge with as much comfort as possible.
At the same time, however, I can assure you that what we're going to
be doing this week is nothing but hard work.

As part of the bridge that we're going to use to make this transition, I have written on the blackboard the basic osteopathic principles you were taught in the colleges. There are four of them: 1) The
body is a unit; 2) The body possesses self-regulatory mechanisms;
3) Structure and function are reciprocally interrelated; 4) Rational
therapy is based upon an understanding of the body unit's self-regulatory mechanism and the body's interrelationship of structure and
function. These are principles you've heard all your practice lives,
from the time you were a freshman in osteopathic college. We all
agree that these are beautiful statements. But how many of you realize, as you hear and read these statements, that we're talking about a
living mechanism? Most of us come away from our schooling seeing
how things apply to the cadaver that's on the table, with the sense
that we can do anything to it we want.

In this week's work, we are talking about a *living* body as a unit, a
living self-regulatory mechanism, a *living* structure and function that
is reciprocally interrelated, and a *living* therapy based on this understanding. These mechanisms are already alive, they are healthy. That
is why we are here today. We now find it necessary to take on the
added responsibility of working with a living mechanism, making it

do the work for us rather than us doing something to it. We are here to learn how this mechanism works for us and that there are rules and regulations that allow us to make it work for us. There are ways to encourage it into an action of cooperation that we can then cooperate with. We don't do something to it, we cooperate with it, because it's already working for us.

So the purpose of this course is to teach health and function as expressed by anatomicophysiological functioning mechanisms. We're here to learn how our body and mind, our various units of function, are working for us in health. We're not here to teach the anatomy and physiology of a craniosacral mechanism; those are just the tools we're going to play with, be taught by, and learn from. We're not here just to learn to diagnose and treat disease and trauma in this mechanism; we're here to learn how health is delivered from within a living mechanism. This requires that we come to understand that we each have a primary physician within, which includes the craniosacral mechanism—you can't separate them, it's all the same unit. We come to understand that there is a primary physician within us that knows exactly what health is and is constantly delivering that health to the surface, provided we will listen to that primary physician.

This living physician within us is always manifesting health. From the time you were conceived until the time you kick the bucket, it is constantly manifesting health for you. For every decade of your life, you have a pattern of life that is right for you. If you're in your twenties, you've got a health pattern that literally is an expression of that decade. It matures as each of us does and gradually changes gears, but it is constantly manifesting health.

Patients come to us for the reason that their health pattern has gotten clouded over a little bit and it's raining on them, but that doesn't change the fact that above that cloud, there's a sun still shining and health is still available. It's up to us to deliver the health pattern from within the traumatic or diseased condition and allow health to be the only pattern left. In this sense, our position as a physician is secondary. It is our responsibility as the secondary physician to work with

4

the primary physician within ourselves and within our patients to allow physiologic function within to manifest its own unerring potency—to bring this health pattern through to the surface.

To practice in this way we have to go deep into another ocean of understanding and allow physiologic function within the patient to literally train us. We seek to learn: Where is health in this patient? How do I get it to the surface? The body physiology of the patient is literally training us. The physician within my patients has been training me for the last forty-eight years, and I'm still a student. This is part of the transition we have to make.

We want to learn to feel and be aware of these mechanisms working within us as well as in our patients. During this week when you are being the patient, allow yourselves to feel these mechanisms at work as the student-doctor attempts to feel those same mechanisms working within you. This is a way to begin to feel function.

To achieve the goals we've laid out here, there are three steps to go through and the first one is the most difficult one. First, you have to accept the fact that the anatomicophysiological function within you and within the patient is living, is already in motion, and is available for your evaluation and use. You have to accept that fact—close your eyes and step across a border and hope there's still some floor there when you touch down on the other side of that border. All of a sudden, you are secondary to the very thing you are working on. The primary boss is inside. The primary boss is in you and in your patients. The secondary physician is going to learn to understand and use it.

Secondly, we need to study the details of the anatomicophysiological mechanism in a living body. We need to understand that the living anatomicophysiological details of the primary respiratory mechanism, of the craniosacral mechanism, are not a separate unit of function or study. We are adding these details to the anatomy and physiology we learned in school. When I went to my first class with Dr. William Garner Sutherland, I told him I had not come to learn his work, I had come to extend my knowledge of anatomy and physiology to include

5

the craniosacral mechanism, which we had not been taught in school. Dr. Sutherland gave that to the profession and now we are giving it to you. You are here to continue your study of the anatomy and physiology of the living body, which includes the primary respiratory mechanism.

The third step is that we have to develop living palpatory skills. To work with living mechanisms in a living body, we need living palpatory skills. It is these palpatory skills that are going to give us the chance to evaluate and make use of the working units of the body to allow them to self-treat the patient. Patients get a self-treatment every time we put our hands on them, if we will cooperate with the mechanisms that are already at work.

LIFELONG STUDENTS

This is an edited transcription of a lecture given in 1986 at a Sutherland Cranial Teaching Foundation faculty development program in Philadelphia, Pennsylvania.

WHAT IS A PHYSICIAN? The role of a physician is to serve mankind. The science of osteopathy begins with the manifesting structure and function of the individual. It is expressed as a fluid drive, motile, mobile mechanism within body physiology. It is expressed as an experience from within the patient, and it is expressed as a self-taught, trained, palpatory skill in the physician. The work of A.T. Still gave us the science of osteopathy. The work of W.G. Sutherland gave us the primary respiratory mechanism with its detailed anatomy and physiology, not as a separate component of the work of Dr. Still but as an integrated unit with the science of osteopathy.

An important point to keep in mind is that from the moment of their respective discoveries, Drs. Still and Sutherland accepted the science of osteopathy as a fundamental living law in body physiology and accepted the need to become lifetime students of the authority vested within the living body physiology. They ceased to be physicians—they became students. They were no longer searching for something, they had found osteopathy; they became students of the science of osteopathy for the rest of their lives. Drs. Still and Sutherland became lifetime students, as all physicians who follow in their footsteps will find it necessary to be—to consent to be used by the same set of living laws in their service to mankind.

We're not here to remember the works of Still or Sutherland; we are here to become students of the laws of the mechanism that was their discovery. These laws are available, they're an open space. Still and Sutherland became students and gave of themselves. They gave the work to their followers, but they only gave clues to their followers, knowing the doctors themselves had to become students of the work. The challenge in the practice of the science of osteopathy is to consider the body physiology as a whole—its structure and function as a unity—to accept this voluntary-involuntary fluid drive, motile, mobile mechanism as a manifesting transmutation from the authority invested in body physiology. As physicians, we need to develop palpatory skills which allow the physician to be used by the physiology of the patient. We need to accept the primary respiratory mechanism as a working unit within the science of osteopathy and incorporate this unit of function into the whole picture of health and/or dysfunction within the body physiology of the patient.

We need to diagnose and treat the body as a whole. We must not separate it into a somatic portion and a cranial portion but instead treat it as a whole, one within the other. The science of osteopathy also shares the function of health and dysfunction as one unit. It's up to the physician to reason with the body physiology of the patient, to learn from it as a unit and learn to avoid the trap of separating the various units of the body. When you're working on any one part, you're in contact with all parts. You're listening and feeling through one part, but you are hearing the whole as you work. If you keep that open-door attitude toward the work, it becomes more than just a unit—it becomes a whole unit.

When you learn to listen to the body physiology of the patient, you may not look like you are doing anything outwardly, but you're working hard; it's hard work to listen for any length of time. But you can learn to do it, and you have the rest of your practice life. Still and Sutherland did it, I don't know why you can't. Dr. Still and Dr. Sutherland were students. They spent their entire lives studying the science of osteopathy, and one of the fundamental things they learned was that there is no time in which you can ever quit learning about the science of osteopathy. They consented to be used by the fundamental laws that are within each body physiology. They learned to know and use the rules of health as they apply within us, and it is these rules that are sought in the restoration to health for any dysfunction, disease, or trauma for which the patient is seeking service. Dr. Still and Dr. Sutherland studied every single mechanism within the body physiology as it applied to a given patient, and they were taught by each individual case the appropriate diagnostic and treatment program. They were taught by that which the body itself was trying to do.

What is new in the science of osteopathy? The answer is simple: the next patient who walks in the office, the one who has been everywhere and tried everything. The body physiology is the teacher and the physician is the student. The mechanism of body physiology offers many doors for experimentation to promote better health. You, as the physician-student, create techniques based on understanding the mechanism, visualizing what you think should be for that area, and then developing techniques as you understand the mechanism for each individual case and each individual patient. In other words, you are allowed lots of room for experimentation, as long as you obey the laws of the science of osteopathy. You get results in proportion to your knowledge and your developing sense of touch. We, as students of body physiology, as physicians, can use and be used by the body physiology of the patient in the care of each individual patient. The future is very bright for those who choose to study and use the works of Dr. Still and Dr. Sutherland. Thank you.

STEPS TO TAKE

These are excerpts from various lecture notes ranging from 1969-1986.

THE FUNDAMENTAL PRINCIPLES OF osteopathy were totally valid in 1874 at the birth of osteopathy and their truths become more valid with each passing decade. Modern-day research is proving the validity of these truths with its increasingly sensitive instrumentation. Even finer instrumentation is going to be required to prove other truths given to us by Dr. A.T. Still and Dr. W.G. Sutherland.

Our job, as osteopathic physicians, is to bring these truths into a workable, practical day-to-day experience wherein we can apply them on a one-on-one basis for each clinical problem and each clinical visit.

The basic principles of A.T. Still are not a give-away program for the instant understanding of a living body physiology in health and in trauma/disease; they are a earn-a-way program for the self-taught physician to develop his understanding of these complex living mechanisms. Each living anatomicophysiological mechanism provides a living demonstration of its innate functioning in health and in trauma/disease

The key to an understanding of the principles presented is that the physician must make the initial change in his whole concept of being a physician. He cannot keep his old concepts as he has practiced them with his patients; he cannot try to adopt these new concepts by simply trying to apply them towards his patients. He must change his way of thinking first and seek understanding within himself, until he

10

is comfortable with his new tools. His second step is to apply them to his patients' needs.

Steps:
1. Accept the Living Mechanism in you and the patient.
   Life is always trying to express health.
2. Surrender comes after acceptance.
   Accept the fact that what the mechanism is telling you is *true*.
3. Develop palpatory skills.
   The body is smarter than you are, so learn to learn from it.

Step one is the hardest, but it is the essential step in the understanding and use of *living* health mechanisms. Seek and learn the mechanisms of living function within yourself first, and it will lead you to understand it in your patients.

Step two is to become a beholder of *living* functions at work. Surrender to the patients.

Step three is to develop a *living* palpatory skill. Palpation is the tool the physician uses to read what the primary physician in each of us is doing to deliver health from within. Learn to *feel* function within, not merely gross or fine movements.

Did you think you came to this course to acquire information? To develop palpatory skills? To become knowledgeable in services to give to your patients and their problems?

No, you have come to *be* the work you are going to understand and to use in your service to your patients.

HELP IS ALWAYS THERE

This is an edited transcription of lectures given in 1988 at a Sutherland Cranial Teaching Foundation continuing studies course and faculty development program in Tulsa, Oklahoma.

I CAME ACROSS A newspaper article called, "Help That is Always There." It is the story of an international organization that has developed a phone network to serve people seeking help. There are various lessons we can learn from the way this organization functions which can, by analogy, be related to the way we treat as physicians. The principles these people use in their work can be adapted to all who are seeking to help others.

The "Help" phone lines are staffed 24 hours a day by trained volunteers who respond to all who call—the young and old, the rich and poor, the ailing, the hopeless, the suicidal, even those who are just plain lonely. The secret of their method is not in what the volunteers say over the phone but in how they listen to those in need.

Volunteers at the "Help" centers learn that listening, even by telephone, is a form of helping. They learn that listening in a particular way to someone in need is, in and of itself, a real response if the person seeking help can, in turn, try to help themselves. The volunteers do not give orders or instructions, they do not preach or teach. They do not say to do this or that or suggest that they know what is bothering the person. Instead, they are taught to listen to what these people are saying without making judgments, to listen to them without trying to analyze them or their problems. In responding to a caller, they speak in a nonjudgmental way. Their goal is to elicit a simple response, something that may help the person to look inside themselves.

In the "Help" method, they also teach that when you are being asked for help, you should try to reiterate the problem as it was expressed by the person seeking help so that he or she can hear how it sounds to other people. Don't assume you understand the problem. Let the person in need express their feelings themselves. Let the person asking for help suggest and move toward their own solution. It is better, for instance, for you to ask, "How are you going to handle this?" rather than to tell them what you would do to handle it. You want to help them find that their own strength is good, no matter how limited it may seem. In this way, the volunteers help callers to use their own best resources and to share their feelings in a more constructive way. Finally, the "Help" method teaches that it is good to empathize and make clear that you do care what happens to the person asking for your help. You do care that they have asked for help and you do care for them as a person.

These are the principles and skills that make the "Help" method work. This method of verbal contact takes training, but its principles are simple to learn and all of us are capable of practicing them in our own lives.

As I stand up here and talk, I want you to listen to what goes on in your mind as you are called on to help. The point to bear in mind is to know your own feelings about the person you are addressing, to accept that person exactly as he is—a person as worthy as yourselves. Listen and respond to him without making judgments about him. People feel a lot freer around somebody who is quietly accepting them for what they are. It is for you to just remain relaxed in the presence of nothing going on. Simply to be present in an atmosphere like that is a healing thing. It is actually this *caring, listening* response, and not a showing or doing response, which makes the osteopathic manipulative treatment work.

Carl Rodgers expressed a similar understanding in his book *On Becoming a Person*. He wrote that, in essence, helping is not giving, it is sharing. He taught that we can help others if we understand and project our real feelings without making judgments and if we accept these people in need of help warmly, as people who are just as worthy as those of us who think we are healthy. People will respond to the value that we place upon them by gaining confidence and moving forward to help themselves.

We have now bridged over from being a volunteer working on a verbal basis to being a physician working in the science of osteopathy. Consider that when a patient walks into the office, she is bringing in a body physiology seeking your help. Instead of verbalizing this help to the patient, we are going to learn to palpate and silently examine the body's physiology. Learn to silently work with that patient, using your skillful sense of touch to allow health to be restored. Instead of simply listening to words, we are silently listening to and understanding the body physiology. Instead of verbally discussing the situation, we are going to physically practice learning how to feel these things, to listen to what is going on within that patient. The patient doesn't need to utter a word, nor do I. I don't need to talk as I am practicing the art of listening to their tissues.

In the analogy of the physician as a volunteer, the physician's secret for success is to train and teach his palpatory skill to listen to the total and specific involuntary mechanisms of a patient's anatomico-physiology that is seeking help. Develop the palpatory skill to literally feel the questions that the patient comes in with. The help the patient is seeking can be matched and coordinated by the listening response that the physician is developing with his palpatory skills. The patient is seeking help, the body physiology is seeking help, and instead of talking about it, we position our hands very carefully upon our patient to find something, work with it, and tease it until we realize that the body physiology of the patient is making some kind of response towards health. The physician must learn to read these things happening within the body physiology, to experience and share the problems of that body physiology, and we do not need to explain it verbally to the patient. The patient is going to feel this contact we have put upon their body, the patient is going to be aware of the fact

14

that health is being shared. When we are a volunteer who listens and allows a patient's body physiology to be the teacher, that physiology will do the talking. In creating changes deep within the patient's physiology, the patient is experiencing these changes, and I, as a physician, am learning from sharing the experience.

It is very difficult to describe what it is we are doing, but it is not so important what we say—it is what we do. I generally don't say anything to the patient during the treatment. I experience them, listen to them, and work with them, not with techniques but with an understanding of the body physiology. The deeper the physician goes within himself to listen to the activity of the body physiology of the patient through his palpatory contact, the greater will be the data shown to the physician in his examination. Accept what is taught to you by the body physiology of the patient. Active listening on the part of the physician arouses the body physiology to go to work. It is going to start helping the patient, and you don't have to think about it or discuss it. You just have to observe it by listening and literally feeling through your palpatory skills. Work very quietly with the patient, be a silent partner, be an active listener.

USING THE ALIVENESS

This is an edited transcription of a lecture given in 1986
at a Sutherland Cranial Teaching Foundation basic course
in Philadelphia, Pennsylvania.

WE HAVE BEEN TALKING about how you have to accept the fact that both you and your patients are alive, and I'd like to discuss briefly the way to use this aliveness as part of your daily practice. I find it improves the efficiency of how I take care of my patients, and I'm going to pass it on to you purely as a suggestion. To begin with, I find it necessary to totally accept the fact that there is a basic primary rhythmic interchange taking place in all that is alive. It is an alternating, beautiful, primary respiratory mechanism-in-action, and I accept the aliveness of this rhythmic motion.

Next, I accept that the sole purpose of any of us being a physician is to learn to serve mankind. In my own practice, I have learned that in order to prepare myself to serve mankind, I first need to quietly still myself within, as part of getting ready to see patients. Having quietly stilled myself, the next step is that I quietly recognize the stillness within that patient I am about to see. This can be done within a matter of fifteen seconds or so, even in the same breath. And all of this can happen while the patient is waiting to see me, before he even gets into the treatment room with me.

Now I have identified, in the stillness that I've sought within myself, a kind of invisible contact with this rhythmic, fluctuating pattern; I am automatically responding to this involuntary movement of the Tide within me. When I tune into a relative stillness within the patient, even before I start working, I am in tune with the very foundation of that patient's being, which is also a similar, tide-like movement. It may not be at the same rate that mine is, but that's not important, it's the same mechanism. In this way, I'm quieting myself so I can silently introduce myself to the patient. I haven't seen him yet, but I'm quietly recognizing that the patient has the same mechanism that I have. Only then do I let the patient into the treatment room. I can then do whatever needs to be done; I work without regard to what I hope to accomplish for that patient. I simply go to work.

This little introduction from within myself, recognizing my own stillness within the patient, is a silent admission that *it is alive*. This is an invisible acknowledgment or realization. Even if you see 45 patients a day, you can allow for this very brief moment to contact a point of silence within yourself and then a point of silence within the patient. Then, no matter how you work with the patient, that's forty-five times a day you have recognized something within yourself and within the patient that is silently going to assist in the program of treatment. What that something is, I have no idea and it isn't important. It's merely the fact of identifying with a mechanism that is in existence within each one of us and putting it to use.

This quieting will guide you as to what needs to be done for that particular day, and I am convinced that the patient doesn't have to consciously participate. I treat a lot of patients who haven't the foggiest idea of what I am doing, but nevertheless they like it because they sense something is happening within themselves. They feel as if, finally, a doctor has gotten ahold of something that belongs to them and is trying to help them. Sometimes they do suspect I am not doing anything, but in the end they know I am because they are making a clinical response.

So this contact acts as a quiet assurance, and it also gives me a few moments break between patients. When you get a case that really tears you apart, and some of them do, you don't want to carry all that garbage with you to the next patient. If you have the opportunity, take a bit longer with this process. Allow three-quarters of a minute to sit down somewhere and just let them wash out, flush them out. You are through with them when they leave the office, you don't even know their name. Then, quiet yourself and ask the next patient to come into the office. Even when it is not a tough case, as a patient leaves, you can also quietly be aware of the fact that something has happened during the time they were in the office. You don't have to say a word about it. This is just a silent interchange between the silence of me and the silence of the patient—no names are involved, no techniques are involved, no nothing's involved. It's just a quiet blending of the fact that you are ready for the next patient, and the patient is ready for you.

I never treat a patient unless they specifically ask for it. I refuse to let a wife make an initial appointment for her husband; the patient has to call me directly to get an appointment. Because if they don't, they often come in with a chip on both shoulders. Occasionally somebody does get pushed into my office; then I'll make a very brief examination and say, "Yes, I find some problems here and there. Go on home, forget it, and if you ever want to do something about it, give me a ring." Maybe six months or two years later, they will finally call me. Then they have accepted the proposition that maybe they need some help. Fifty percent of the fight is getting them to admit that they need some help. Once they accept that fact, by the time they enter the office, they've already started to work on their own problem; they've accepted the idea of getting a treatment in the first place.

Although I said this quieting will guide you, I don't use this silent quieting to make a diagnosis—it only sets the stage. It's simply accepting the fact that there is an aliveness, a livingness within the patient's body, so why not challenge it? We're not asking it to make a diagnosis, we're not asking for anything except the pure fact of including the aliveness. In trying to serve patients, I get better results knowing that the aliveness within them is there just as much as it is within me. This is not a matter of learning something; this is a matter of using something, using an unknown factor which is going to contribute to your health and the patient's health. You will have to see if this invisible action of quietly setting things up makes a difference in your practice. I'm convinced it does in mine and I'm comfortable doing it.

RELAX, THERE'S NO HURRY

The Mechanism Has No Problems

*This is an edited transcription of a lecture given in 1986
at a Sutherland Cranial Teaching Foundation basic course
in Philadelphia, Pennsylvania.*

I'D LIKE TO TELL you an interesting story about one of the experiences I had with Dr. Will Sutherland. At a course in Denver, Colorado studying the science of osteopathy, one of the physicians in the class brought a patient to the course for consultation. The man had been in a tractor accident and had developed a pattern of convulsive seizures. The doctor had been working on the patient but believed they weren't really getting anywhere, and so the doctor asked Dr. Sutherland to check the patient and see what else could be done to help the patient.

Now, Dr. Sutherland was a very taciturn type who never bothered to waste ten words when he could say it in one. He examined the patient and finally turned to the doctor whose case it was and said, "I think you're on the right track, just keep up the good work." Then, as Dr. Sutherland started to leave to go back to his chair, the doctor in charge of the case said, "Dr. Sutherland, just a minute please. What would you do if the patient were to have a convulsion while you were trying to help him?" Dr. Sutherland simply said, "Lock him up," and kept on walking. Well, I happened to be sitting where I could see the audience, and there were thirty blank faces. "Lock him up" was all he said. He expected us to go back to our patients' mechanisms and figure out what he meant. So he was a great man to teach you the mechanism by allowing the mechanism to teach you itself.

So we can relax, rejoice and quit worrying about it. We have to accept the fact that life is already functioning in both the physician and the patient, so we might as well relax. We're not going anywhere and your patients are also going to be around. The patient has to take the responsibility and come in to see you, and they're not going to run away unless you really louse them up badly. They're going to be around, and most are going to be willing to come back again for another visit. So I mean it sincerely—relax.

You're here at this course to spend five days learning about what these patients are carrying around in their mechanisms, which happens to be what you're carrying around in your own mechanism. I don't see any particular reason to hurry, to rush into this knowledge that you've been gaining this week. Accept the fact that you're already here. You and your patient already are at work, quietly doing the things within that are required to be done to maintain the health pattern. Patients aren't in any particular hurry. They may act as if they're in a hurry, but their mechanism isn't in any hurry, not one bit. I don't worry about the fact that the patient may have to come back again for another visit just because I didn't hear the mechanism as clearly as I should. Perhaps I didn't get quite the results I was supposed to get. Nevertheless, I am permitted to see that patient again in the next office visit, and so I can relax and enjoy and try to work from that which is in front of me.

The mechanisms within the body physiology have no problems whatsoever, none. They are literally at work within each one of us. They're doing the best job they can to keep us alive. Even if they acquired a problem through an accident, birth trauma or some environmental pattern and their mechanism isn't in accord with what it's supposed to be, they are also bringing the solution for that problem. Some problems do require outside help; they require surgery, complicated medicine, or other supplemental help. But the mechanism itself is not aware of this. If it has some strain patterns within itself, it very quietly also has the tools with which to allow itself to be corrected again. So we, the physicians, should be the willing servants who will take ahold of this mechanism within a patient and cooperate in this effort to help itself.

The mechanism itself will teach us. Yes, patients do have problems—they wouldn't be in our offices if they didn't. But we don't have to hurry or rush to find out what is and what isn't, where it's going and what it's doing. We have to quietly accept the fact that both the physician and the patient are alive and functioning, and the rules for the game are built into the patient's mechanisms. Patients don't think in these terms. They think in terms of symptoms, they think in terms of suffering, they think in terms of this, that, and the other. But the mechanism isn't suffering, it's quietly doing its work. If there is a strain pattern—for example, an occipitomastoid type of lesion in the base of the skull—brother, that is a problem, but the occipitomastoid lesion does not realize it is a problem. It's busy practicing being an occipitomastoid lesion. So we've got to go to that occipitomastoid lesion and quietly ask it, "Look, you may enjoy life as you see fit, but that body you're living in isn't enjoying it too much. Now, why don't you consider allowing me to get my hands on you in such a way that you can modify your approach and cease to be a so-called lesion complex?"

We are given the right, the privilege, and the mechanism within us to understand that occipitomastoid lesion within the patient. We have an occipitomastoid mechanism within our own head which may not be in lesion, but we can understand this mechanism we're studying from within us. We are certainly going to understand it better as we get our hands on the people who come to us.

The very mechanisms that require health are also the mechanisms that can express health. They work and are in constant motion; they are always working towards the very goal we have within us. We fight— we live—in order to express health within ourselves. All we're asked, all we're being told by the next patient who walks into the office is, "That's all I'm asking for, Doctor. I would like to express health within me, and I've been told that you understand the mechanisms within you and within myself that will allow me to restore myself to health." We do not have to hurry about it. We can answer, "We've got 'x' number of minutes for the visit this time. We'll do what we can; we'll give a little direction here, a little direction there, and now you go take that home with you and you put it to work. Quietly just live your daily life, follow some suggestions, come back again next week, and we will continue our efforts to help each other." Quietly, the patient kind of joins with the mechanism within me, and I quietly join with the mechanism within the patient; we quietly try to work in an atmosphere in which we mutually exchange ideas and capacities for function, and we then just quietly ease on.

When you go home from this course, all these mechanisms within you are going to work on the mechanisms within the patients, and both of you are going to have fun. Take care.

Getting Started

This is an edited transcription of a lecture given in 1976 at a Sutherland Cranial Teaching Foundation basic course in Milwaukee, Wisconsin.

NOW, I WOULD LIKE for you to just sit quietly for a moment or two and let what you have had for the last four and a half days at this course soak into your system as something that has occurred for the total internal, involuntary, physiological mechanisms of your being. Quit thinking about the details of what you have learned for a moment. Sit up straight in your chairs, focus your attention on your own Sutherland fulcrum, and quietly feel four and a half days work in your own being.[1] Let it soak into your being and also let it return back to where it came from. We've brought you materials, understanding, and concepts; we've brought you a lot of things, and it has to be returned to where it came from. So let it return right back to the source from whence it came because that's the thing that's making it work anyway. Just sit there and just idle at the interchange between that which has come in and that which should be returned—this settles it down, it's a stillpoint.

Fine. Thank you. Now, why did we do this? What I want you folks to do when you go home to your practices is not to take this vast accumulated knowledge and charge into practice as if, "Now I've got something!" Take this information, this knowledge, this experience back into your practice and do exactly what you've been doing in your practices; look at your patients exactly the way you did before you took the course. Unfortunately, you won't be able to, but allow this information just to be there.

When you go home and decide to do something for a patient, first consult the stillness within your self, and immediately, as fast as a snap of the fingers, something happens. In this way, as you lay your hands on this patient, you discover your hands and your mind and their body are beginning to integrate, and you will begin to better understand what you need to do for this patient that day. Consult your own Sutherland fulcrum when you contact this patient–consult your own Sutherland fulcrum and the stillness.

Let's get back down to earth. When you get home to your practice, allow this knowledge to become a part of what is available to meet the needs of the patient. Don't project it out–the patients themselves are going to show you the need to try what you have learned. It's like when you study for a state board exam. You study like crazy, cramming all kinds of information in, and you're not certain where it is going. You just study and read and soak it into your being. Then you throw all the textbooks out the window and go to the exam, and somehow the information flows out that you need for that examination.

So allow a few days for this course to soak into your being before you attempt to use it–use it comfortably. Let the knowledge of the motion of the temporal bones; sphenobasilar patterns; individual, specific, membranous articular strains; condylar parts; the fluid dynamics of the living fluctuation fluid; the to-and-fro movement of a reciprocal tension membrane; and an articular mobility of a bony skull and a sacrum between the ilia–let those things just kind of soak into your being for a few days. Introduce these new diagnostic tools to yourself gradually. The patients who will be walking into your office when you get home are the same patients you have been treating for the "x" number of years you have been in practice, and if they have not had the benefits of this approach before, a few days more isn't going to make that much difference.

---

1. The "Sutherland fulcrum" is the name given to the area of the straight sinus, where the falx cerebri adjoins the tentorium cerebelli. It is considered the fulcrum for the dural, reciprocal tension membrane.

BE STILL AND KNOW
A Dedication to William G. Sutherland, D.O.

This paper was presented on September 22, 1965 in Philadelphia,
Pennsylvania as the Sutherland Memorial Lecture. It was then printed
in the December 1965 newsletter of The Cranial Academy.

THE THEME OF THIS paper is the continuous recognition of the necessity of "being still in order to know" through the most direct Channel possible, that of being closer to your Maker than mere material breathing. It should have as a better subtitle, "A *Re*dedication to William G. Sutherland." When one thinks of a dedication to a man who has given a great service to mankind, there is a tendency to think of it as something that happened when he was alive and that this is a new day and filled with new discoveries. A rededication, on the other hand, is a living thing, a continuing experience, an unfolding understanding, and the promise of greater truths to follow. Such was the work of William Garner Sutherland. He brought to us an understanding of the Breath of Life as a healing principle and demonstrated it to us by his work as a man and as a physician, by experimentation upon himself until the truths he gave us were verified, by his service for his patients, and by the classroom instruction he left with his students.

How often in this day and time do we hear reference made to the Master Mechanic of the human body, the Grand Architect, the Master Architect, God, Deity, Creator, or other terms of reverence for the maker of the human temple in which we reside? These are the terms of the science of osteopathy as envisioned by Dr. Andrew Taylor Still. Dr. Sutherland told us, "I have often said that we lost something in osteopathy that Dr. Still tried to get across, that was the Spiritual that he included in the science of osteopathy." Dr. Still was closer to his Maker than mere material breathing in his development of the science of osteopathy; he was guided by a Spiritual Fulcrum and so was

Dr. Sutherland. If we, as students of the science of osteopathy, are to understand osteopathy, we will find it necessary to reawaken our knowledge of the Deity that centers us, make it our Spiritual Fulcrum for our guidance, and learn to think, feel, and use the Creator in our daily practices. Through his knowledge and use of the science of osteopathy, Dr. Sutherland gave us the guideposts to follow. Let us compare, for a moment, this dedicated type of reasoning of the early 1900's with the science of today. I read an editorial in a recent publication written by a renowned scientist who was trying to reconcile spiritual and scientific truths. It was his conclusion that science and the spiritual are not incompatible but rather that the great truths of each are more or less parallel to each other—in other words, that each reaches toward that unknown understanding that is necessary for known understanding. That thought does not strike me with a sense of agreement. How can one reason that this is a scientific truth and that this is a spiritual truth? I would place my confidence in a scientist who is reaching for scientific understanding through a Spiritual guidance rather than trying to raise a separate superstructure.

I like the thought of a biologic scientist who was discussing the phenomena of life when he stated, "In fact, the life sciences are not only much more complicated than the physical sciences, they are also much broader in significance, and they penetrate much farther in the exploration of the universe that is science than do the physical sciences. They require and embrace the data and all the explanatory principles of the physical sciences and then go far beyond that to embody many other data and additional explanatory principles that are no less—that are, in a sense, even more—scientific. The point is that *all* known material processes and explanatory principles apply to organisms endowed with the phenomena of life, while only a limited number of them apply to non-living systems." The osteopathic concept concerns a living system and includes the cranial concept. Dr. Sutherland told us, "The cranial concept is not a specialty unit set apart from the science of osteopathy. In truthful realization, the concept was envisioned by Dr. Andrew Taylor Still." Again, I say, the total osteopathic concept requires the search for all explanatory principles, universally speaking, to bring it into understanding, and this includes the Creator who brought it into being.

There are several roads one may follow in giving a memorial lecture to the man we honor today. We could recount the history of his development of osteopathy in the cranial field in the chronological manner, but this would only serve to limit it to the days and years in which he lived it. This is not enough; the truths he gave us are steppingstones to greater truths yet to be unfolded. We could discuss in considerable detail the functioning anatomy and physiology that he learned in his years of study, but this would only serve to give us information and would not point towards the path that the Master Architect offers in acquiring *knowledge* of the functioning of all the anatomical-physiology he discussed. We could develop hypotheses to explain the principles he gave us, but in the end they would remain hypotheses and we will have ended nowhere. I am reminded of a quotation I read concerning theories, "One of the tragedies of life is the murder of a beautiful theory by a brutal gang of facts."

Rather than travelling any of these roads, I believe it is in order to discuss the work of W. G. Sutherland as he worded it, with the emphasis on learning something about a Spiritual Fulcrum and its clinical application in the daily care of our patients. With this thought in mind, let us take the terms he used—Highest Known Element, Potency, Fulcrum, Stillness, Tide, and Breath of Life—and try to read between the lines to find a practical fulfillment of these basic principles. Throughout this discussion, let it be remembered that Dr. Sutherland was guided by his Maker, whom he affectionately called Dad. This was not a term of irreverence but one that allowed him to feel close to his Maker on Whom he depended for guidance and from Whom he received the necessary urging to "dig on" when the road was difficult to follow. This is no mere fancy. This is a reliance on a Great Wisdom from Divine Mind.

It will be necessary to define function as it is used in this theme. Physiological function is the special, normal, or proper action of any part or organ of the human body. We are not concerned with the end products of functioning but with the mobility and motility that accompany functioning within body physiology, its tissues and its fluids. We are concerned with the movements the body makes in response to its internal and external environments, with its voluntary and involuntary actions, and with those factors we can learn to feel through the use of thinking-feeling-seeing-knowing fingers.

When we place our hands upon a patient who has good health, we feel an overall sense of wellness. We feel the respiratory cycle of his breathing. We feel the flexion and extension of his midline sutures in their functioning. We feel the alternate external and internal rotation of his bilateral structures in their functioning. We feel any voluntary motions he may make and many involuntary motions from different organ systems within the body. If we have our hands upon his cranium, we can feel the movements of the cranial articular mechanism, the to-and-fro movements of the reciprocal tension membrane, and the fluctuation of the cerebrospinal fluid as an integrated functioning mechanism. Throughout the whole body we can sense something else not ordinarily mentioned in the anatomy and physiology texts of today. This is an overall tidal movement of the whole body, a coming in and ebbing out. It is as if the whole body, functioning as a unit, is responding to a force similar to that moving the tides of the ocean. It is a rhythmic movement within all the fluids of the body. It is more powerful, in its quiet way, than any other physiological functioning within the body mechanism, more important and more powerful than the respiratory cycle, the voluntary, or the involuntary movements, or any of the other movements we ordinarily consider. Our knowing touch learns to discern all of these factors operating in integrated functioning in any part of body physiology which we are examining. This is a rhythmic Tide in physiological functioning with its Highest Known Element and its innate Potency.

As we go deeper into our understanding of body mechanisms, we learn that all normal functioning of the individual units of the body— whether they be bone, ligament, membrane, fascia, organs, or fluid—

seem to operate through automatic, shifting, suspension fulcrums. The Sutherland fulcrum, where the falx cerebri adjoins the tentorium cerebelli, is an automatic, shifting, suspension fulcrum for the reciprocal tension membrane. The sternal end of the clavicle is an osseous fulcrum for the functioning of the entire upper extremity. The atlas is an osseous fulcrum for the condylar parts of the occiput during childbirth. There are fluid fulcrums throughout the body for all kinds of fluid functioning. We can bring the cerebrospinal fluid tide down to that short rhythmic period wherein we reach a stillpoint, a pause-rest period, and we know that we have arrived at a fulcrum point for the cerebrospinal fluid for that moment in time. We are told by Dr. Sutherland that it is at this moment that there is a transmutation from the Highest Known Element that creates an interchange between all the fluids of the body, even within all the living bone cells of the body. As the body responds to this transmutation process and unfolds itself towards more normal body functioning, we can note that there is a change in the tidal movement of the total body mechanism as compared to that which we observed at the beginning of our examination.

We are told by Dr. Sutherland that the motive power for functioning is at or in the fulcrum, not at the ends of the lever. We are instructed by him that it is the fulcrum point you read in the body mechanisms, to listen and feel the functioning at the fulcrum points, to get the tone quality at the fulcrum points, to note the rhythm at these pause-rest periods. They are automatic, shifting, suspension fulcrum areas, yet they are a still point of balance, an important balance point which we can seek in working with the tissue elements and their fluid contents with our knowing touch to bring them to this functioning balance point. When we have reached this pause-rest period, in comes the Potency of the Tide for the transmutation process that brings normalization to body functioning. As human engineers, as physicians, we are dealing with the most powerful force within the human body when we learn to use the tidal movements of body physiology, tidal movements designed by a Master Mechanic.

It was from research work done upon himself and detailed study of all the parts of the primary respiratory mechanism that enabled Dr. Sutherland to state, "The rule of the artery is supreme, but the cerebrospinal fluid is in command." To further clarify this thought, he said, "The breath of Life in the cerebrospinal fluid Tide is the fundamental principle in the primary respiratory mechanism." And then he gave us detailed instruction on how to develop thinking-feeling-seeing-knowing fingers in order to bring this Tide down to its stillpoint, its pause-rest period, in order to control its functioning in body physiology. It is important to know we are not limited to the craniosacral mechanism in learning to control the Tide. As we seek balance in tissue and fluid elements in any part of the whole body during our search for disease or disabled conditions, we are learning to bring the Tide into its balance point or fulcrum area. In doing this, a transmutation process can take place to reduce the lesion mechanics, correct pathology, and regain health for that individual. This is the healing principle of the Master Mechanic at work within our patients; and we, as physicians, can develop our awareness and observe its workings in the tissues of the patients.

In our discussions up to this point, I have referred to the functioning of the Tide of the body and to the many fulcrums that operate in the body physiology. It is time to refer to something else that Dr. Sutherland gave us in developing our understanding. This is the stillness of the Tide—not the up-and-down fluctuation of the waves of the Tide but the stillness found at the fulcrum point within the Tide. There is a Potency within this stillness. The idea of stillness can confuse us in our thinking in trying to understand this work. How can there be a Potency or Power or Energy in stillness? Dr. Sutherland used to give us the illustration of transmitting a vibration to a glass of water and observing the surface of that glass of water forming a still point in its center. And he called attention to the fact that this was a fulcrum point within that glass of water and compared it to the fulcrum point we reach in bringing the cerebrospinal fluid fluctuation down to its stillpoint in compression of the fourth ventricle or any other of the Tide control techniques. "It is the stillness of the Tide we seek," he would say, for in that stillness is the Potency of the Tide.

Those of us who were privileged to be in his classes while he lectured on this subject have observed and shared in the experience of feeling the whole classroom becoming still. He would call it to our attention and would tell us that it was something that frequently occurred when the Potency of the Tide was being discussed. It occurred spontaneously and was not something that was planned or predetermined. Those who experienced this could feel the stillness, and his comment would be, "Can you feel the change in the Tide?" This is something that occurred in a moment of time and then it was gone. So we are discussing something that occurs in a vital mechanism in a time sequence when all of the factors that lead to its appearance are properly tuned for it to happen. Does this stillness have an inert feeling of lifelessness or absence of vitality? No. It is a living thing that has the feeling of power and Potency within it. It cannot be explained for I have no words to describe it, but it does happen and it is beneficent.

There have been times within your own offices when this has occurred while you have been treating a patient. You are suddenly conscious that the whole room in which you are working seems to become a pause-rest period, and there is something there, a Stillness, that is above and beyond anything you can explain to yourself or to the patient. There is a feeling of being close to your Maker. When asked about this point, Dr. Sutherland said, "We know we have a Potency. We need not worry about where it comes from; nor where it goeth."

Nature has given us many examples of the Potency and power within the stillness of her functioning. The eye of the hurricane is a tremendous center of stillness and yet it is a potent stillness. It is also an automatic-shifting-suspension-fulcrum site as it moves across the ocean. The winds that blow over the surface of the earth cannot blow everywhere at once. There must be a point of calm. The axle of a wheel has to have a still point around which the wheel moves. And we could go on and on. Are these living systems in nature that I have cited? We do not classify them as such. But in dealing with the body physiology of biologic systems, we are dealing with principles and "laws not framed by human hands," and we do find there is power and Potency within the stillness of the Tide within body functioning. We are not dealing with a static mechanism in which we say we are still as we sit here in our chairs. Our bodies are a dynamic flux of energy operating from the moment of conception throughout life, and within these energy fields are moments of time—moments of Stillness within these energy fields, fulcrum points in time for various physiological needs—and all centered with the Potency of Stillness as the motive power for the action that follows. We must understand the mechanism of this Stillness and use it in the care of our cases, and we do not need to have a full explanation as to what it is or where it comes from or where it goes after it has served us at this moment of using it—the stillness of the Tide in body physiology.

Up to this point I have discussed function, automatic, shifting, suspension fulcrums, and the Tide, Stillness, and Potency that operate within all of these facets within body physiology. It would appear that I am trying to develop a theological hypothesis to explain this work. That is not true. I am trying to point out to you that the Creator of the human body and its mechanisms is more than a passive terminology to whom we give lip service but do not use. The science of osteopathy includes the active use of the Creator in its daily service. It is an acquired art as well as a science, and I like the quotation I read somewhere, "Therefore be at peace with God, *whatever you conceive Him to be*, and whatever your labors and aspirations, in the noisy confusion of life, keep peace with your soul." Therefore we need tools in understanding and using a Spiritual Fulcrum in our daily practices.

What are some of these tools? First, I would say that a physician should develop an objective awareness. He should know anatomy, physiology, and pathology and all the integrated, interrelated, and intrarelated functioning that is manifest between these elements in body physiology. He must be able to evaluate and determine diagnostic and prognostic insight from the day of his initial examination of the patient until he discharges that patient. He should be able to coordinate the tissue changes taking place through using the Potency within the tissues with the objective progress of that case toward normalcy or recompensation. He should be guided by the objective findings he makes in determining the care for each case.

Secondly, the physician should have a subjective awareness of the potential for using the healing principles discussed herein. He should be able to sense the degree of possibilities for reversing pathological conditions within the patient and the degree of potential recovery that can be made within the tissue units. He is dealing with the subjective phenomena of life itself and he will share in the subjective changes that take place within the patient through his seeking to evaluate them. He must know the anatomical-physiological needs of each patient's problem and subjectively work with them in addition to objectively watching their progress.

Thirdly, he should develop thinking-seeing-feeling-knowing fingers that can literally follow the moment-to-moment changes that take place within disabled tissues as they work with the Master Architect in reconstructing their normal or recompensated pattern of health. This *knowing* touch is not easy to acquire. It takes months and years of patience and patients to make it a working, efficient tool for use in diagnosis and treatment. Every patient is a challenge to further improve his skills and there is no point at which a physician can say, "I know all there is to know about this particular problem." The very next visit of that patient opens new doors for further investigation.

There are many other factors that can be discussed, but these three points are the main ones that primarily concern the physician in learning to use the healing principles of the Highest Known Element in his diagnostic and therapeutic approach to his patient. In addition to these three points is the fact that, at all times, he should accept one thought each time a patient comes to him for his services. This is the objective, subjective, and knowing awareness of a Potency within himself, within his developing, knowing fingers, and

32

within the patient—a Potency to which the physician quietly submits himself for guidance and understanding. I am not suggesting that this approach produces an instantaneous healing each time the patient submits himself for treatment, although the results obtained will frequently surprise you. I am trying to tell you that working with the Master Mechanic each visit will permit the physician to give the finest, the most efficient, and the most skillful service in any of the healing arts available to the patient. It is a scientific approach that includes all the principles of those "laws not framed by human hand," that includes "*all* known material processes and explanatory principles endowed with the phenomena of life." It is a living application of the science of osteopathy.

We have been exploring some rather deep water. It is time to change the pace and explore some of the lighter moments that occur in our clinical experience in using these truths. One of the first things I would suggest for the physician is the development of a sense of humor. The most common statement I hear in my practice is, "He didn't do anything, but.... All he did was put his hands on me and sit there and when he was through, I felt better." There is always need for a good patient-doctor relationship and for allowing physiological function within to manifest its own unerring Potency for the motive power for correction rather than the use of blind force from without.

After you have secured good results in someone who has made the rounds of routine care, including manipulative osteopathy in some cases, you will have a patient who likes to send his or her friends to you, and it is interesting to see how they prepare that potential patient for your services. The new patient is told, "When you go to my doctor, don't be surprised as to how he treats you. You are going to think he is not doing anything, but you will feel better when he is through and if he says he needs to see you again, you stay with him and he will get you well." I have a very fine gentleman in my practice who has sent me many patients and he tells them, "You go see my doctor with the magic hands. I don't know how he does it, but he can help you."

Patients come back and send their friends because you are able to produce good results in problems that have not been solved by medicine, physiotherapy, or any other form of examination or tests. As your skill continues to develop, you will get more and more complex cases that have made the rounds and are still seeking help for their problems. About the time the physician thinks that he has seen as tough a case as it is possible to see in a busy practice, a new case will come in from one of his many patient referrals that makes all the previous tough cases seem simple. Utilizing the unerring Potency as the motive power for diagnosis and treatment attracts complex cases to the physician's office as flowers attract bees. This is why this work is continuously interesting. There is always something new to be learned from the physiological picture of the patient's body. The physician will always have a need for greater insight with which to help the patient.

"You are getting back to: Cause," said Dr. Sutherland. "If you understand the mechanism, your technique is simple." Think, for a moment, of the many implications these two statements present to the physician. In this world of effects, the problem cases we see are effects piled upon effects until the effects overbalance the causative factor–cause, in these cases, being the initial injury or disease that started the syndrome. Now we are being guided to a Creator within this disabled condition, a Cause that will penetrate through the effects and allow health to reappear within the patient. We are seeking the revitalization of health within the patient, not the mere symptomatic relief of the effects. Within the overall Cause is health and it is our job to help the patient bring it through for his recovery.

What wealth of insight there is in the few words, "If you understand the mechanism." It embodies all that we have discussed. The physician should have a knowing awareness of the Creator within himself and within his patient. He should be aware of the Potency and its rhythmic capacity to function within the Tides of body physiology and how to work with those Tides throughout the body to make use of the Potency within them. He should have a working knowledge of functioning within body physiology and with a knowing touch be able to sense the tissue and fluid changes taking place. He should have a working knowledge of all the anatomy and physiology as is found in our present-day texts and then be able to go beyond this point and be open-minded and opened touch-wise to accept those experiences that come to him through the unerring Potency within body physiology as it does its unseen work. It is an invisible force, to be sure, but it is manifest through anatomical-physiological elements, and it is something that the physician can learn to feel and to interpret for his diagnostic and therapeutic care in his cases. He should develop an understanding of fulcrums, automatic, shifting, suspension fulcrums in body physiology. He should develop his understanding of the Potency within the stillness in these fulcrum pause-rest periods as they function in their moment in time, when all is in tune for their time sequence to unfold.

He will find it necessary to develop a different patient-doctor relationship, for the physician has largely ceased to be the doer in the treatment program and is allowing physiological function within to manifest its unerring Potency rather than applying blind force from without. He is going to be subjected to many questions and much questioning within many patients' minds. Fortunately, this point is easily overcome by the positive results he obtains in a high percentage of his cases and by the positive remarks about his treatments that his patients make in referring other cases to him. However, the doubtful patient is a point to consider, and this does create an interesting challenge in using this type of work. In addition, the physician should have an objective awareness, a subjective awareness, and a thinking-seeing-feeling-knowing touch. It is possible to summarize these qualifications in Dr. Sutherland's few words, "If you understand the mechanism, your technique is simple." And it is simple. This was and is the science of osteopathy as enunciated and practiced by Dr. A. T. Still, by Dr. W. G. Sutherland, and by many other leaders within our profession. Today, we are concerned with the truths, and demonstrations of those truths, as brought to us by Dr. Sutherland.

Now is the time to consider what all of this means to us who practice in this year, 1965, and in the future years ahead of us. Our profession is a highly qualified profession, and we need every service within it that we now use. We need our hospitals, our surgeons, our internists, our pediatricians, our obstetricians, our psychiatrists, and all of our specialty groups. We need every modality that modern medicine can give us for the routine care of our patients. There is room for all of these and there is room for something in addition. There is need for at least 2,000 men and women who will take the time to teach themselves the disciplines necessary to make the truths of Still and Sutherland available for use in their daily practices. I have been told that not every physician is capable of acquiring these particular skills, that he must be gifted in some way before he can obtain them. I do not feel this way about this ability. I feel that it takes perseverance, time, and a great deal of work on the physician's part to acquire this art and science. If any physician is willing to devote time and effort to the basic premises of "being still in order to know" as the means of getting closer to his Maker than mere material breathing, his path will lead him to the necessary acquisitions of becoming a man or woman skilled in those principles and practices given to us by Dr. A. T. Still and Dr. W. G. Sutherland. Frankly, I would like to see 2,000 men and women practicing this type of osteopathy because those physicians will be giving a service to many thousands of patients who have been told, "We have done all that is possible for you. You will have to learn to live with the problem as it now manifests itself." A high percentage of those thousands can be led to a much higher degree of health than is now available to them. I am concerned for the patients who can be helped. Thus, there is born the need for those who can help them to come forward and develop their personal skills in this area. At present, there is but a handful in this country who have taken the words and work of Dr. Sutherland to heart—his concept of osteopathy as a whole unit—and who are trying to become this type of physician.

There is another point to be made here that has not been touched upon. The physician who takes it upon himself to acquire this type of practice is going to become a research physician within his own office. Just as Dr. Sutherland spent many a long year in learning the truths he gained from work upon himself and from observations he made in his patients, just so will every physician find avenues for exploration and study that cannot be found in the textbooks and periodicals of today's literature. The Authority for many of the problems to be solved will be found within the complexities of the body physiology of each patient and within the physician's astute awareness of the potential for learning from those problems. The guideposts and work given to us by Dr. Sutherland are but the beginnings of further insight, which will broaden the platform of existing knowledge and bring forth new truths that will need testing and retesting until they can be brought forward for the use of all of us.

A young patient of mine, who has now entered his freshman year in one of our colleges, told his mother that he plans on getting his D.O. degree, coming back to Dallas, and studying under my guidance until he can acquire the principles and the means of implementing those principles in his own practice. Then he told her that he plans to do a better job than I do. His mother said she felt this was a form of conceit on his part. My reply was that he should be able to do a better job than I do, that the experiences I have gained will shorten the time he needs to acquire the skills it takes to produce the results I obtain, and that he should be able to stand on my shoulders and become a better man in the years he has before him. I applaud him for his attitude. I think it is high time we all stand on Dr. Sutherland's shoulders by first, becoming as skillful as he was in his work and second, by using that skill and understanding to further his work and that of Dr. A. T. Still. Herein is our role as research physicians in the science of osteopathy. It was Dr. Sutherland's wish that this be so. Are we ready to accept the challenge?

"Be Still and Know;" "You are getting back to: Cause;" "The Breath of Life is the fundamental principle in the science of osteopathy." These are the thoughts that Dr. Sutherland left us in his dedication to the science of osteopathy. I would like to close with a quotation from a letter he sent me many years ago. I wrote him in reference to certain aspects of osteopathy in the cranial field, although his reply could be expanded to include all of the total body physiology in the science of osteopathy. However, I will quote him as he gave it to me:

> Closer to me than breathing is the Creator of the cranial mechanism.... Closer to the patient is the Creator of his or her cranial mechanism.... My thinking-feeling-seeing-*knowing* fingers are guided *Intelligently* by the Master Mechanic Who designed this mechanism. It matters not what interpretation one may apply, providing one's mental trolley is on the *Wire*.

Let me repeat, "It matters not what interpretation one may apply, providing one's mental trolley is on the *Wire*."

Understanding
The Mechanism

THE INVOLUNTARY MECHANISM
This is an edited transcription of excerpts from four lectures given in 1976 at a Sutherland Cranial Teaching Foundation basic course in Milwaukee, Wisconsin.

LET'S TALK ABOUT THE nature of the primary respiratory mechanism, which is a simple, basic, primary, rhythmic unit of function. It is totally involuntary in nature; it incorporates the whole of anatomy and physiology; it is palpable to the trained physician in any part of the body; and it provides the physiological evidence of health within the whole body physiology as well as evidence of less than health for any areas of dysfunction. It can be used as a diagnostic tool as well as being a tool for treatment, and it is a manifestation of life within the patient that the physician can use in his service to restore health to the patient.

The primary respiratory mechanism has been broken down into five components for teaching purposes, but it remains one unit of function. All these components are part of this simple, rhythmic, primary unit of function within body physiology. Note that I did not just say "within the primary respiratory mechanism" but "within the body physiology." The whole unit has this factor. Everything obeys the laws of flexion/external rotation and extension/internal rotation of anatomicophysiology. We are totally dependent on this simple, rhythmic, fluid drive, mobile, motile mechanism.

All of the body has an involuntary mechanism. Your psoas muscle, even if it is sick, is designed to go into external and internal rotation. Your foot is designed to go into external and internal rotation 10 to 12 times a minute, not because of this primary respiratory mechanism, but because the primary respiratory mechanism can only function this way; that's why we have to learn its rules and its regulations.

Let me read you a quotation that contains the theme for a point or two I want to make. This was written by Loren Eiseley in a book of essays. If you haven't read Loren Eiseley, you should; if you want to learn how to palpate, get ahold of one of his books. As you read his books, you share the experience of his fossil hunting. You share the experience of going back in time and being alive to the things he is describing. You can palpate it as well as be aware of it with your whole being. I have found it very useful. The quotation is as follows:

> Imagine for a moment that you have drunk from a magician's goblet. Reverse the irreversible stream of time. Go down the long dark stairwell out of which the race has ascended. Find yourself at last on the bottom-most steps of time, slipping, sliding, and wallowing by scale and fin down into the muck and ooze out of which you arose. Pass by grunts and voiceless hissings below the last tree ferns. Eyeless and earless, float in the primal waters, since sunlight you cannot see. Stretch out absorbing tentacles towards vague tastes that float in the water. Still in your formless shifting, the view remains. The sliding particles, the juices, the transformations are working in exquisitely patterned rhythm which has no other purpose than your preservation—you, the entity, the ameboid being whose substance contains the unfathomable future. Even so does every man come upwards from the waters of their birth. Yet if at any moment the magician bending over you should cry, "Speak, tell us of that road," you could not respond. The sensations are yours but not, and this is one of the great mysteries, the power over the body. You cannot describe how the body in habit functions, or picture or control the spinnings that are the dance of the molecules, or why they chose to dance into that particular pattern which is you, or again why up the long stairway of eons they dance from one shape to another. It is for this reason I am no longer interested in final particles. Follow them as you will, pursue them until they become nameless, protein crystals replicating on the verge of life. Use all the great powers of the mind and pass backwards until you hang with the dire faces of the conquerors in the

hydrogen clouds in which the sun was born. You will then have performed the ultimate deception that our analytic age demands. But the
cloud will still veil the secret, and if not the cloud, then the nothingness
into which it now appears. The cloud in its turn may be dissolved. The
secret, if one may paraphrase, lies in the age of night.

Now, after eons of development, the body has become what it is
today. Following the dictates of its origins, it has to have an involuntary mechanism to make it move, to keep it alive, in order for it to be
what it is as a mind/body structure, an anatomicophysiological, functioning mechanism. We have many involuntary systems in our body—
circulatory, digestive, and the like—but there is one particular involuntary mechanism of the human body that is key. Every single cell of
the body, every single individual cell residing within the fluids in
which it is being made, is being flexed and extended, externally and
internally rotated 10 to 12 times a minute.

So, if we have a patient who is in health—whether sitting quietly,
walking, sleeping soundly, running, in full activity, or at total rest—he
has, inside, this involuntary, physiologic motion of function throughout. The neurocranial and sacral mechanisms happen to be the parts
we focus on as manifesting this mechanism—this involuntary motion.
But the neurocranial and sacral axes of activity, their physiologic functioning, is more or less the drive shaft, if you will, in the system,
through which all of the wheels, pulleys and everything clear out to
the very doors of the factory are made to do their job—flexion/exter-
nal rotation and extension/internal rotation. So there is no way you
can make the neurocranial and sacral mechanism a separate entity
from the total body physiology. We are dealing with the largest, most
important involuntary system in the human body every time we put
our hands on a patient. Every single time we touch that patient, whether
we choose to do it in relation to one tiny joint in the finger or whether
we grab ahold of a whole leg, we have to start tuning into this involuntary, physiological mechanism.

Voluntary mechanisms are anything the decision-making part of this brain decides to do with this involuntary thing. I choose to walk, stand, or sit; I choose to talk, eat, and think (or think I am thinking); I choose to do a million things. I choose to have emotions, mental thoughts—these are all voluntary. They are activities that we can use intelligently, trying not to insult them, starve them to death, or overfatigue them. We just use them in normal day-to-day life, and as soon as we quit using them, they simply sink back to wherever they came from, and our involuntary mechanism continues to support us until we give orders that we want the voluntary to do something else. It's the voluntary side of life that gets us into trouble, not the involuntary.

When a patient comes in with some pattern of stress or strain at whatever level—mental fatigue, emotional shock, or physical effects of disease or trauma—as I quietly sit there and work with the problem they present, as my hands quietly search in and out and through the cellular structures, the fascias, the fluids, and the mechanics of that human body, I realize that even before I have ahold of that mechanism, it was automatically trying to wash this problem out through its involuntary mechanism. As I quietly get ahold of that mechanism, I tune into that involuntary mechanism, the involuntary physiologic motion beneath this trauma. I try to sense through into the involuntary mechanism within which this trauma has occurred. And then I try to work with getting balance at the minute, micro level necessary to find the point at which this involuntary mechanism can break the fetters embarrassing it. At that point, I can feel this little change take place within the patient that says, "Yes, now I can try to do something for this problem," and as it goes through its fulcrum point, its stillpoint, its balance point, it shifts into a pattern of being that no longer is restraining the involuntary mechanism for that particular part of the body. When it can stick its head out and say, "Alright, I can get to work," it's like dropping a pebble into a quiet pool of water; you see the waves of this involuntary activity beginning to spread, not only from the site at which you're working, but throughout the entire involuntary systems throughout the body—you can just feel it expand outward and outward and outward.

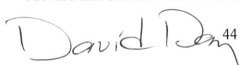

44

After this shift has occurred, I discover that when I go back to check and see how the voluntarily induced trauma or process is behaving, if it wasn't too bad in the first place, it isn't there anymore. In all this process, I never pay any attention to the strain itself until after I get the involuntary mechanism to wake up. Then, usually, what's left to be corrected is so minor, it's practically nonexistent and takes very little effort to make a correction.

Now, what is this shift that takes place in this involuntary mechanism? How long does it take to bring it about? A beautiful illustration is that Escher drawing with the stairs. Are the stairs going up or down? Study it until you can see them shift. In a nanosecond, they shift in your perception from stairs going up to stairs going down. That is the shift that Eiseley is talking about, the myriads of patterns, from one state of function to another in the involuntary mechanisms you work with. That's how long it takes; that's the period of time it takes to shift. Our job as physicians is to quietly tune, from within ourselves, into an understanding of this thing. Our understanding comes from something we cannot explain, though we can sense it. What we feel, by virtue of the fact that we can sense it, is an effect. But, still, we can be aware of the fact that in that nanosecond, something takes place. We can observe what pattern there was before and we can observe the pattern afterwards, and in our intelligent understanding of that involuntary mechanism, (because we have studied the details of the physiological movement of every part of this involuntary mechanism, not only in the craniosacral axes but throughout the entire system), we are in a position to make this a clinical entity of function and use.

A Universal Design

THERE IS AN ASPECT of universality in this craniosacral mechanism and in the total anatomy and physiology of the whole body. It has taken something like ten-thousand generations or three million years to build up the human body as it is designed today. And it's basically designed to function as a voluntary and involuntary mechanism. The only reason we are sitting here today is because we are the product of "x" number of generations of people who managed to survive. So the mechanisms within us as a total body are those that nature said should survive.

In other words, the fundamental principle of the healing arts (deliberately, I did not say "osteopathic profession" because all the healing arts should understand this) is that the body is a beautiful mechanism from the top of the head to the bottom of the feet, and although it has many parts, it's designed as a universal unit; it is a universal design for function. The more clearly we can understand how it functions within us as a total mechanism, including both the voluntary and involuntary, the more accurate can become our diagnosis and certainly, the more skillful can become our treatment.

Yesterday, the faculty talked about the architectural principles of the neurocranial bones. All of us have temporal bones, all of us have an occiput and a sphenoid, all of us have two parietals, and all of us functionally have two frontals. It makes no difference who they belong to—they are the same in everybody in terms of the fact that they are an anatomical principle of function. There's an automatic tendency for those of us in the healing arts to look at somebody and say, "Ah, he's got a lesion. I can see his face is askew, therefore that means he's got trouble." But our first thought should be, How is that area of that skull designed for function in that man? What is its pattern of health, what is its basic principle for working within this physical mechanism?

The same applies to an arm. When somebody comes in with a complaint of tennis elbow (lateral epicondylitis), he has an appendicular mechanism in which he's produced a strain. Our first thought should be to consider what design that mechanism would be in if he had not come in with a strain pattern. How should the muscles be, what are the basic principles for the function of those muscles in that arm, the forearm, the wrist, and the shoulder? How are they designed in this particular person for health? Then, when we take ahold of it, we can understand how it is functioning within the particular problem that patient comes in with.

#1 How would the system work in health.

So our basic purpose for being here at this course is not to learn the pathologies of these areas we are discussing and putting our hands on. Our job here is to learn what the basic principles are for this mechanism. What is this or that thing supposed to be doing within this patient? The question is not, what are they doing? What they are doing is only the diagnostic clue that they may have a problem. The question is, what are these mechanisms supposed to be doing in this patient? And I'm not just talking about the craniosacral mechanism, though this course is focused on that. The principles of the anatomy and physiology of the craniosacral mechanism are identical with those principles of every other system in the body—including the musculoskeletal, digestive, cardiovascular and respiratory.

So we must ask ourselves, how is this universal design manifesting and working in this patient? This universal design has an individual name in every individual, and it has an individual pattern for every patient walking around with it. Each person has an individual design around which he works, but the parts of him are universal. Each component of the craniosacral mechanism has principles that function universally in all of us and are then individualized within the individual it belongs to.

Now this broadens our horizons considerably because we are not looking for pathology when we study in these courses, we are looking for the principles that make this mechanism work. So you are here to study, not the so-called normal but the *principles* involved in the so-called normal for the individual you are going to be working on.

DNA Pattern

IF YOU COULD EXAMINE someone's involuntary structure, without any interference from the voluntary, you would find that there is an individualized pattern of health for each individual person on earth. Their anatomicophysiological, involuntary mechanism from the vertex to the feet is following a pattern instilled into them, created for them, by the DNA present at the time of conception and around which they built their pattern for health. It is endowed with energy to create that

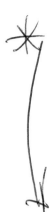

pattern. It takes nine months to get into the world and 90 years to get out, but all the time, the involuntary structure is being constantly rebuilt cell by cell with only the DNA pattern for that particular body to create the inside mechanism that makes it a working, involuntary system.

When you tune into this patient with your hands with the intention of finding problems, you are finding problems imposed by voluntary stresses, disease, or trauma—something the patient did from the outside, in. But instead, if you can work through what has been imposed upon this thing and keep the totality of the involuntary pattern in focus, you are calling upon the most powerful energies in the world—DNA and its pattern or template—which say, "This is what I want to be." That pattern is individually designed for that one soul, that one individual.

So when I take ahold of this cranial mechanism, or I take ahold of whatever it is I'm trying to treat, as I focus my awareness on this patient's mechanism, I try to read underneath, asking, What does this involuntary mechanism want to do? Where is it and how can I get it up to the surface for function? Since I know it has this energy powered from birth or beyond and that energy is available, then as I focus on that, it can come through and express itself in the area I am treating. When I feel it stick its head up and say, "Okay, boss, I've found this neutral point and now I can go to work," I know something has happened at the involuntary level, and I can go back and check the voluntary mechanism strain I originally found. In this process of simply focusing, a lot of strains correct themselves.

A Deeper Relationship

LET'S ASSUME WE'RE back home in practice, and we have the usual physician-patient relationship. We take a careful case history, do a physical examination, run lab tests, take X-rays, call in specialists to get consultations, and we finally arrive at a diagnosis and consider a treatment program. We may use medications or surgery; we do whatever is indicated to the best of our knowledge in this physician-

48

patient relationship.

But now suppose we want to have another, deeper layer of relationship—to have a little closer union, a more one-on-one relationship. Instead of the usual, objective physician-patient relationship, let's have a little more subjective approach; let's bring our physician and patient into one unit.

The physician and the patient have a similar physical body. They both have the same anatomicophysiological mechanism within their own body. This mechanism has no ego, it has no name—it's name isn't Becker, it's name isn't Jones. They both have an energy body that's making them alive, a mental body of intellectual capacity as well as emotional capacity and spiritual capacities. They're the same thing, there is no difference. It's the same body; there is no difference, none at all.

You, as students, we, as faculty, have identically the same mechanism as I've described. None of us has any ego as far as this mechanism goes.

The mechanism has no ego. Doctor, patient, student all have the same mechanism.

MOTION—THE KEY TO DIAGNOSIS AND TREATMENT

This paper was presented in 1979 at a Cranial Academy conference sponsored by the Sutherland Cranial Teaching Foundation.

MOTION IS NOT LIFE. Motion is a manifestation of life. The miracle of life expresses itself in motion and movement from the flow of electrons about a nucleus to the animated beings we call viruses, bacteria, fungi, plants, animals, and mankind. This life can be found in the sea, on land, and in the air—perhaps even in outer space. Mankind has lived, or adapted himself to live, in all of these environments.

Webster has defined motion as "the act or process of moving; the passage of a body from one place to another; movement; the act of moving the body or any of its parts; in mechanics, a combination of moving parts; mechanism."

Dorland's definitions include 30 descriptions for movement. Several are: 1. An act of moving; motion. 2. Active m., a movement produced by the person's own muscles. 3. Automatic m., a movement originating within the organism, but not by an act of the will. 4. Communicated m., one produced by a force acting from without. 5. Passive m., any movement of the body effected by a force entirely outside of the organism. 6. Reflex m., an involuntary movement provoked by a remote external stimulus acting through a nerve center. 7. Spontaneous m., one which is originated within the organism. 8. Index m., a movement of the cephalic part of the body about a fixed caudal part. 9. Brownian m., the dancing motion of minute particles suspended in a liquid. These nine descriptions are the important ones needed for this discussion. For example, definition number eight, "Index motion, a movement of the cephalic part of the body about a fixed caudal part," is a very clear definition of the clinical condition we find in a whiplash injury or after a severe fall on the buttocks wherein the locked involuntary movement of the sacrum contributes to a movement of the cephalic part of the body about a fixed caudal point.

As physicians, we are concerned with motion and movement within a patient on a one-on-one basis. In health, he has no need for our services. His life and manifested motion and movement within and without his environment and his anatomicophysiological mechanisms are in a freely functioning state of being. All of his internalized systems, both voluntary and involuntary, are working to maintain his homeostatic balance of functioning from within, and he is responding and reflecting a natural interrelationship and intrarelationship with the specific environment of his external world of motion and movement.

In our training to become physicians, we have dissected this body in which we live both anatomically and physiologically. We have given names and descriptions of function to all parts of a complex system of cells, fluids, and mechanisms of bodily parts and their motion and movements. In reality, our anatomicophysiological body has not divided itself into the many parts we know as physicians. This physical and functioning body has not defined its many parts and actions. It has no name, really, not even the name given to us by our parents. This no-name body, which we use in our walkabout on earth, is working on a simple one-on-one relationship both within itself and with its environment.

This is an important point. We, as physicians, need the detailed knowledge of anatomy and physiology we have acquired for our analytic awareness of our patient's needs. Our patient's body has no such need for this detailed knowledge. Life in the body and its manifested motion and movement is working as a unified whole mechanism to manifest health, to resist and combat disease, and to correct or adapt to trauma.

We talk about holistic medicine and holism, but in actual experience, it is largely a matter of verbalization not put into practice. My no-name body and that of my patients—no-name because it is experiencing holism—gives me, the physician, an opportunity to practice clinically applied holistic principles in both diagnostic and treatment procedures. The resources of my no-name body and that of my patients, with their manifested motion and movements, both gross and finite, powered by an inherent potency, permits me, the physician, to allow physiological function within to manifest its own unerring potency rather than using blind force from without in the care of my patients.

Our no-name bodies have other resources that add to, complicate, enhance, and reinforce the total functioning of our internal and external environments. We have a name, given to us by our parents. We have an ego, a mind, and emotions. These three—ego, mind, and emotions—are also manifestations of life as motion and movements at different frequencies than that of the physical and physiological structure of our no-name body. All three are inherently part of our holistic nature and must be included in the total being of our existence. Ego, mind, and emotions create fields of manifesting motions and movements with as many variables with the aptness and likelihood to change or vary as there are people on earth. Here, again, our no-name body is responding and reflecting a natural interrelationship and intrarelationship with the many variables of these fields of ego, mind, and emotions.

Witness the body of a man expressing anger throughout his whole being as compared with the body of a person experiencing the serenity of one who is in a total state of surrender in meditative silence. Witness the influence of a frightened mother when her child is injured. A baby was brought to me who fell from a highchair and was unconscious. The mother was sitting across the room while I examined the baby. I checked the baby carefully while he was still unconscious and found nothing physically injured. I said, "There is nothing to worry about. Your child is all right." She exclaimed, "Thank God!" and she relaxed. Instantly, the baby responded by beginning to cry and move about normally. The mother's fear had contributed to the child's immobility.

We have briefly discussed the total unity of manifested motion and movement in a no-name body inherently capable of responding to and reflecting its internal and external environment as a unit of function within itself. We have added to it the multiple variables that the ego, mind, and emotions can contribute to it with their form of motion and movements. These are not cause and effect relationships. This is a total individual, whether it be physician or patient, in internal and external interrelationship and intrarelationship with the individual environment.

There is one more factor to be included in our clinical holistic approach and that is life itself, which manifests the motion and movements of the no-named body and the variable fields of the ego, mind, and emotions. If you have life as a factor that manifests itself in motion and movement at all levels from gross motion and movements to minute electron levels within cellular function or fields of ego, mind, and emotion, then life as a factor should be studied and developed until it, too, can be a clinical experience synchronous with the clinical development of motion and movement as the manifesting patterns of life.

Call it Life, Potency, or whatever term that is comfortable to you as a physician. It is a factor individually present in me, the physician, and in every living creature on earth—the patient at well. The factor of life can be developed and used by the physician and within the patient on an individualized basis. It is interesting to note that the relationship of the physician or patient to life as a factor is again on a one-on-one basis, as was the one-on-one basis of the no-name body. Life is without the variables of ego, mind, or emotions. Life is. The individual physician seeking to understand and use life as a factor in active participation in clinical application must develop his own understanding as a self-taught experience. I cannot teach you, you cannot teach me, how to include this factor of life in our daily use and in our individualized patient after patient relationship. It is something that can be learned but apparently has to be done by an individual effort.

In summary, we have discussed motion and movement in a no-name body physiology and in a named body physiology which includes ego, mind, and emotions. All motion and movement are effects, whether they be thought processes, emotional experiences, or body physiological mechanisms. In order to have motion and movement, it is necessary to include the automatic, shifting, suspension still points or fulcrums that allow these motions and movements to exist. Motion and movements are perceptible to the sensory input of the physician. The coexisting, shifting fulcrums that center motion and movements require the use of the physician's conscious awareness of their existence. It is important that the physician has clinical, conscious awareness of existing fulcrums as well as sensory experience of motion and movements in his diagnostic and treatment programs in the care of his patients' needs.

The following criteria for physician and patient can be found in body physiological functioning. Our no-name body physiology has four major patterns of motion and movement, five sensory inputs for the physician's use, plus his conscious awareness in diagnosis, and five basic principles of treatment potentials.

The four major patterns of motion and movements are:

1. Neuromusculoskeletal motion and movements; one might say the voluntary mechanisms of body physiological functioning.

2. The secondary costal respiratory mechanisms which move all tissues of the body during the respiratory cycles of breathing.

3. The inherent involuntary craniosacral fluctuation of the cerebrospinal fluid and the total lymphatic system at a rate of 10 to 14 times per minute in health, in rhythmic motility and mobility. Dr. William G. Sutherland has described this total rhythmic motion and movement as a tide-like phenomenon. This means that in any ten-minute period, the entire bodyphysiology has gone through a flexion with external rotation and extension with internal rotation cycle of motion and movement 100 times. This is a powerful diagnostic and therapeutic tool.

4. A large tide-like motion and movement that occurs about six times in a nine-minute period of time, a fluctuant mechanism, taking approximately one and a half minutes for each rhythmic cycle. I first noticed this large tide within my patients ten years

ago, and I have no idea as to its source or its basic nature. It is a more massive-feeling tide with a gradual, welling expansion of the whole body physiology and a gradual, receding movement to be followed by another gradual, massive expansion in rhythmic balanced interchange within and throughout the total body physiology. I have counted it in two patients simultaneously, and it was present in both but was individualized for each of them. It is a powerful therapeutic tool, as will be discussed later.

The total resources of body physiology, including the four major patterns of motion and movement, respond to and reflect the creative tensities of normal functioning through the involuntary membranous articular mechanisms of the primary respiratory mechanism and the fascial-ligamentous articular voluntary and involuntary mechanisms for the rest of body physiology. These same creative tensities are also found in the patterns of stress or strain associated with specific problems within the patient's body physiology. In other words, it takes reciprocal tension balance to maintain a homeostatic state of health, and it takes reciprocal tension balance to maintain a specific pattern of stress or strain within the no-name body physiology.

In addition to the physician's conscious awareness, he has the following five sensory inputs for evaluating motion and movement:

1. Sense of smell for odors.
2. Sense of taste for chemicals in food and liquids.
3. Sense of hearing for listening to motion and movement in tissue functioning.
4. Sense of sight for observing motion and movement.
5. Sense of touch and palpation for feeling motion and movement in the no-name body physiology.

All sensory inputs are given to us from birth, and we use them without conscious effort. However, we can consciously train any of them to perform at a much deeper level of perception. Witness the sense of smell of a perfume maker, the sense of taste of a wine or tea merchant, the listening experience of a musician, a cardiologist, or a lung specialist, and the sense of sight of an artist.

To truly develop the touch and palpatory sense requires months and years of conscious awareness and experience. It takes patience and patients over a long period of time to learn to feel the many gradations of motion and movement in the no-name body physiology. The art and science of palpation can be enhanced in both quantity and quality by learning to consciously project the sense of touch from the sensory area of the brain through to the hands by way of the proprioceptive neural pathways as well as the tactile endings, rather than passively waiting for sensory input to be transmitted from the hands to the sensory centers in the brain.

Another important factor is to recognize that the development of a palpatory skill is a one-on-one experience in quantum mechanics. It is impossible to be a detached observer. We are in fact active, consciously developing participators, sharing the experience of motion and movement at all gradations of functioning, from the simplest positional movement of articular mechanisms to the deepest level of voluntary and involuntary motion and movement in the total physiology of the patient.

The more sensitive our palpation becomes as a participator, the more awareness we develop for appreciating the inherent capacity and resources of our patient's voluntary and involuntary mechanisms to give us diagnostic evaluations and to provide the therapeutic mechanisms for treatment of the many problems presented to us as physicians. The opportunities are without limit.

The concept of motion and movement in therapeutics in the healing arts covers a wide field and many disciplines including all the medical and surgical approaches, psychology, radiology, physiotherapy, nursing, and any other supplemental care. All of these disciplines are based on sets of principles specifically oriented for the use of each type of service and to meet specific problems in securing a working diagnosis and a working clinical therapeutic restoration towards health. Our discussion will be a continuation of the criteria we have established for some of the major motion and movements found in a no-name body physiology and the physician's use of conscious awareness, his projected sensory inputs, and his sensitive motor skills to coordinate with his palpatory findings as a participator.

The therapeutic principles involved in using motion and movements are: 1. Exaggeration, 2. Disengagement, 3. Direct action, 4. Opposing physiological movement, and 5. Compression.

The art and science of palpation for diagnostic evaluation, when consciously serving as a participator, cannot be separated from the therapeutic principles, as it is a synchronous process in no-name body physiological functioning when the physician is working with the problem in the patient. The reason is simple. The no-name body of the patient has developed a problem that brings the patient to us. Our careful evaluation, using our participatory palpation and motor skills, gives us the experience of the motion and movement pattern within the patient. We are guided by the motion and movement. In our evaluation, we employ the principles, not the techniques, of exaggeration, disengagement, direct action, opposing physiological movement, compression, or a combination of these principles in order to localize and bring into focus the specific nature of motion and movement for the patient's complaint. These are also the initiating steps we use to treat the problems. The treatment process goes one step further in that we seek the point or points of balance for this motion and movement disability, and then we allow the inherent physiological resources and the potencies of the no-name body to secure the corrections available for the day's treatment.

A treatment could, perhaps, be described as follows: Our hands, our sensitive motion and movement palpatory skills as a participator in quantum mechanics, provide fulcrum points of reference for the no-name body physiology of the patient to awaken and use its motion-and-movement, internal resources to do the work of correcting its problems and guiding its mechanisms towards health. Through conscious awareness, palpatory skills, and sensitive motor skills, we seek the motion-and-movement patterns' points of balance for the specific strain or strains; we support the tissues at these points of balance; we feel the tissues and fluids go through a period of tensities to resolve the problem; we become aware of a quiet period, a stillpoint, a shift of the reciprocal tension balance or fulcrums specific to the problem; and we feel the gentle resolution in the tissues of restoration towards health following the correction. The no-name body physiology has done the work available for this day's treatment. One or several areas may be worked on in any given treatment session depending on the needs of the patient.

The five principles of treatment are principles and not techniques for the reason that any one or combination of them in their application initiates the no-name body physiology into action. What are some of the resources initiated? Any disability is going to modify the four major patterns of motion and movement: the neuromusculoskeletal voluntary motion, the secondary costal respiratory mechanisms, the inherent rhythmic involuntary fluctuation of cerebrospinal fluid and lymphatic system, and the large tide-like motion that has a rhythmic cycle of approximately one and a half minutes. It is these resources, and probably many more, that provide us with the tools we need to diagnose and treat using the five treatment principles.

It is, again, interesting to experience that when we have reached the point or points of balance and are supporting the tissues so that they will go through the treatment cycle, the creative tensities of the no-name body demonstrate exaggeration, disengagement, direct action, opposing physiological movement, and compression—or a combination of them—from within the body itself as it seeks and goes through the quiet period of the reciprocal-tension-balance shift of correction. The no-name body is using, within itself, the same set of principles we as physicians employ to find the point of balance that allows the body to go through its treatment cycle.

A brief comment about the large tide-like motion and movement as a therapeutic tool. It is not always clearly perceptible in every patient. When it can be monitored, it is a more massive feeling, with a gradual welling expansion of tide-like fingers of fluid infiltrating the bundles of membranous and fascial envelopes throughout the whole body. If one lived on a sea shore and saw the incoming tidal fingers filling up the nooks and crannies of an estuary, one would get the idea of this large tide's way of functioning. During the receding pattern, the tide-like fingers retreat from the membranous and fascial bundles to again return on the next incoming rhythmic cycle. It is a powerful therapeutic tool, as one can feel dozens or hundreds of minute membranous articular and fascial-ligamentous articular corrections taking place—a connective tissue that has enriched itself from some source that puts it to work at its most efficient phase of living function. The participating palpatory and sensitive motor skills can learn to find and use this large tide, not necessarily in every case or treatment but often enough to make it interesting and productive when it does show itself to the physician.

In conclusion, I, as a physician, and my patient, as an individual, are endowed with life, which manifests itself as motion and movement. We experience the resources of this endowment at all levels of our being in our spiritual awareness, egos, minds, emotions, and no-name body physiological functioning. As physicians, it is self-evident that we can use this manifested motion and movement as keys to diagnosis and treatment in the care of our patients. I would like to leave you with a question, "What is the key to motion?"

ANDREW TAYLOR STILL:
PHYSICIAN - ENGINEER - HUMANITARIAN
This paper was presented in 1985 as the Scott Memorial Lecture in Kirksville, Missouri.

THE SCIENCE OF OSTEOPATHY is a study of the human body as it functions in health.

Physician

Dr. Andrew Taylor Still announced his discovery of the science of osteopathy on June 22, 1874. This took place after years of intensive study, observation, skepticism, sorrow associated with death in his family, and service as a physician in the Civil War and as a midwest frontier doctor. Dissatisfied with the current medical care of his era, he sought for a new, living knowledge of detailed anatomicophysiological study of functioning in all structures in the human body. His laboratory was the patients he served in his day-to-day practice as well as the observations he made in the animal forms of his frontier life. He was an engineer and a physician seeking truth in the function of living forms. His "discovery" was the culmination and synthesis of his lifetime of study.

Twenty-five years later, he published his autobiography in which he confirmed his discovery of the science of osteopathy as a viable, living experience within each individual seeking a return to health. Dr. Still's role in this process was his detailed knowledge of anatomy and physiology as it functioned in health for the individual as well as his ability to use his hands and skills to guide and direct the resources of the living patient's mechanisms toward a return to health functioning in response to that patient's need.

In 1910, after 35 years of practicing the science of osteopathy, Dr. Still published his book, *Osteopathy: Research and Practice*, and reconfirmed all that he had found as truths in his discovery in 1874. Anatomy, understood; physiology, understood; innate vitality in each living individual, understood; and physician's use of this basic anatomical-physiology within the living patient to restore health, understood. Thirty-five years were spent in experiencing the demonstration of these principles. It was Dr. Still's ability to know the basic anatomy and physiology of the living body, to be able to get a mind's image of health mechanisms within the individual, and to develop a skilled manual corrective approach to the patient's body physiology to guide its return to health functioning. Dr. Still knew these principles and, more importantly, used these principles and observed the results—the return of health from within-out in the patients seeking his service.

The principles that Dr. Still discovered 110 years ago are as applicable and true today, in 1985, as they were in 1874. The term, "principles," is defined in the dictionary as: "1) The ultimate source, origin, or cause of something, or, 2) a natural or original tendency, or endowment." These definitions describe the fundamental concepts Dr. Still put forward.

It is refreshing to read the works of Dr. Still, and it is easy to find hundreds of quotations concerning the direct, one-on-one relationship between Dr. Still and his individual patients. Dr. Still was given an insight from his discovery into the fact that these active principles and concepts are inherently living in the mind, body, and soul of each patient; that it is the first object of the physician "to find health" for the individual, "anyone can find disease;" that the resources of the living body are available to the perceptive physician for the use of a mind image and palpatory skills to evaluate body physiology in health as well as disease and/or trauma; that the living body of the patient has the inherent tools with which to promote and induce the self-healing principles available from within the patient.

Engineer

The preface of Dr. Still's *Osteopathy: Research and Practice* provides this quotation:

Osteopathy is based on the perfection of Nature's work. When all parts of the human body are in line, we have health. When they are not, the effect is disease. When the parts are readjusted, disease gives place to health. The work of the osteopath is to adjust the body from the abnormal to the normal; then the abnormal condition gives place to the normal and health is the result of the normal condition.[1]

Here is an engineer's dream, a living machine capable of being in health through many decades of life, a machine available for the engineer's use. Each decade of life for the individual provides an evaluation as to the status of "normal" for the particular period in which the patient is seen. From an engineer's viewpoint, what is the health for this man or woman in their teens? How does it differ in these same individuals in their thirties or forties?

Normal health in body physiology is a state of being that defies definition. Normal is normal and is a living experience and a principle in life. If normal health cannot be defined, it can be described as two levels of function: One is basic involuntary mobility and motility in body physiology throughout life, and the second is voluntary mobility in body physiology as we live our daily life. Motion is not life. Motion is a manifestation of life. The engineer-physician has the opportunity to examine both involuntary and voluntary mobility in the body physiology of his or her patient and to determine the quality of health mechanisms in that patient. In other words, the manifestation of "normalcy" from within the patient provides the motion and function called health to demonstrate itself to the observing engineer. Since the goal of every patient is to return to normal, it is important that the physician knows what is health functioning from within for the patient seeking his service.

The emphasis in the quotation from Dr. Still is on the normalcy of health in the living human body. This primary focus on health is found throughout all his writings. The second lesson to be learned from this quotation is the fact that the presence of any disease and/or trauma in body physiology is an effect only, a departure from the normal in position and function in the areas wherein disease and/or trauma is found.

Health is a living principle in the living body, and it cannot be defined. Cause and effect is a principle in body physiology that can be defined in the presence of disease and/or trauma.

For example, a patient presents with a severe ankle sprain with possible torn ligaments. The ankle is experiencing symptoms and disturbed functioning, but these are only effects, not a cause of the disability. Perhaps the patient tried to catch himself with his outstretched hand or hands as he twisted and turned during his fall. There can be a departure from the normal at a number of sites in the patient's body, and each of these sites is a contributing cause to the final development of the sprained ankle. There can be an abnormal twist of a knee or acetabulum in either the right or left leg, a strain pattern in the psoas muscles, or a ligamentous articular strain in the arm and hand as they struck the ground during the fall. The accumulative results of these separate causal sites add up to being the cause of the ankle's injury. Each one of these sites must be evaluated and corrective treatment administered to restore health functioning at causal sites as well as at the ankle. With return to normalcy, health is again demonstrated in the ankle, and even torn ligaments will make a more complete resolution of tissue functioning.

Disease is another entity of departure from health and, like the ankle injury, is an effect only. Disease may take many forms, from long-standing problems, such as rheumatoid arthritis which lasts for years, to a relatively short-term illness, such as lobar pneumonia. The sick lung, in the case of lobar pneumonia, is not the cause of anything. It is a series of effects that runs a specific pattern as a departure from normalcy. Health returns to the lung when all effects are dissipated. To give corrective evaluation and treatment for cause in a disease state is to work on the sites of body physiology that allowed the lung to lower its resistance to disease and permitted the pattern called lobar pneumonia to develop. The effect is the sick lung. The sites of cause that contributed to this effect are to be found in the fluids, flesh, and bony relationships that control blood supply to the lung, the venous and lymphatic drainage from the lung and thoracic cage, the autonomic nervous system control of secondary respiratory mechanisms, the functioning of the excretory organs, and the awakening of the immune systems influencing the sick lung. In other words, corrective treatment is designed to work through causal sites to restore health in the effect area of disease, not merely the relief of symptoms.

Literally thousands of books and papers are prepared each year on symptom complexes, clinical syndromes, disease states, diagnostic and treatment programs for traumatic problems, and suggestions for health. There are multiple laws, principles, and concepts expressed to explain these entities. Cause is a term used to give support to other explanations for the clinical problem under discussion. The material printed is valid within the framework of knowledge as described by the authors involved. The mass of data is almost overwhelming in this day and age.

Dr. Still, on the other hand, offers the physician-engineer two basic principles from his 1874 discovery: 1) The principle of health within a living body physiology in bone, flesh, and fluids; 2) The recognition that disease and/or trauma are effects only and obey the principles of cause and effect in body physiology in bone, flesh, and fluids. To understand Dr. Still, it is necessary to practice his work as he discovered it and use the principles he promulgated.

Humanitarian

"Humanitarian: A person devoted to promoting the welfare of mankind, especially through the elimination of pain and suffering." In applying this dictionary definition to Dr. A.T. Still, it is necessary to go deeper into the definition by adding the phrase, "especially through the restoration of health from within."

Dr. Still's work began the hour he turned his back on the ineffectual health care of his day and age. Describing his discovery of the science of osteopathy on June 22, 1874, he states:

...I was shot—not in the heart but in the dome of reason. That dome was then in a very poor condition to be penetrated by an arrow charged with the principles of philosophy. ...Part of the time upon that day I withdrew from the presence of men to meditate upon that event, wherein I saw by the force of reason that the word, "God," signified perfection in all things and in all places. I began at that date to carefully investigate with the microscope of mind to prove an assertion that is often made...that the perfection of Deity can be proven by His works.[2]

Dr. Still took it upon himself to investigate, experiment, study, test, think, feel, and work with all the hidden factors that the principles of the science of osteopathy implied. It was an abrupt break for a man to shift from "an elimination of pain and suffering" to the "restoration of health from within."

There are many facets of knowledge and understanding to be learned from the *living* body physiology of the patient. There are many *living* diagnostic and treatment skills that can be used with development of perceptive coordination of the *living* physician working with a *living* patient to achieve a correction towards health.

The emphasis on the word *living* is intentional. Dr. Still's discovery includes his recognition that the human body is a machine run by the unseen force called Life. It is the "livingness" of the human body that permits it to respond to tests and techniques and tools of medical science, from the highly technical advances of computerized scanners and magnetic resonance imaging to the development of vaccines that have eradicated some of mankind's killing diseases to the refinement of antibiotics and other drugs to sophisticated heart surgery and so on. More advances have been made in the past six to ten years than have been made in the past 50 years. Many thousands of lives have been saved as a result of these advances.

Medical science and osteopathic science are not in competition with each other. Both depend on the "livingness" of the human body with its inherent life principle. One does not get a response to any diagnostic or therapeutic measure unless there is a "livingness" within the human body to make such a response. The quality of this "livingness" determines the results obtained. For example, a dose of a given medicine will respond poorly in a body with lowered vitality. It takes a relatively healthy body to respond correctly to any drug used in a diagnostic or treatment program. Another example is from an actual case many years ago. A patient had experienced a severe case of rheumatic fever that left him with a cardiac valvular disability and a murmur to indicate its presence. When the day-to-day "livingness" of the patient's body was good, his murmur could be heard loud and clear. When his vitality was low as a result of misuse in his way of life, the murmur weakened to the point of barely being able to hear it. With osteopathic treatment to restore his "livingness" toward health, his murmur would come back full strength. In his case, it took a strong heart to produce a good murmur. These two examples demonstrate that "livingness" is a function in body physiology that can be evaluated and used by the living physician in his work with his living patient.

In considering the applications of the science of osteopathy, think of the thousands of whiplash cases that have been restored to health and of osteopathy's role in preparing patients for surgery with pre- and post-operative osteopathic treatment to facilitate the return to health by utilizing the patients' resources from within. Think of the osteopathic care given in thousands of traumatic cases with major and, more often, minor injuries that contribute to less than normal health for the patient. Think of the osteopathic care available to hundreds of patients with disabilities who have been told, "Nothing can be done for your problem." Osteopathic diagnosis and treatment in these cases has demonstrated that "livingness" in body physiology functioning does have resources with which to arouse a path towards health from within.

There is an unseen quality in the work given to us by Dr. Still that is difficult to define or discuss but which should be touched upon in words and transformed into a learning experience in the physician's day-to-day practice. The definition of a humanitarian will perhaps serve to explain this quality of service. The Dr. Still of pre-discovery time was working as a physician for mankind, "especially through the elimination of pain and suffering" from without-in, with the medical art and science of his day. He was dissatisfied with the results he obtained, as a humanitarian should be, and he sought answers and skills with which to improve himself. At the moment of his discovery, "something happened," an unseen factor, a step into the unknown. The quality of his life as a physician was changed, transformed, or could the word, "transmutation," be used to explain what took place? As a result of this "silent" event, he became a humanitarian whose primary interest was service to mankind "through the restoration of health from within." He, himself, now understood the meaning and experience of the "livingness" of his own being and the same "livingness" from within his patient as one unit of life. He accepted this quality of "livingness" given to him without question and made it serve him in knowledge and use as a physician, engineer, and humanitarian in his daily practice.

What took place at the time of his discovery is something which has happened hundreds of times to individuals who have been involved in many disciplines. It is part of a learning process in those self-taught individuals deeply seeking answers to their specific needs. It occurs at the moment of its choice, not by intention.

Dr. Still gave the world the science of osteopathy and two clear, basic principles that could be used to serve mankind's needs: 1) the principle of health in body physiology that can be used as a principle in itself, and, 2) the principle of cause and effect that can be used in the care of disease and/or trauma in body physiology wherein any such problem is only an effect that can be diagnosed and treated through causal sites to restore health processes. Both principles are available for use for the living physician in working with a living patient.

The following quotation from Dr. Still provides an insight into his depth of knowledge and into the quality of his experience in the use of his work:

> I am fully convinced that God, of the mind of nature, has proven His ability to plan (if plan be necessary) and to make or furnish laws of self, without patterns, for the myriads of forms of animated beings; and to

thoroughly equip them for the duties of life, with their engines and batteries of motor force all in action. Each part is fully armed for duty, empowered to select and appropriate to itself from the great laboratory of nature such forces as are needed to enable it to discharge the duties to its office in the economy of life. In short, that the all-knowing Architect has cut and numbered each part to fit its place and discharge its duties in every building in animal form, while the suns, stars, moons, and comets all obey the one eternal law of life and motion.[3]

Thus, a physician's knowledge, an engineer's applicability, and a humanitarian's response towards health are the universal keys to the work given to us by Dr. Andrew Taylor Still.

1. A.T. Still, *Osteopathy: Research and Practice*, p.vii.
2. A.T. Still, *Autobiography*, p.258.
3. *Ibid.*, p.148.

STILLPOINTS

This is an edited transcription of a discussion held in 1986 at a
Sutherland Cranial Teaching Foundation faculty development program
in Philadelphia, Pennsylvania.

YOU HAVE ASKED THE question, What occurs at a stillpoint? That's a
good question and I'll try to elaborate, but this isn't the answer—
because there is no answer for what occurs at a stillpoint.

By shifting the relative functioning of a lever over a fulcrum, you
go through a stillpoint. You're creating a total interchange between
the two ends of a lever.

Now, don't let this throw you, but I gave up using the stillpoint; it
is not a goal I am seeking in a treatment. I even gave up looking for it.
I found a million stillpoints—before, during, and after...and eventually I gave up. I just get myself out of the road as far as necessary for
whatever to happen.

A stillpoint is a physiologic balancing act that the body physiology of any patient is going through. It can occur anytime, anywhere,
anyhow. It probably occurs spontaneously in patients during a good
night's sleep or something like that. It's the body's attempt to release
itself back to a total motile mechanism. In a treatment, it is an observable event that the physician can recognize as having taken place within
the body physiology but not one that he deliberately is seeking nor is
he trying to evaluate it. It is an anatomicophysiological change the
body is making, and I have nothing to do with it as a physician. I
don't even have to recognize it. The fact that it does take place indicates that the body physiology chooses to use it, and I am a simple
observer and not a goal seeker.

Often, stillpoints will happen in front of you, but you can also
frequently have the experience of them occurring at some distance.
You're quietly working on, listening to, some area in a patient, and all

of a sudden, you're aware of something happening elsewhere. Well, it had to have gone through a stillpoint for that to have happened. But you weren't in the area at the time it took place. You can be aware of the fact that the change took place, that something went through a stillpoint, but you weren't the author of it.

SITTING WITH YOUR MECHANISM

This is an edited transcription of lectures given in 1976 at a Sutherland Cranial Teaching Foundation basic course in Milwaukee, Wisconsin.

Internal Sensing Experience

IN THIS COURSE, WE started with the skull bones on the outside, went inside through the reciprocal tension membrane, brought in the coiling and uncoiling of the central nervous system, and introduced a fluid drive, the cerebrospinal fluid, into the neurocranial mechanism. We saw that this mechanism has the capacity to do certain things and create certain patterns–torsion, sidebending-rotation, vertical and lateral strains, and compression. We found that it can have specific membranous articular strains and that it has a great number of joints, and today we hung a face on it in detail.

Now for just a few minutes, I'd like you to sit up straight in your chairs and tune into your selves; we're going to reverse the process of the training program this week. I want you to very quietly, without effort, consciously be aware of the fluctuation of the cerebrospinal fluid taking place within your head–the fluctuation of the fluid drive. Quietly feel the cerebrospinal fluid, the fundamental principle of the primary respiratory mechanism. Whether you can actually feel it or not, simply be aware of it. I'm not asking you to actively feel it, just be aware of this as a fluid drive, rhythmically fluctuating, ebbing and flowing like the tide of an ocean, coming in and going out within your total craniosacral mechanism, going out along the cranial nerves, along the spinal nerves, drifting into and becoming part of the lymphatic system–your whole body becomes a coming-in and going-out of the cerebrospinal fluid.

Now see that fluid as a fluid drive rocking the Sutherland fulcrum. Imagine yourself at this fulcrum and see the dura reaching forward as

71

the falx cerebri, the tentorium cerebelli, the diaphragma sellae, and see it going down along the neural tube to the sacrum. All are part of that dural membrane lining the inside of the neurocranium. Feel it gently rocking back and forth within your own mechanism, within everybody's mechanism. It's the same in all of us, there's no difference.

See the central nervous system coiling and uncoiling rhythmically, the temporal lobes coiling around. There is a general movement forward over the parietal lobes towards the frontal lobes, towards a kind of fulcrum point, if you want to call it that. The coiling and uncoiling moves towards and away from the third ventricle. See the brain stem and the cerebellum, widening and narrowing; see the spinal cord coming down from the brain stem. Feel the fluid drive influencing the central nervous system, influencing the reciprocal tension membrane, rhythmically, in unison.

Now try to be aware of all these units very gently rocking the sphenobasilar synchondrosis into flexion and extension, the temporal bones into internal and external rotation, the parietals, frontal(s), and facial bones into internal and external rotation. Feel the sacrum; feel the pull of the dura on the sacrum. Feel the sacral base moving posteriorly during flexion of the sphenobasilar synchondrosis and anteriorly during sphenobasilar extension. Feel the whole mechanism at work.

Study this thing from the osseous skeleton inward, as a total involuntary mechanism within us, and then start back where it begins from the inside, with the fluid, the central nervous system, the reciprocal tension membrane, and the osseous skeleton. Feel the influence throughout the fascias of the body, the flexion-extension at the base of the skull influencing the cervical fascias to go into flexion-extension, while the ribs are going into external and internal rotation as are the arms, the legs, and the pelvis. Everything in your body is going into external and internal rotation, flexion and extension. Feel the whole thing working. Quietly. Without effort. This most powerful mechanism is a dynamic, total mechanism working towards health. Thank you.

Meditation

I'm GOING TO do something this morning I've never done—I don't know whether it's going to work, but it's an interesting thought. In Dallas, we have quite a large number of yoga groups, and because the yoga students are westernized bodies attempting to sit in non-western positions, they come to me with physiological strains they have induced from attempting to sit and meditate over a period of time. I'm not talking about yoga exercise, I'm talking about sitting for meditation. But I have also had contact with at least two people who are leaders of meditation groups and have become very adept at sitting in the posture that is called for in yoga meditation, and I believe there is a physiological reason why they use that position.

When they sit in the lotus position, they are sitting in such a way that they are not sitting down on their backsides the way you are now, leaning back into a chair and putting pressure on your sacrum against the seat, restricting the primary and secondary respiratory mechanisms. Instead, they are sitting up and forward, with their spines straight, sitting on their ischial tuberosities and thighs. What does this do? They have suspended their primary respiratory mechanism in mid-air—their entire mechanism from the cranial vault down to the sacrum is literally hanging in space.

Because this involuntary mechanism is rhythmically moving to and fro, the fluid, the reciprocal tension membrane, the central nervous system, and the articular mechanism can just hang there in suspension and allow the potency within the cerebrospinal fluid to nourish every single cell in the body. It allows the reciprocal tension membrane to gently rock the fascias into flexion/external rotation and back again; it allows the bones, ligaments, central nervous system, and everything else to shift and modify their pattern at a microlevel, which permits them to shift back towards a more normal physiological mechanism. They are literally in a state of self-treatment when they are in that position; they are making this mechanism a living factor of function.

Now, sit in your chairs with your feet on the floor, straighten your spines, and shift forward slightly so you're sitting on your pelvic bones

73

and not leaning back in your chair at all. Then, quietly, for a moment, with your eyes closed, think of a potent cerebrospinal fluid expanding and contracting rhythmically. This is an internal feeling—quietly within yourself try to feel a body of fluid that comes to a still point and expands, comes to a still point and ebbs, comes to a still point and expands, comes to a still point and ebbs, rhythmically every five to ten seconds. Fuse that feeling with the to-and-fro rocking of the reciprocal tension membrane by focusing on the straight sinus, the fulcrum of the reciprocal tension membrane. Don't worry about the ends of the levers, look to the fulcrum. Focus your attention, not your mental brain but your awareness, on the reciprocal tension membrane at the Sutherland fulcrum. Quietly. Quietly. Still...be still and sense this life in motion.

The
Cerebrospinal
Fluid Tide

THE CEREBROSPINAL FLUID
This is material from a written lecture dated 1977.

AN UNDERSTANDING OF CEREBROSPINAL fluid in the anatomicophysiology of the whole body offers concepts rich in anatomic detail, physiologic detail, and more importantly, in philosophic detail. Dr. A.T. Still has stated that "...the cerebrospinal fluid is the highest known element that is contained in the human body, and unless the brain furnishes this fluid in abundance, a disabled condition of the body will remain. He who is able to reason will see that this great river of life must be tapped and the withering field irrigated at once, or the harvest of health be forever lost."[1] W.G. Sutherland added that the arterial stream is supreme but the cerebrospinal fluid is in command, and its fluctuation within a natural cavity can be observed by palpation. The key to understanding cerebrospinal fluid is that it can be *used* by the physician for both diagnosis and treatment by way of its fluctuation patterns and, more importantly, as an anatomicophysiological entity within a living body in integrated function with the whole body. One might say that through the understanding of cerebrospinal fluid and its fluctuation patterns, one is dealing with the rechargeable battery of life and health in human physiology.

Anatomic Considerations

The discovery of the cerebrospinal fluid is generally ascribed to Domenico Cotugno, but the first serious study of cerebrospinal fluid was made by Francois Magendie, a French physiologist, in 1825. It is now widely accepted by most observers that the greater part of the cerebrospinal fluid is elaborated by the choroid plexuses, although there are still some questions as to whether it is formed by secretion or by dialysis. In addition, there is evidence that small quantities of cerebrospinal fluid are made by cerebral structures in the perivascular spaces and from structures in the central canal of the spinal cord.

The choroid plexuses are tufts of small capillary vessels of the tela choroidea which are fringe-shaped and which are covered by a very fine layer of ependymal cells. In other words, the capillary beds of the choroid plexuses are not in direct contact with the cerebrospinal fluid but are separated from it by this thin curtain of ependymal cells. A choroid plexus is found in each ventricle of the brain. The venous drainage for the choroid plexuses of the lateral and third ventricles is by way of the great cerebral vein of Galen, which passes through the junction of the falx cerebri with the tentorium cerebelli—the Sutherland fulcrum of the reciprocal tension membrane. The venous drainage of the choroid plexus in the fourth ventricle is by way of other venous sinuses in the floor of the occipital portion of the cranial base.

The circulation of cerebrospinal fluid has been determined by radionuclide studies. These have demonstrated the flow of the cerebrospinal fluid from the lateral ventricles through the foramen of Monro into the third ventricle, down the cerebral aqueduct of Sylvius to the fourth ventricle, and from the fourth ventricle through the foramen of Magendie in the roof of the fourth ventricle into the cisterna magna or through the two lateral foramina of Luschka into the lateral recesses. From these three openings in the fourth ventricle, the movement of cerebrospinal fluid proceeds into subarachnoid pathways towards the apex of the brain, where resorption takes place principally in the pacchionian granulations along the superior sagittal sinus. Part of the cerebrospinal fluid descends down the spinal canal to then reascend and rejoin the general circulation. The greater absorption of cerebrospinal fluid is by way of the pacchionian granulations, but in addition, there is slow absorption by way of the perineural spaces of the cranial and spinal nerves into the lymphatic system. This is particularly true of absorption into the lymphatic apparatus of the neck from the subarachnoid space through its relation to the olfactory bulb, the first cranial nerve. It is generally accepted that the cerebrospinal fluid (the third circulation in the central nervous system) is absorbed into the lymphatic system (the third circulation in the whole body). The total quantity of cerebrospinal fluid in the ventricular and subarachnoid spaces varies usually between 125 and 150 cubic centimeters.

Editor's note: An article reviewing the various pathways of cerebrospinal fluid distribution is "Recent Research into the Nature of Cerebrospinal Fluid Formation and Absorption." J. Neurosurg *1983, 59:369-383.*

Physically, cerebrospinal fluid is a living fluid, the water content of which is somewhat greater than that of blood. Its protein content is very low in comparison with blood and its sugar content, moderately reduced. Other substances such as creatinine, uric acid, urea, inorganic phosphate, bicarbonate, hydrogen ions (pH), sodium, potassium, magnesium, calcium, and lactic acid are present in spinal fluid in quantities equal to or generally less than that found in blood plasma. Spinal fluid drawn by spinal tap will vary slightly from that found in the ventricles.

In addition to the circulatory patterns of the cerebrospinal fluid described, there is reference in some studies to an ebb and flow within the cerebrospinal fluid, a characteristic of a fluctuation. When it is referred to in these writings, it is not a clear-cut acceptance of this phenomenon but rather an observation made, which finds such a pattern to exist but has no explanation for it. Since most of these studies were trying to determine circulatory factors in cerebrospinal fluid, their primary interests were on that subject rather than the finding of a fluctuation pattern and its significance.

Physiologic Considerations

A 1975 editorial from *Lancet*, "Cerebrospinal Fluid: The Lymph of Brain?", contains the following quotations worthy of note:

A function of the lymphatic system is to clear the tissue spaces of substances that pass out of blood capillaries, or originate in the tissues, and are not reabsorbed into the blood stream. The meninges and nervous tissue of the brain lack lymphatic channels; does their absence mean that there is no problem of disposal?

...besides the bulk flow of CSF back into blood through the arachnoid villi, substances may be cleared from CSF by the choroid plexuses. This conception seems bizarre if attention is limited to the plexuses in the lateral ventricles; producing CSF as they do, how from upstream could they remove constituents from it? But these are not the only plexuses; the third ventricle has its plexus, and the stream of CSF emerging from the ventricular system passes through the fronds of the fourth ventricle's plexus. Certain organic acids can be actively absorbed by this route; and a considerable range of other substances, some (such as noradrenaline and serotonin) of obvious interest because of the neurotransmitter function, are accumulated by isolated choroid plexus preparations, so that they too may be absorbed there, or else from the cerebral subarachnoid space. So there is a route from CSF back to blood other than by bulk flow through the arachnoid villi.

...Another component which enters the brain readily is CO_2; it is of course also produced there, and lactate and pyruvate may originate within the brain itself. CSF is poorly buffered; it contains about as much bicarbonate as plasma, but little protein and few cells. Thus its flow can serve to convey information about excess CO_2 or increased acid formation within the brain, since CSF pH will fall. The information is sensed on the ventrolateral surfaces of the medulla and the response consists in increased pulmonary ventilation—a tenfold rise in man for a CSF pH change of 0.05. The stabilizing effect on CSF pH is evident—provided that the respiratory system is normal and capable of excreting more CO_2. The arrangement is much faster and more effective than simply waiting for the slow flow gradually to wash the brain clean again. Lymph flow clears the extracellular fluid in the body generally; CSF flow seems to do the same for the brain more precisely and efficiently.[2]

The clues offered by this brief discussion from the editorial in *Lancet* indicate that a study of the substances and metabolites within cerebrospinal fluid is a very complex subject, one which has occupied the minds of many researchers over many decades and will occupy a great many more minds in the years to come.

An interesting, though now historical, use of cerebrospinal fluid was made by A.D. Speransky, a Russian physiologist, and described in his book, *A Basis for the Theory of Medicine*, published in 1943.[3] One section contains the following chapter headings: "The Connection of the Submembranous Spaces of the Brain with the Lymphatic System," "Our Investigations on the Connection of the Submembranous Spaces with the Lymphatic System," "The Movement of Cerebrospinal Fluid within the Medulla and Submembranous Spaces," and "On the Penetration of Various Substances into the Nerve Trunk and their Movement Along It." These chapters indicate some of the directions of thought by Speransky and his colleagues.

In his chapter on "Rheumatism," Speransky describes a method of "pumping" the cerebrospinal fluid: "Pumping was performed by means of lumbar puncture, usually in a sitting position. For the operation we used a 10.0 cc 'Record' needle. The withdrawal and reinjection of the fluid was repeated from 8 to 40 times. The last portion of fluid was removed. The operation must not be carried out too slowly or too rapidly. Rapid extraction, especially during the second half of the operation, always produces headaches, which do not pass off until the evening and sometimes persist until the following day. In isolated cases, vomiting occurred."

This gross mechanical pumping of the cerebrospinal fluid within the dural sac and subarachnoid spaces was used in a number of neurodystrophic processes or diseases. The methods he used were not without danger, to say the least. Speransky's work created a great deal of controversy during his time and for many years.

His opening statement in Chapter XXI, "This book cannot have a conclusion," is significant. There may, indeed, be no conclusions other than that the knowledge concerning cerebrospinal fluid is most complex. Cerebrospinal fluid interchanges ions, metabolites, and trophic factors with the choroid plexuses, the neurons of the central and peripheral nervous system, the autonomic nervous system, the pituitary-hypothalamic axis, the pineal gland, and the lymphatic system. In addition, its thin film of fluid in the subarachnoid spaces combined with the cisterns act as water beds for protecting the brain and spinal cord.

Philosophic Considerations

To *use* cerebrospinal fluid in a diagnostic and treatment program requires more than a synthesis of anatomicophysiological detail and more than the study through laboratory procedures of the cerebrospinal fluid's characteristics as it is found in health, trauma, or disease. It requires the art of palpation to bring to the physical the experience of working with this living fluid within a living organism, the human body.

When we talk about palpation, I like to think of it in two phases working concurrently. There is the input of sensing the activity from within the body as recorded by palpation and there is a motor output, which I choose to call applied palpatory skill, wherein I work with the activity sensed by palpation to achieve a change within the activity or pattern of functioning. To me, an applied palpatory skill as a motor output is more sensitive and subtle in its application than a so-called manipulative technique. Any work done with the cerebrospinal fluid in clinical application as a living fluid already in motion requires sensitivity on my part as a physician, if I am to achieve maximum efficiency in my clinical use of cerebrospinal fluid dynamics. The subject of palpation brings up another feature worth noting. Palpation involves the use of energy, both for sensory input and motor output, and it can only be explained by quantum mechanics. An article in *Science News* summarizes this point:

> Mechanistic philosophy of classical science: A thing has an objective reality of its own. The basis of science is objectivity...In the quantum domain, maybe not. Thus quantum mechanics makes the observer a participator. Not only in Heisenberg's sense that the observer disturbs what he measures, but in the more profound sense that his choices of what to measure will determine what he finds. Reality has no objective existence apart from the act of observation. Wheeler says, "In some strange sense, this is a participatory universe. What we have been accustomed to call 'physical reality' turns out to be largely a papier-mache construction of our imagination plastered in between the solid iron pillars of our observations. These observations constitute the only reality."

Wheeler concludes: "Until we see why the universe is built this way, we have not understood the first thing about it.... We can well believe that we will first understand how simple the universe is when we recognize how strange it is."[4]

My point is this: When I, the physician, am working with the living cerebrospinal fluctuation patterns within the patient, I am a participator with that fluctuation pattern and am sharing the experience of that which I observe through palpation by sensory input and that which is changing within the patterns as a result of palpatory skills as motor output. The only reality permissible to consider is that of continuous change—changes taking place as I observe the patterns, changes taking place as applied palpatory skills modify patterns, and changes that take place within the anatomicophysiology of the patient after my diagnostic and treatment program continues that day's work. The role of the physician as a participator in his palpation of cerebrospinal fluid functioning is most important.

I like the thought of being a participator rather than a third-person observer in taking care of problems within the patient's body, whether it be a musculoskeletal dysfunction, a fascial strain pattern, or one associated with the primary respiratory mechanism. In either a diagnostic or a treatment program, I have the feeling I am experiencing the changes taking place within the patient and thus have better diagnostic insight as to the nature of the dysfunction. I am, therefore, able to better control the results of treatment for the corrections available for that day's work. I find it necessary to accept the thought that I am a participator and to maintain this awareness throughout my diagnostic and therapeutic survey. I get a much deeper quality of experience and results as a participator than when I am merely a third-person observer.

Working with the natural resources within the body, including cerebrospinal fluid, and using our sensory and motor qualities of awareness require three definitions and two sets of principles for a more complete understanding of the mechanisms involved. The definitions include self-organization, fluctuation, and transmutation. The two sets of principles are the Breath of Life and the breath of air.

Self-organization: the innate capacity of the individual to express life physically, mentally, emotionally, and philosophically.

The individual has a dual set of mechanisms working concurrently throughout life—a voluntary capacity to work, play, and rest and a complex involuntary mechanism designed to maintain health and adapt to trauma and/or disease. In 1932, Cannon described this self-organization of the body as homeostasis, a dynamic equilibrium in which all the body processes are maintained in their respective equilibria. This is definitely not a static process but a continuous living process. A.T. Still's autobiography speaks of it in this way:

> I hope all who may read after my pen will see that I am fully convinced that God, of the mind of nature, has proven His ability to plan (if plan be necessary) and to make or furnish laws of self, without patterns, for the myriads of forms of animated beings; and to thoroughly equip them for the duties of life, with their engines and batteries of motor force all in action. Each part is fully armed for duty, empowered to select and appropriate to itself from the great laboratory of nature such forces as are needed to enable it to discharge the duties peculiar to its office in the economy of life. In short, that the all-knowing Architect has cut and numbered each part to fit its place and discharge its duties in all buildings in animal forms while the suns, stars, moons, and comets all obey the one eternal law of life and motion.[5]

Most of us, as physicians and patients, rely on this self-organization within us blindly, without asking questions, for maintaining health and combating trauma and/or disease. I have a question. How much more could we as physicians and surgeons accomplish for our patients if we would develop and use our awareness for the potentials of this self-organization within ourselves and within the patients every time they come to us seeking our services? Each of us, as an individual, must ask our own questions and seek our own answers.

Fluctuation: the movement of a fluid contained within a natural or artificial cavity, observed by palpation or percussion.

Cerebrospinal fluid fluctuates rhythmically within a natural cavity, the neurocranium, and it can be observed by palpation. Because the body is basically fluid in composition, and in addition, cerebrospinal fluid is absorbed, in part, into the lymphatic system of the body, the fluctuation of cerebrospinal fluid can be observed throughout the body.

The basic rhythmic patterns of cerebrospinal fluid fluctuation which can be observed by palpation are longitudinal, alternating lateral, and spiral patterns. There are probably many other patterns or combination of patterns not so easily observed because of their minute character. A more specific rhythmic pattern of cerebrospinal fluid fluctuation can be palpated by directing the cerebrospinal fluid across the long diagonal of any portion of the body.

The accepted rate of cerebrospinal fluid fluctuation in health is 10 to 14 times per minute, although this varies according to various states of dysfunction within the individual. It can be very slow in chronic disabilities and increased in the presence of fevers.

The quality of the fluctuation patterns is far more important than the rate. In health, there is a palpatory sense of full amplitude, a sense of vitality and living dynamics. In rheumatoid arthritis, due to stasis of all connective tissues and lymphatic fluids, there is a sense of a thin, watery, low amplitude; in cases of post-meningitis or post-encephalitis, there is a sense of a dull amplitude because the reciprocal tension membrane has lost its physiological tone quality. These are but a few of the more obvious illustrations of the variability of the quality of cerebrospinal fluid fluctuation patterns. This living cerebrospinal fluid with its manifest fluctuation is meeting the challenges of hour-to-hour, day-to-day health patterns within the individual and will show changes of quality and rate to reflect those needs.

We are told by Dr. Sutherland that the fluctuation of cerebrospinal fluid comes first, as a phenomenon in and of itself, and I am in complete agreement with this thought. There are those who disagree and seek to associate it with the contractility of the central nervous system or the rhythmic inhalation and exhalation of the respiratory system. There is obviously an interrelationship with all of the living tissues and their rates of rhythmic function, a motile central nervous system, a to-and-fro rocking of the reciprocal tension membrane, a rhythmic respiratory mechanism, and others, both voluntary and involuntary, and these modify the fluctuation of the cerebrospinal fluid and are modified by the fluctuation of cerebrospinal fluid. Nevertheless, if we, as physicians, with our awareness and palpatory methods, will work with the cerebrospinal fluid dynamics with the thought in mind of it being the primary phenomenon, we will do better work in our diagnostic and treatment programs. As an analogy, I listen more intently to the heart knowing it is the primary pump in the cardiovascular system. This goes back to what was said earlier: We are participators with a living entity in a living body in the application of our skills.

Here is another form of fluctuation pattern. Within the craniosacral mechanism, the fluctuation of the cerebrospinal fluid, the motility of the central nervous system, and the motility of the reciprocal tension membrane produce rhythmic flexion and extension of the midline articular mobility of the cranial bones and sacrum associated with external and internal rotation of the bilateral bones. These rhythmic patterns are not confined to the craniosacral mechanism. They are present throughout all the anatomicophysiological mechanisms of the body, and this micromovement within every bone, cell, and fluid of the body is one of the essential factors of the self-organization of the body for health. It is an involuntary movement throughout the span of life for the individual that contributes to Cannon's homeostasis and to Still's "one eternal law of life and motion." It is an involuntary movement that is present during all voluntary movements of the individual, working, playing, or resting. It can be sensed by palpation.

At this point, I would like to suggest two diagnostic tests that utilize this involuntary movement and self-organization of the body:

1. The patient has an area of somatic dysfunction you, the physician, wish to correct. Using an alert but quiet palpation, check the quality of the involuntary flexion/external rotation, extension/internal rotation pattern anywhere else in the patient's body, then check it in the area of somatic dysfunction. Check it again after the corrective treatment has been made for the somatic dysfunction. If you can feel approximately the same quality of involuntary movement in the area of somatic dysfunction as you felt in your test area, you can rest assured your correction will continue to unfold towards health for that problem. If you do not feel the improved involuntary movement after the correction in the area of somatic dysfunction, you may have secured mobility for the area, but its innate function has not been obtained for immediate use by the body.

2. With an alert but quiet palpation, be aware of all the components of self-organization involving the quality of the fluctuation of cerebrospinal fluid and the involuntary movement within the body. Palpate to assess the total vitality of the patient's anatomicophysiological mechanisms. While this vitality is not necessarily electrical in nature, I like to compare it to a voltage reading and make an estimated reading for each patient. In other words, the average patient should feel as if their vitality is 110 volts. In cases of dysfunction, such as a chronic nervous system breakdown, the voltage may be down to 60, 50, or less. The same is true in cases of rheumatoid arthritis. It can be low in acute fatigue within the patient, but this voltage reading feels as if it is temporary and will probably correct itself with a good night's sleep. The voltage reading for professional athletes is not 110 volts but a physiological 220 volts. It would have to be to take the punishment these people get in their sports.

This is a useful test because it gives you a sense of the quality of the vitality you are working with in diagnosing and treating problems. Adequate voltage means adequate vitality with which to make a correction and have it continue to unfold as you would like it to do; low voltage indicates your attempted corrections should stay within the capacity of the patient to use the correction because an over-correction, in this lessened vitality state, will not last and adds to the patient's local and general fatigue already present.

This test is not to be confused with counting the cranial rhythmic impulse (CRI). The test I have given you is more sensitive and informative. Both of these tests require further elaboration, but enough has been said to bring them to your attention.

Transmutation: the change of one thing into another; the change of one chemical element into another.

Transmutability is a natural phenomenon occurring within the body throughout life. The rhythmic fluctuation of the cerebrospinal fluid involves transmutability and creates rhythmic balanced interchange with the choroid plexuses, the physiological centers in the floor of the fourth ventricle, the neurons of the central and peripheral nervous system, the pituitary-hypothalamic axis, pineal gland and other hormonal glands throughout the body, the lymphatic system, and, in fact, with all the cellular and fluid systems of the body.

This transmutation factor in the fluctuation of the cerebrospinal fluid can be enriched, revitalized, and maximized in the patient by the physician. By use of his awareness, palpation, and applied palpatory skills, the physician can apply a controlled compression to the existing patterns of fluctuation of the cerebrospinal fluid—whether it be a longitudinal, alternating lateral, or spiral pattern—to bring it down until it reaches a brief rhythmic period in its functioning, a "stillpoint." By bringing it down to and through this stillpoint, an immediate and instant rhythmic balanced interchange occurs between all the bodily fluids. It is far-reaching in its physiological effects.

A dramatic example is found in two case histories. In 1947, a nine-month-old baby was brought to me, screaming and crying. The baby's skin, from the top of its head to the soles of the feet, was a continuous dermatitis—cracking, weeping, and blood tinged. The dermatitis had been present for eight months, and the baby had been seen by a dozen physicians without control or relief. What could I do for this child? I didn't know. I gave it a treatment using compression of the fourth ventricle. Within 18 hours after this first treatment, the baby had grown a complete, new skin without a blemish on it. Three days later, when the child was brought back to me, it still had an intact new skin with a minor breakdown in isolated spots over parts of its body. It continued to improve during the succeeding months.

Equally dramatic was the case of a 55-year-old man whose rheumatoid arthritis had reached the chronic stage of disability, but without pain. I told him nothing could be done for his "arthritis" but that I would give him a treatment since he was in my office. Due to the peripheral resistance of the lymphatic stasis throughout his body, it took me 45 minutes to apply a compression of the fourth ventricle and bring the fluctuation down to and through its stillpoint. He came back a week later and insisted on another treatment. He showed me his legs from his knees downward (I had not examined them before), and they were covered with a dry exanthematous crust, which he told me had been weeping for years. A second application of compression of the fourth ventricle was given which took 30 minutes. The skin of his legs completely healed within another week and stayed healthy.

Howard Lippincott, D.O., describes the results of compression of the fourth ventricle as follows:

It is hard to appear conservative in considering the uses of compression of the fourth ventricle because this potent fluid, activated by the technique, produces results that justify enthusiasm.

There is a beneficial effect upon the entire circulatory system, with reduction of congestions, ischemias and edemas, such as in the realm of possibility without surgical interference.

Metabolic processes are improved, including nutrition to the tissues and the gradual absorption of fibrous and calcium deposits that are not physiological or compensatory.

It enhances organic function, and in the presence of infection immunity is increased through effects upon the spleen, pancreas and liver.

The endocrine system is regulated to the immediate needs of the body.

The cerebrospinal fluid is in command of the metabolism, much of the involuntary operation, and the autoprotective mechanism of the system.

Dr. Sutherland calls attention to the fact that secondary osteopathic lesions become less perceptible under the influence of compression of the fourth ventricle. So it is of value in determining the primary lesion.[6]

As indicated, the involuntary mobility of the body with its micro-movement of flexion/external rotation and extension/internal rotation is revitalized. Furthermore, the battery of life, as expressed by the suggested voltage indicator, is immediately transmuted towards that which is physiologically ideal for that patient, whether it be 110 volts or 220 volts.

Controlled compression of the fluctuation of the cerebrospinal fluid, bringing it down to and through its short, rhythmic period or stillpoint, can be applied through the parietals, the frontal(s), the temporals, or the sacrum. It does not have to be solely applied as compression of the fourth ventricle. In fact, it is necessary to apply this technique by way of the sacrum in severe head trauma or suspected cranial fractures.

What is this transmutation factor? Dr. Sutherland said that when the fluctuation of the cerebrospinal fluid is brought down to this short, rhythmic period, the stillpoint, there is a rhythmic balanced interchange with the Breath of Life. He did not have an explanation for this transmutation factor nor did he explain why the fluctuation of cerebrospinal fluid is primary in itself. The results of changes in all the bodily fluids can be measured before and after using these techniques for cerebrospinal fluid, and the tests will speak for themselves. The Breath of Life principle, which enters into and is the fundamental transmutation factor within the self-organization of the body, remains invisible and is not measurable. The awareness of the physician can accept this principle of transmutation as a fact the physician can use in working with cerebrospinal fluid. The physician can measure the results with his palpation and applied palpatory skills and his laboratory tests.

The following case histories present the use of repeated compression of the fourth ventricle technique as the sole treatment for each type of case; some of these were purely experimental:

My daughter was three years old in 1945 and came down with lobar pneumonia. In three days, she went through the whole disease process and her lungs were clear. In eight days, her vitality was that of physiological health. Similar results were obtained in a number of adult cases of lobar pneumonia.

In 1955, my 20-year-old son came down with a severe case of mononucleosis. In 30 days, his total pattern was that of health, including his differential blood counts. He recovered his full health long before his classmates who fell ill at the same time. This was duplicated in a series of such cases.

In a series of over 50 cases of nervous system breakdown with thin, watery, low amplitude, low voltage reading fluctuation patterns, compression of the fourth ventricle was applied once a week over a period of six to nine months. A physiological, self-sustaining fluctuation health pattern was restored in each case, although the results were slow to manifest during the first half of the period of treatment, and it took a lot of persuasion to keep some of the patients coming long enough to achieve the results they were seeking.

An equal number of rheumatoid arthritis cases made a similar clinical response and regained their inherent vitality. Although the disabled appearance of the involved joints remained, their pain was much less. Again, it took six to nine months. I also had two cases which made an inadequate response, but even they were improved. As described earlier, it took a long time to get down to the stillpoint at the beginning of their treatment program, but this phase improved as the weeks went by and as they responded to the rhythmic balanced interchange taking place in their congested tissues.

Many cases of terminal cancer, including some with inoperable brain tumors, were kept relatively pain-free and their lives made more bearable during the last few weeks and months before their passing.

I have used the application of controlling the fluctuations of cerebrospinal fluid, bringing it down to its short rhythmic period, in many ways and in hundreds of cases to meet varying needs. I do not use it in every case that comes through the office. I use it whenever my awareness of its need arises. It always meets the challenge within the patient, generally with a lot less drama than some of the cases already described, and I am aware, through my palpation and applied palpatory skills, that it has met and fulfilled the needs for that day's treatment.

Breath of Life Principle: Dr. Sutherland has stated that the Potency of the cerebrospinal fluid might be considered as a fundamental principle in the functioning of the primary respiratory mechanism. He has also referred to it as the Breath of Life, an Invisible Element, and in other terms that would attract our attention to its importance in the functioning of cerebrospinal fluid. Dr. Sutherland spent years developing his understanding of all elements and components of the craniosacral mechanism: the cranial articular mechanisms and sacrum, the reciprocal tension membrane, the motility of the central nervous system, and the fluctuation of the cerebrospinal fluid. Working in solitude, he performed experiments using compressive bandages on his own head to produce extension, flexion, sidebending-rotation, and torsion mechanisms; he produced membranous articular strains, some of them quite severe, and corrected them. With these compressive bandages, he studied the intense response of working with the cerebrospinal fluid, of bringing the cerebrospinal fluid down to its short rhythmic period, its stillpoint, and he observed the milking effect on the lymphatics and bodily fluids throughout his entire body. He worked with his own thinking-feeling-seeing-knowing fingers upon his own mechanisms to *know* the intricate functioning of all elements of the primary respiratory mechanism before he began using this approach for the problems within his patients. His understanding, terminology, and concepts are based on a participating knowledge from within himself and not solely upon clinical observations in testing for these findings in other individuals.

We, as physicians, can develop our participating awareness, our palpation and applied palpatory skills. It is a painfully slow process for most of us to develop our own thinking-feeling-seeing-knowing fingers so as to experience within our patients that which Dr. Sutherland gave us concerning all phases of the primary respiratory mechanism.

I do not find it necessary that Dr. Sutherland should have given us an explanation for the fact that the fluctuation of cerebrospinal fluid comes first as a phenomenon in and of itself nor for the phenomenon of transmutation and interchange with the Potency, the Breath of Life, or whatever you choose to call it (I have my own private name for it), which takes place during the short, rhythmic period, the stillpoint, as well as an immediate rhythmic balanced interchange that takes place physiologically in all bodily fluids. Dr. Sutherland gave us his terminology many years ago. Modern science is still seeking terminology and understanding in all disciplines of science, as Wheeler exemplified in the statement quoted earlier: "We can well believe that we will first understand how simple the universe is when we recognize how strange it is." Dr. Sutherland proved his concepts from within himself; we prove it in our clinical experience within our patients.

Breath of Air Principle: Just as the Breath of Life principle provides us with the information that cerebrospinal fluid is a fluctuating rhythmic entity of function for interchange with a life force, so does the breath of air principle provide us with information concerning all anatomicophysiological circulatory and rhythmic systems of function for our walkabout on earth. We require a lot more than just a life force to manifest as an individual. We require food, water, air, light, darkness, mobility, motility, and other factors; we have whole sets of internal systems, some voluntary and some involuntary, designed to modify each other and to be modified by each other in performing their circulatory and rhythmic duties and functions; we have something called a mind, consciousness, or awareness, to allow us to realize we are a product of a total environment, and not merely our own (even if we do think it is the most important), and that we must be in rhythmic balanced interchange with that environment. These are some of the elements for the integrated function of the self-organization of life for the individual in maintaining health and adapting to trauma and/or disease.

As physicians, we are given a continuously developing, massive array of diagnostic and therapeutic tools with which to evaluate and treat the individual who comes to us with a problem. One of the most valuable tools we have is our own awareness, palpation and applied palpatory skills to participate with the internal milieu of the patient for either primary care or as supplemental care in a diagnostic and treatment program.

For the purposes of discussion, I have divided the self-organization of the individual into a Breath of Life principle and a breath of air principle, but in reality they are one: one in the innate capacity of the individual to express life physically, mentally, emotionally, and philosophically. As a physician, I can utilize all the available resources of modern medicine and surgery to give aid to the patient who seeks my service; and as a participator, through my awareness, palpation and applied palpatory skills, I can work with the innate capacities to achieve balance in functioning within this dynamic homeostatically controlled body as it obeys the "one eternal law of life and motion." Cerebrospinal fluid, as one of these innate capacities, still provides an open-door challenge to explore its potentialities.

1. A.T. Still, *Philosophy of Osteopathy*, p. 39.
2. "Cerebrospinal Fluid: The Lymph of the Brain?", *Lancet*, 1975, 2:444-5.
3. A.D. Speransky, *A Basis for the Theory of Medicine*, ed. and trans. C.P. Dutt (New York: International Publishers, 1943).
4. "Quantum Mechanics," *Science News*, Vol 109, No. 21, May 22, 1976.
5. A.T. Still, *Autobiography*, p. 148.
6. W.G. Sutherland, *Contributions of Thought*, pp. 152-3.

THE POTENCY OF THE TIDE

*This is excerpted material from written lecture notes
dated 1985 and 1969.*

THE CEREBROSPINAL FLUID HAS a Potency within it, a Breath of Life principle, a Highest Known Element—a fluid within a fluid. This invisible factor is found at the midway point between inhalation and exhalation, a fulcrum point in the tidal shifting from flexion/external rotation to extension/internal rotation. This Potency is found at the point of balance for the cerebrospinal fluid tide.

The cerebrospinal fluid tide can be used and controlled by modifying its existing rhythmic pattern, bringing its fluid movement (with its inherent Breath of Life) down to and through a stillpoint. During this stillpoint, there is an immediate shift within the tide and an interchange between the cerebrospinal fluid and all the fluids of the body—a transmutation between the dynamics of the Potency, with its Breath of Life, and the vitality of every living tissue and fluid in the body. It is a point wherein a transmutation takes place between the Potency and its manifesting, visible physiological functioning in the whole body.

The various types of cerebrospinal fluid fluctuations (tides) can be observed by palpation, and the quality of the tide for each individual can be evaluated. It is also possible to observe the changes taking place when the tide is brought down to and through its stillpoint as well as the therapeutic response in the primary respiratory mechanism and body physiology. In this response to the stillness of the tide and the transmutation, the effects go beyond a simple release of somatic dysfunction to a release which initiates a return to health functioning. Knowledge and use of the cerebrospinal fluid tide provide an example wherein one "allows physiological function within to manifest its own unerring potency rather than the use of blind force from without."

Dr. A.T. Still did not invent the fundamentals of the science of osteopathy; he discovered them. He states this in his autobiography. Dr. W.G. Sutherland did not invent the cranial concept; he discovered its fundamental principles. He discovered that the cerebrospinal fluid interchanges with what he chose to call the "Breath of Life." When the cerebrospinal fluid fluctuation is controlled by bringing it down to a relative still point, there is an immediate transmutation, an interchange between the highest known element and the cerebrospinal fluid, that contributes a nourishing factor, a "Spark" and "bioenergy" factor, and other factors yet to be discovered, between the cerebrospinal fluid and the central nervous system, the capillaries of the choroid plexuses, and wherever cerebrospinal fluid is found in total body physiology. Complicated, inanimate machinery—such as an automobile, an automatic dishwasher, a moon rocket—needs a spark in its systems to initiate action and to keep it running. Biologic systems have had a "Spark" and "bioenergy" system built into their mechanisms for eons. This is not an esoteric or religious fantasy; it is a simple, bioenergetic, physiological fact.

THE FLUCTUATION OF THE CEREBROSPINAL FLUID
Its Nature And Therapeutic Use
This is an edited transcription of a lecture given in 1976
at a Sutherland Cranial Teaching Foundation basic course
in Milwaukee, Wisconsin.

WE ARE TALKING ABOUT something here that reaches up and beyond our ordinary experience or thinking. Because of that, I don't know how to put it exactly, but we'll dive in and try to find our way out. Dr. Sutherland, in his teachings, did not give instruction in the use of the cerebrospinal fluid to the students of the early years because he felt they were not ready for it. He knew about the cerebrospinal fluid from his thirty years of research, and he used it. He used it within his own mind, within his own hands, and in his own patients for many years. He did not, however, give the use of the cerebrospinal fluid or fluid drive to the instructors to teach in the class until about 1947. Because of this, some have said he did not discover the cerebrospinal fluid until 1947; that is not true.

Dr. Will Sutherland and I came to know each other well, and I know the cerebrospinal fluid was an integral part of his understanding from the very beginning of his development of the detailed anatomy and physiology of the primary respiratory mechanism. It was simply his judgement that the class participants in those first few years were having sufficient problems allowing for the idea of cranial bones moving, let alone talking about the motivating factor that allowed them to move. So he gradually worked us from the outside in: He began with the osseous, articular mobility of the cranial skull; then he gradually worked us into the reciprocal tension membrane that was working as a unit to unite and move the bones; then to the motility of the central nervous system; and finally to the fluid drive.

There's no way to separate this mechanism into separate units of function; that isn't the way it works in the body. It works as one unit—it has five divisions which we teach, true—but it works as a single unit of function. Your entire body is going into anatomicophysiological flexion/external rotation and extension/internal rotation, from the top of your head to the bottom of your feet in its involuntary mobility ten times a minute. A micromobility throughout the total pattern of function of the whole body.

I have a voluntary body I choose to move around, let rattle, and do what I want to do with it; and all the time I am doing that, all the time I am standing here, I have this involuntary flexion/external rotation, extension/internal rotation taking place throughout the entire mechanism of everything we own.

While we may lack "scientific, laboratory proof" that the primary respiratory mechanism is responsible for this total involuntary system throughout the whole body, we can say categorically—we can very definitely make this statement—that this is the only way the primary respiratory mechanism works. There are no muscular agencies or other voluntary mechanisms within the primary respiratory mechanism to cause it to do this flexion/external rotation, extension/internal rotation—but this is the only way it does work.

It is a mechanism and that means we have to study it as a mechanism. We have to study the bones, the membranes, the central nervous system, and the cerebrospinal fluid as the working units of a something that is already doing what it does because that is the way it was designed and it's the only way it can function.

My assignment now is to discuss the cerebrospinal fluid portion of this mechanism. Dr. Sutherland made the statement that the cerebrospinal fluid is the primary, fundamental principle in the primary respiratory mechanism. Dr. A.T. Still said it's the highest known element in the human body, and he made other references in his writings indicating something was there that was different than in other fluids within the body, there was something going on within the cerebrospinal fluid that represented a fundamental principle. It is a fluid drive, it fluctuates and shifts, and it doesn't require the coiling and uncoiling of the central nervous system to make it fluctuate. It fluctuates, period. Accept that fact. I've accepted it ever since the first day I heard Will Sutherland say it. I assumed this was true, and I have never found any proof in my patients to suggest otherwise. I care less than nothing about what makes it a fluid drive—I simply want to put it to work—it's a principle.

The cerebrospinal fluid has an automatic fluid drive that permits things to happen. Dr. Sutherland said it was blessed with a Breath of Life. Now, what did he mean by that? Well, you can figure that one out for yourself. It has an invisible spark, a potency, it has something that loves to become a fluid drive. It has something that makes it what it is, a fundamental principle. It has a nourishing factor. A nourishing factor that bathes the entire central nervous system including the 12 pairs of cranial nerves. It also goes down around the spinal cord and in the central canal of the spinal cord. It goes out through the dural sheaths and follows out along the peripheral nervous system, and through the peripheral nervous system and the ganglia that connect to the autonomic nervous system, it bathes and nourishes the autonomic nervous system. As it goes out, it eventually becomes part of the lymphatic circulation; this is where it finally terminates. This has been demonstrated scientifically. In this way, there is absorption of the cerebrospinal fluid, not only by way of the pacchionian bodies into the venous drainage but also into all the lymphatic fluids of the body.

Editor's note: An article reviewing the various pathways of cerebrospinal fluid distribution is "Recent Research into the Nature of Cerebrospinal Fluid Formation and Absorption." J. Neurosurg 1983, 59:369-383.

So we have something here that has a universal presence in the lymphatics (the third circulation of the body). We have something that has a universal presence in and around all the most vital structures that deal with human life—the central nervous system with the pituitary body, the hypothalamic axis for the hormonal system, the physiological centers in the floor of the fourth ventricle, and the central autonomics. We have a nourishing factor that brings something from this spark or this Breath of Life that is apparently what the body needs. At least my patients demonstrate it and I sure use it.

An example of using the cerebrospinal fluid principle in treatment came up in a patient of mine who was having recurrent headaches. I found she had a long, narrow, extension-type head, and she had this, that, and the other besides. But the thing that was the most striking was that she had a torsion pattern you wouldn't believe. In testing for this, I started the mechanism into the torsion right pattern, and she wound up until it felt like I myself had been twisted right around. I tried initiating a torsion left, and it stopped before I could even get started. Now, what would a marked torsion of that degree do? The central nervous system would have to be twisted into torsion, the reciprocal tension membrane would have to be twisted into torsion, and the osseous elements would have to be twisted into torsion. She had enough torsion mechanics that the aqueduct of Sylvius was twisted like a hose, and she couldn't interchange the fluids between the third ventricle and the fourth ventricle comfortably. She probably had a torsion mechanism all her life, but she had done something—fallen or twisted or sat down too hard or something—and she aggravated her torsion mechanism into more torsion.

To correct this, I took her into the right torsion pattern, exaggerated it, and then held it out there. In this way, we were starting the whole mechanism—the fluid drive, the motile nervous system, and the reciprocal tension membrane—to treat this torsion pattern. What constituted the completion of the treatment for that particular day was when the central nervous system quieted down until there was practically no movement, when the reciprocal tension membrane quieted down to practically no movement, and the cerebrospinal fluid quieted down to a point of infinite quietness. It went through a stillpoint for the fluid, the nervous system, and the reciprocal tension membrane. When it went through the stillpoint, her head began to unwind itself comfortably back to a mechanism that was right for her. Afterwards, when we checked it again, she was still in a pattern of marked torsion right, but now the tube, the cerebral aqueduct, could do what it was meant to do. It could let fluids through, and that was the end of her headaches. The point I am making is that we had to carry the cerebrospinal fluid through a stillpoint for it to function correctly, to get the correction.

This is also what we try to do with compression of the fourth ventricle (CV4) technique. We are interested in bringing this fundamental principle down to a point in which it can shift gears within itself. In doing this, it is meeting the physiologic needs of the patient. It is bringing its potency factor into existence. It is interchanging with the fluids of the body. It is going clear down to the lymphatics of the toes. When we bring it down to a stillpoint, it can shift gears in all these things, and we have influenced the total physiology.

When we're talking about a CV4 (or lateral fluctuation), we're talking about controlling the cerebrospinal fluid tide to bring it down and through a stillpoint. We're going to experience different types of responses in different types of people, and these are some of the points I would like to call to your attention. As we bring it through this stillpoint, we're going to influence the lymphatic system completely so that the lymphatics can automatically detoxify toxins flowing through them. We're going to be able to put a charge into a nervous system that has had a nervous breakdown. Doing these cerebrospinal fluid techniques to bring the fluctuation down to a stillpoint gives any sick tissue the chance to recharge.

Meningitis: CV4 has effects in cases of post-meningitis or post-encephalitis. Just recently, I had a case of a man who had encephalomeningitis thirty years ago and reported a vague bunch of symptomatology. I took ahold of his mechanism to test it, and the meninges felt as if they were about as thick as wet cardboard and had about the same tone quality–the meninges were sick. I saw him for a treatment once a week over a period of about four or five months and kept using the CV4 type of approach on him (we happened to do it through the parietals and not the supraocciput). We went through a stillpoint every time he came back, and gradually over a period of time, the meninges began to absorb their waste products and become thinner.

101

They lost their wet cardboard feel and became wet paper; then they developed some tone quality, and then we got it. One day, he came in for a treatment and said, "I don't know what happened, but something happened after the last treatment on the way home; I never felt better in my life." And I took ahold of him to assess, and he had made all the necessary corrections. The membranes had their tone quality back and he was done; we could fire him. So in cases where you have chronic meningeal involvement, you're going to have a different tone quality in the meninges. Use the cerebrospinal fluid tide as a way to allow it to correct itself.

In both acute and chronic encephalomeningitis, the clinical problem is of a meninges that is hurt and insulted. In the red-hot, acute cases, it has all the tone-quality of wet Kleenex and in the chronic cases, of wet, thick cardboard. Suppose I had also found a cranial strain in that patient and tried to get a membranous articular correction. Forget it. Sick membranes don't make good corrections, they can't. There's no tone-quality in that reciprocal tension membrane; it's there, yes, but it's not functional.

So, for several weeks or months, depending on the chronicity of the problem, your CV4 as a regular part of your treatment will gradually restore the total tone quality and function of the reciprocal tension membrane and gradually bring back the normal tensity and thickness of it. Having this corrected, you not only get better corrections, you make a live patient out of them.

In severely involved cases, patients always ask how long it is going to take. I tell them, "You can forget how long it's going to take; we'll be at it until you're tired of me and I'm tired of you, and you're not going to see any change for six months. If you don't want to do it, don't start." Given this, maybe one out of three takes the treatment. The one who does gets results.

Nervous Breakdown: There are people who have complete nervous breakdowns—and I am not talking about psychosomatic cases—I'm talking about people who come in who have physiologically had a nervous breakdown. You take ahold of their mechanism, and they've got no charge in it. They barely get up to 20 volts (when they should be at 110 volts)—it's a sick nervous system. They have had a nervous breakdown. It is a weak, tired, low-energy mechanism. It's chronic, it's been there for years; it had some months that were better and some months that were worse, but it's a lousy mechanism. The nervous system is sick. It has no charge.

What charges them? A CV4 once a week for about as long as it takes to take care of a rheumatoid arthritic (six to twelve months). You have to tell them, "You're not going to feel better for some time, and I'm not going to try to prove to you that you are getting better. This mechanism has to prove to both of us that you are feeling better." After about two or three months, all of a sudden, instead of 20 volts, it feels like 25. The next time they come back, it's back to 23, but it goes up to 27. Eventually, one day, they walk in and the thing is charging. And finally, one day, they walk into the office (the corrections usually take place between treatments, not while they're on the table), and you put your hand on their mechanism, and it says, "110 volts—fire her." So I do, and that's the end of that nervous breakdown.

I had one woman who did exactly what I'm describing to you, only when she finally made the final major correction, it just happened to be when she was taking the treatment at the office. It was intense; she threatened to get off that table and clobber me because she didn't like what was going on. What she was feeling in that moment of change was the same thing she had felt six or seven times over a period of years at the point just before she had to go back into the hospital. She could have made this correction in between treatments, but she didn't. She coincidentally made it when she was in the office, so I observed it. My point is that whenever that correction takes place, the next time they walk into your office, you know their mechanism is well. At that point, I said, "I don't need to see you anymore." Afterwards, she went through the death of her husband and two or three other episodes that ordinarily would have dumped her into the hospital, and it had no more effect on her than it should have. She had maintained her full charge of 110 volts and was able to handle life.

So we have a physiological approach to some of these people who truly have a physiologic nervous breakdown. There's something that took it down in the first place—not a disease, I don't know what— something took it down, but it can be rebuilt.

When you take a patient who has a lot of problems and they have a certain amount of chronic disability which you know needs help, include all the factors that are in that patient. If they have a bad history of multiple accidents or multiple illnesses, even as far back as early childhood, include all the factors into your sense of touch so that when you are reading those tissues, you stay within the tolerance available for diagnosis and treatment for that particular day. These patients have been around for a long time—so there's no sense in rushing in and projecting your magnificent discoveries on them and creating more problems than they already have. Stay within the tolerance of multiply-damaged or ill people as you start your program, and allow time for things to build up; it's much more satisfactory, and it is a lot more fun.

Rheumatoid Arthritis: I assume that all my rheumatoid arthritics are seeing other physicians, and they're coming to me for what I know about the science of the human body, and that's what they're going to get from me to the best of my ability. In my rheumatoid arthritics, I treat with the CV4, period. I don't use those techniques where you work with the individual joints and so forth. To me, rheumatoid arthritis is a connective tissue, collagen disease from the top of the head to the bottom of the feet. Everything is in stasis. Say you want a method whereby you can influence the total collagen system in the shortest, quickest way possible, and you want to instill within it the desire to interchange all the fluid and cells of its being so it can be that which it is supposed to be, and you want to do it from the top of the head to the bottom of the feet—including all the sick joints. What type of physiologic medicine would you give? CV4, period.

This is an edited transcription of a lecture given in 1976
at a Sutherland Cranial Teaching Foundation "advanced"
course in Milwaukee, Wisconsin.

CV4: Compression of the Fourth Ventricle

The contact for our hands should be on the lateral edges of the supraocciput inside the occipitomastoid suture. We then apply a mild compression at these areas to gently compress the fluid, the brain, the reciprocal tension membrane, and everything in the area beneath the tentorium cerebelli. We're gently compressing and slowing down the motility of the central nervous system, we're slowing down the movement of the reciprocal tension membrane, we're slowing down the fluctuation of the cerebrospinal fluid, and we're slowing down the mobility of the cranial articular mechanism until we get the cerebrospinal fluid tide to go through its stillpoint.

When giving a treatment, you can't be thinking about next week's golf game. You've got to concentrate and feel that which is taking place within this fluid drive when you work with it and use it intelligently. It has intelligence; join yours to it and carry it through the treatment program with conscious awareness. This makes the correction much more secure for the patient and avoids reactions.

You can get tremendous results in the supplemental care for your rheumatoid arthritics by using compression of the fourth ventricle. But you have to sit there and actually do a fourth ventricle technique on them and that can be a challenge. Cases of rheumatoid arthritis are sick from the top of the head to the bottom of the feet. Every connective tissue in their bodies is saying, "I am loaded with molasses as thick as it is in January, and if you think I'm going to make any changes for you, you are mistaken." With the rheumatoid arthritics, I don't get involved with their medication management; I just give them a CV4 every week. In a new patient with rheumatoid arthritis, it can take a long time, sitting at that supraocciput, to bring the cerebrospinal fluid tide down to a stillpoint. There is trouble in every tissue of the body, in all the fascias of the body, in all the lymphatics of the body. So, I am not just doing a CV4 in the area of the fourth ventricle, I am doing a CV4 that is influencing the total cerebrospinal fluid pattern throughout the entire body.

In one case, it took 45 minutes of sitting there waiting for this fluid to come to a stillpoint and go through it before that supraocciput got hot. The next time he came back, it only took 40 minutes, and the next time it was down to 30 minutes, so we were headed in the right direction. In about six to twelve months, we'll have it back to the normal seven minutes, and he will be alive. He'll still have rheumatoid arthritis—that's not the point—but he will be alive again.

My point is that the CV4 is a living treatment. You've got to read the quality of the fluid within the mechanism and read the quality of the tissues. Every CV4 is not just a routine of putting your hands here, do this, and it's going to happen. Read the quality of the whole mechanism when you are using a CV4.

How much pressure you use on the supraocciput varies from patient to patient and from treatment to treatment—some are tougher and some are milder. You can get reactions in using CV4 at the supraocciput, particularly if a patient has an occipitomastoid lesion, and it doesn't matter whether the lesion has been there for 25 years or 25 minutes. These patients already have a compression of the supraocciput on the temporal bone on the side of the lesion, and now you apply more compression to it. Occipitomastoid lesions are notorious for kicking off reactions; you can get into a problem by doing a CV4 at the site of an occipitomastoid lesion if you just blindly apply the same force from both sides of the supraocciput.

I will give you a little hint, but it's going to vary with every single patient, and it's not going to work the way I talk about it on every patient; you will need to shift its gears according to the quality and need for each patient. Since this supraocciput has already been driven

106

up inside the temporal, it already has all the compression you would want for that side in giving a CV4. So, you just support the side on which the supraocciput is in an occipitomastoid lesion, and you apply your compression on the opposite side until you can bring the cerebrospinal fluid tide down through a stillpoint for the CV4. In this way, you're putting the occipitomastoid lesion to work; you're compressing only the opposite side of the thing until it goes through its stillpoint. You're not applying pressure bilaterally, equally. This will avoid a reaction. It's just a suggestion.

Patients with extension-type heads also require extra care. If you force them into extension, there is a tendency for them to stay in extension after the CV4, and the patients complain of depression and low energy. To avoid this, in doing the CV4, you compress the supraocciput neutrally; you do not pull it back into extension. In these extension types, the operator should make sure that the patients' occiputs and temporals resume full flexion/external rotation after doing the CV4. Having them take a few deep breaths can help with this expansion.

We can enhance the CV4 procedure by having the patient exhale and hold their breath to the limit. We can also enhance this by having the patient extend their feet to encourage the sacral base and the occiput to go into extension—anything that will retard and slow down the existing fluctuation. Gradually things quiet as we continue our observation, and within three to seven minutes, there is a sudden shift within the cerebrospinal fluid fluctuation pattern that takes place when it's ready. Following that, we can see a number of clinical effects that allow us to note that something has happened. We can note a sense of warmth, an idling of the secondary respiration, or sometimes a fine perspiration on the forehead or skin. We get a number of clinical effects that allow us to note that something has happened.

Instead of applying the CV4 approach to the supraocciput, you can take ahold of the parietal bones and very gently encourage internal rotation and still the fluctuation by that route with your attention on the body of the cerebrospinal fluid in the lateral ventricles. But there is an awful lot of fluid there, and you may not have as much control as you do down by the fourth ventricle and the supraocciput.

You can also do this procedure by way of the sacrum, and this is important to know. You do it by tipping the sacrum into its extension phase position and holding it until you sense the cerebrospinal fluid response of stilling to a point where it changes its fulcrum within itself. The sacral approach is used in all cases where you suspect there's enough cranial trauma that you don't dare get on the head, yet you would like to do something therapeutic for the patient. We know that stilling the cerebrospinal fluid creates fluid balance interchange; it stimulates the vital, physiologic centers; it modifies the tensity in the intracellular spaces of the fascias and the ligaments; it arouses an immunological response; it does a lot of things. So if we can still the cerebrospinal fluid by way of the sacrum, we can do a lot of good, and we don't have to worry about creating more problems in a potential fracture of the skull or some other traumatic injury.

Lateral Fluctuation

We have a technique for creating lateral fluctuation. We're going to take ahold of the temporal bones like we do for examining the motion for the temporal bones—our hands are around the base of the skull, thumbs along the mastoid processes and the mastoid portions, with our fingers located under the neck area. If we then very gently roll our fingers, our middle fingers, we automatically will gently turn one temporal bone into external rotation and the other one into internal rotation, and the body of cerebrospinal fluid will start a fluctuation pattern of going from side to side. We barely roll our middle fingers until we feel this lateral fluctuation going over and coming up the opposite side. As soon as we even sense that we have this thing going from side to side, we decrease the amount of roll from side to side so that we begin to restrict it. We started something and now we start retarding it—gradually slowing it down. In other words, the fluid wants to go over here, but we don't quite let it, and we start bringing it back. We gradually retard this fluid fluctuation until it comes down to a shift in the fulcrum within the cerebrospinal fluid. When done this way, it's a palliative thing. It quiets down reactions you may get from treatment, and it's an important one to understand and use in your practice.

If we have a patient in dire need of a flow of energy, in cases where the cerebrospinal fluid mechanism in the body feels as if it's half dead, there's nothing going on, we can use this same lateral fluctuation technique to incite it, to start it up, and make it be more active. If we do this, however, it is always wise to have the sensitivity to know how much it should be incited. And if all you do is just incite it and let the patient off the table, you're liable to leave them feeling drunk. We want to have an effect on their energy by creating a new interchange in the system; after inciting it, we then bring it down to a stillpoint so that the shift in the fulcrum within the cerebrospinal fluid will correctly distribute the beneficial needs you aroused by incitation.

THE CEREBROSPINAL FLUID AS A MECHANISM

This is an edited transcription of a lecture given in 1986
at a Sutherland Cranial Teaching Foundation basic course
in Philadelphia, Pennsylvania.

WE, AS INDIVIDUALS, LIVE a life of voluntary mechanisms and involuntary mechanisms. There are a million different mechanisms within the total body physiology of the patient. Our voluntary mechanism allows us to do everything from jog down the street to sleep quietly. This action mechanism varies in each individual according to how their whole quality of life is behaving.

On the other hand, the quiet primary respiratory mechanism is a totally involuntary unit of function, physiology, activity and livingness that allows us to be an active, living voluntary mechanism. We never give a thought to the changes that take place in function within the so-called cerebrospinal fluid fluctuation and the primary respiratory mechanism; they just are. We accept life for what it is; we accept the fact that our mechanism is at work; we don't think about it. When we get together and start talking about it, then it becomes a topic for conversation, but ordinarily, we don't give a thought to the fact that we're a primary respiratory mechanism. The involuntary mechanism is the thing that keeps us alive and functions as a manifestation of life.

The cerebrospinal fluctuation is one part of the primary respiratory mechanism that also includes the central nervous system motility and the mobility of the reciprocal tension membrane, cranial bones, and sacrum. We can't separate any of them—they're all one unit. Any trauma or disease that happens anywhere in the body is going to affect the primary respiratory mechanism, and any restoration towards health, the correction of dysfunction within the body's voluntary mechanism, has to include improving the function of the primary respiratory mechanism—it's a unit of function. It is also a mechanism.

110

The fluid drive is a mechanism. The water in the conduit of a turbine is a mechanism, the tide in the ocean is a mechanism, the fluctuation of the cerebrospinal fluid is a mechanism, and even the potency within this cerebrospinal fluid is a mechanism. Mechanisms, both voluntary and involuntary, are a matter of life and function. When we are checking for the to-and-fro, rhythmic, cerebrospinal fluid fluctuation, we are looking at a mechanism. We study these mechanisms and learn how they work in health and how we can guide our patients back towards health. We are silently in contact with the primary respiratory mechanism, which is assisting us in our correction and bringing things back to normal.

There are various kinds of tides within the body physiology and within the cerebrospinal fluid. The easiest one to find is the longitudinal, 8-to-12-times-per-minute, cerebrospinal fluid tide. It is like the tide in an ocean; twice a day, the tides move in and the tides move out. In our own body mechanisms, it is a basic rhythm of 8 to 12 times a minute. We use the word, "tide," simply to get the thought into our minds that it is coming in and going out rhythmically. This tide-like movement of cerebrospinal fluid is a mechanism constantly in motion, and we call it a fluid drive.

The longitudinal tide is the one with which everything in the body, rhythmically, is going into a simple flexion and extension for midline structures and external rotation and internal rotation for bilateral structures, 8 to 12 times a minute. The total body cells—the cells of the heart, the lungs, the osseous structures, everything, the whole thing as a unit of function—is going into a slight flexion/external rotation, extension/internal rotation rhythm throughout life. The longitudinal tide is the one that is with us all the time or most of the time. When we lay our hands upon a patient, it's the one we usually find—longitudinally reaching from the top of the head to the bottom of the feet.

There are lateral fluctuations in which the cerebrospinal fluid, together with the total units of the body, will rhythmically go from side to side. We can induce this type of pattern within our patients, meeting specific needs, or it may occur spontaneously, in which case, it can be palpated and diagnosed as a lateral fluctuation. There are also spiral fluctuations. These are little eddies of coiling and uncoiling, perhaps in various portions of the central nervous system.

These things I am talking to you about are things that can be observed by any physician who understands the mechanism and learns to read the things coming from the patient through to the palpatory skills. The longitudinal tide and the lateral tide are relatively easy to find; they're big and the whole body goes with them. The spiral tides are like those little animals that crawl along the shores of the beach or like the times you can see the spiral in the swaying of the seaweed near the shore. They don't bang at you; these spiral tides are possibly part of local changes taking place.

Then, there are what I call rip tides. A rip tide is a tide which can be adapted by the physician to secure a change, as a motivation to get the existing tidal mechanism of the patient to change its pattern of functioning. Through its use, we are going to modify that tidal mechanism within the patient slightly. If we have the patient lie on his back and dorsiflex his feet, this is tipping the total body unit mechanism towards flexion. Then, if we initiate a lateral fluctuation while the patient is holding his feet in dorsiflexion, pretty soon we have two tides working in the body: one, longitudinal with this lateral tide superimposed on it. Of course, this is all done under the control of a physician who has learned how to work gently with the mechanism, who can slowly initiate the fluctuation, reading what he palpates carefully and allowing these things to happen within the patient. Work with it some and then try to figure out for yourself why you might want to use it.

There is another tide which came to me from outer space, I think. I had a patient with a rather severe, generalized, complicated problem, and I was quietly trying to read this fluid drive, working within the content of this patient's body physiology, and all of a sudden, I was aware of the fact that there was this larger tide superimposed on the one going 8 times a minute. Here was a large tide which felt as if it was coming in from somewhere, and it began to expand, stop, expand, stop, expand, stop. It took a full minute and a half for this larger tide to come in and be part of the body physiology of the patient, and then it drained away just as slowly as it came in. Where it came from and where it went to, I don't know, but its influence was certainly modifying the trophism of every cell of the body to do something. For that patient, that trophism was certainly a help because the clinical response was that of an improvement in the areas of dysfunction.

Since that first appearance, I have observed this long tide on occasion. It's not something you do or look for, but in giving osteopathic treatment by way of the primary respiratory mechanism and utilizing it as a tool, it may show up. When it first appeared, I was quietly working with something that needed quiet help. This thing only shows up when it's needed and you happen to be still enough and the patient's still enough for it to show up. It's not necessary to order it.

The quality of the cerebrospinal fluid fluctuation can also be used in a diagnosis. Just quietly lay your hands on a patient and ask yourself, does this mechanism of tidal movement feel alive or does it feel tired? You can learn to judge this by comparing the sense in several patients over a day's time. Regardless of what the rate of the cycle is, ask, What's the quality of that tide? Does it feel alive? When you find one that just doesn't have any particular spunk—it doesn't feel like it's supposed to—you can use that as a guiding point for what you're going to do in the treatment phase.

The patient who has a tired primary respiratory mechanism, measured in terms of the quality of the tide and the involuntary units of the body functioning, does not have the energy with which to make major corrections. Sometimes results won't hold; there isn't the quality of life available to keep them working following your corrective treatments. So you learn to treat within the framework of the vitality of the tide within the patient, the vitality of the primary respiratory mechanism. Learn to work within that frame of reference, and the corrections you make will be more satisfactory to you and certainly more corrective to the patient.

When assessing a patient, first lay your hands on her and very quietly get a sense of what she feels like as an involuntary unit. How does she react, what is her response? Now that you've gotten an idea of the whole patient, lay your hand under the area of complaint. In the case of a psoas spasm, get a hand under that spastic lumbar area and put the other hand on the abdomen above it so you've got the problem between your hands. Now feel for that cerebrospinal fluid tide involuntary mechanism that you felt in the total body. Do you find it the same in this area of strain? No, it's restricted, there's enough obstruction present to interfere with the fluctuation pattern, you're aware of the fact that you're not feeling the same vitality as you did in the whole person. Note what that dysfunction feels like.

Now go ahead with your treatment. Give that patient a treatment for that particular day and that particular problem; use whatever technique you want, it doesn't make any difference. When you're through with your treatment and you think you've made your corrections or whatever you thought you did, lay your hand under that lumbar area again and feel for that same tide that you first felt in the whole body. If you sense that this lumbar area you just treated is better able to express involuntary motion, that means the treatment you gave for that lumbar spasm actually did secure some corrective results because the "Boss," the total involuntary mechanism, is now also available locally in that area. You can feel it, it happened, something's going on.

If instead, when you go back and check, you find the same local sense of dullness that you did before you treated that patient, I guarantee you didn't accomplish much. By the time she gets to the front office, she will already be back to the same messages she came in with. So this tide can be used as a little, invisible diagnostic clue; we can use this silent, involuntary mechanism as a clue to guide us in our treatment programs for the rest of the body.

With each patient you see, quietly ask yourself, What is the quality of this primary function of life within this given patient? What is the quality in the areas of health, what is it in the area of strain, what is it before and after each office visit? As you work with the strains and dysfunction in your patients, always be quietly aware of the fact that this fluctuation pattern, this whole unit, is constantly your silent partner and is helping you to secure corrective changes in the lesion areas because your goal for this given patient is to restore health. The patients are not there purely to get their lesion popped or corrected. They are there to release the tensities, the loss of function, the disturbance of motion—to unlock and permit the doors of life to go in and go out freely, the way they're supposed to. You have a silent partner within the fluctuation of the cerebrospinal fluid, and you have the right to learn to understand it, to use it, and to test it.

When you go to the tables to practice now, take a simple vault hold and very quietly work to simply identify yourself with the patient as a whole, quietly feeling and seeing between your hands. You could say you are looking at the patient from within by looking right through your hand contact and patiently waiting for a few minutes. Wait for the expansive phase of the parietal bones coming slightly outward into external rotation with the welling up of the fluid within that mechanism, and then gradually wait for it to go back towards internal rotation. A rhythmic motion, a tide-like movement, coming in and going out, expanding and contracting the body as a unit. Dr. Sutherland chose to call this movement the fluctuation of the cerebrospinal fluid. (The term "cranial rhythmic impulse" was developed by others purely for the purpose of counting.)

Sharing the experience of the fluctuation of the cerebrospinal fluid is a dynamic, living function, and function is what we are studying this week. We want to start playing with it, to feel this little, rhythmic tide coming in and going out. You can feel it in the head; you can feel it in the rest of the body. You can palpate and feel this flexion-extension mechanism anywhere in the body when you have trained your sense of touch. You can feel it in the ankles, you can feel it in the big toe, you can feel it in any part of the body you can get your hands on. We don't want you just to focus on the head; we're trying to get you to be aware of the whole picture so you can use the whole mechanism for diagnostic and therapeutic care anywhere in the body.

TIME, TISSUES, AND TIDES
This paper is dated September 1983.

"To FIND HEALTH SHOULD be the object of the physician. Anyone can find disease." This is a dictum given to us by A. T. Still. Health is far more than the mere absence of disease or trauma; it is a living, dynamic experience of anatomicophysiological functioning, physically, mentally, and spiritually.

Certain basic principles are accepted by the osteopathic physician:

1. The body is a unit.
2. The body is a self-regulatory mechanism.
3. The body has the inherent capacity to heal itself.
4. Structure and function are reciprocally interrelated.

Based on these principles, time, tissues, and tides are the working tools the body is using to express health or to express specific areas of trauma and/or disease.

The Body Is a Unit

The body is designed to be in existence for a given period of time; it is a complete system of tissues and fluids in constant mobility and motility; it is endowed with voluntary and involuntary mechanisms that allow it to be used for day-to-day living and for the maintenance of health. Dr. Still gave us the science of osteopathy with which to understand the body as a unit, including the cranial concept. Dr. Sutherland frequently stated that his contribution of the detailed anatomy and physiology of the craniosacral mechanism was a continuation of the science of osteopathy as envisioned by Dr. Still. One body—one unit of function.

The Body Is a Self-regulatory Mechanism

To understand the body as a unit is to understand it in health. One must come to recognize and accept the self-regulatory mechanisms by actively observing them and listening to them where applicable and learning to palpate them with a trained sense of touch as they function in health.

One of these self-regulatory mechanisms is a pattern of mobility and motility throughout the body physiology that is involuntary in nature, that is present throughout the life span of the individual, and that is easily palpable. All of the body's midline structures, fluids, and tissues rhythmically move alternatively into flexion and extension while the bilateral structures, fluids, and tissues move into external rotation with the flexion phase and into internal rotation with the extension phase. The timing for this pattern of inherent, involuntary mobility is 8 to 12 times per minute in health. The quality of this movement as well as its mechanical mobility can be a diagnostic clue as to the vitality of the patient, indicating his or her health status, as well as a clue for consideration in trauma and/or disease states.

The fluid portion of the rhythmic flexion with external rotation, extension with internal rotation is an innate fluctuation of the cerebrospinal fluid. It is a tide-like movement that permeates the whole body. While the cerebrospinal fluid is basically formed from the choroid plexuses of the ventricles of the central nervous system, it is reabsorbed into the circulatory system by venous channels, and most importantly, it is also reabsorbed into the general body fluids by way of perineural channels into the lymphatic system. Thus, the cerebrospinal fluid-lymphatic fluid system rhythmically interchanges with all the tissues of the body in a tide-like pattern of self-regulatory functioning during each 8-to-12-times-per-minute cycle of fluid movement.

There is another tide-like movement that occurs in body physiology besides the one that is 8 to 12 times per minute. This second tide permeates the entire body unit as a massive, involuntary flexion with external rotation, extension with internal rotation tissue and fluid

117

pattern showing itself approximately six times in a ten-minute period, or about one and a half minutes for each rhythmic cycle. This tide, coming in and ebbing out, can be observed by palpation in all tissues of the body during its rhythmic movement *when* it begins to manifest itself. I do not know its origin; I do not feel it occur in every patient, and I do not induce it to begin its rhythmic pattern. It showed itself to me several years ago while I was treating a patient and observing the 8-to-12-times-per-minute tide doing its work within the patient. I have observed this massive tide many times and can report that it is not universally the same in every patient; that it is individualized for each patient; that I do not know when it will make itself manifest; and that I do not know where it disappears to when it ceases its work within a given patient.

There are hundreds of self-regulatory mechanisms in the body physiology, but at this time, emphasis will be upon the involuntary mobility of the fast tide, 8 to 12 times per minute, and the slow tide, 6 times in 10 minutes. Both tidal movements can be palpated with the development of a trained sense of touch. Palpation for the presence of these tides is preferably as a participator, as in quantum mechanics, a process whereby the physician tunes in with his sensory input to participate with the movement of either tide as it does its work within the physiology of the patient. Both tides are present in health and also in trauma and/or disease. The quality of tidal movement will vary in the presence of health, trauma and/or disease, sometimes only locally in a given problem or as a whole body unit of tissue functioning.

Both tides are innate, inherent, and involuntary self-regulatory mechanisms whose primary goal is the maintenance of health—to be contributing factors in the body's efforts to heal from trauma and/or disease. The reciprocal balanced interchange that takes place between the fluids and tissues of the body is a result of and is augmented by the fast and slow tides, which are continuously working during the life span of the individual.

The Body Has the Inherent Capacity to Heal Itself

The rhythmic, involuntary mobility of the tissues and fluids and the various tides are all totally integrated with each other and with the body as a unit. They are contributing factors to the self-healing capacity of the body and should be recognized and accepted as self-functioning mechanisms. They also can be considered innate tools within the body physiology of the patient that can be used by the physician to augment and reinforce the body's effort to heal itself.

Midline-Bilateral Movement: This involuntary movement, present throughout the life span of the individual, can be used as a diagnostic tool by the physician before and after each treatment session to evaluate the corrective process of a given treatment at the time it is administered and for each subsequent visit. The midline-bilateral movement is present throughout the total body physiology, and although small in degree of motion, it can be palpated anywhere in the body.

Here is the process for using this as a diagnostic tool. A patient comes in with a complaint of somatic dysfunction in a given area of the body. The physician places his observing palpatory hands on the area of stress and then on a comparative area of relative health away from the somatic dysfunction. He evaluates the midline-bilateral movement in the two areas, the one of relative health and the one of stress. The rhythm of the two areas will be the same, but the quality in the area of health and in the area of stress will be distinctly different. Following the corrective treatment for that given day, the two areas should be rechecked. If the two areas show the same pattern as before the treatment, very little has been accomplished in initiating a corrective change at the site of somatic dysfunction. If the midline-bilateral structures in the somatic dysfunction show a definite return towards that experienced in the health area, the physician can be assured he has initiated a self-corrective change in the somatic dysfunction. The next office visit will confirm this self-corrective measure. A body physiological change towards health functioning has been initiated by the treatment, not mere mobilization, and the test for midline-bilateral movement in the area of relative health and in the area of somatic dysfunction will provide a diagnostic tool to record this event. The time it takes to make this evaluation is very short, once the physician has taught his sensory input to feel this innate, involuntary, small movement.

The Fast Tide: The 8-to-12-times-per-minute fluctuation of cerebrospinal fluid is one of the fluid components of the midline-bilateral involuntary mobility. The cerebrospinal fluid and its tide-like fluctuation has been studied for years. Its fluctuation patterns can be modified to meet physiological needs within the patient. An understanding of some of the uses of the cerebrospinal fluid and its fast tide may give some understanding of the slow tide in its functioning. A tide within a tide.

The cerebrospinal fluid is one component of the primary respiratory mechanism, an involuntary mechanism that includes fundamentally that highest known element, the cerebrospinal fluid, within which dwells that invisible Breath of Life. The science of osteopathy recognizes and accepts all the physiological mechanisms that create and maintain health for the individual and, certainly, the vitality factors of the fast and slow tides are fundamental aspects of these health principles.

The fluctuation of the cerebrospinal fluid can be observed by palpation. The existing fluctuation pattern of the fast tide can be modified by gently, intelligently, and gradually restricting the movement of the cerebrospinal fluid in its rhythmic ebb and flow until its fluctuation is reduced to and through a stillpoint. As it goes through this stillpoint, there is a change that takes place in its rhythmic fluctuation that is of physiological benefit to the whole body physiology—a brief but potent transmutation from within the cerebrospinal fluid.

Dr. Howard Lippincott has described what occurs as a result of a carefully applied compression of the fourth ventricle technique (retardative longitudinal fluctuation technique) for modifying the cerebrospinal fluid fluctuation:

> It is hard to appear conservative in considering the uses of compression of the fourth ventricle because this potent fluid, activated by the

120

technique, produces results that justify enthusiasm.

There is a beneficial effect upon the entire circulatory system with reduction of congestions, ischemias and edema, such as is in the realm of possibility without surgical interference.

Metabolic processes are improved, including nutrition to the tissues and the gradual absorption of fibrous and calcium deposits that are not physiological or compensatory.

It enhances organic function, and in the presence of infection, immunity is increased through effects upon the spleen, pancreas and liver.

The endocrine system is regulated to the immediate needs of the body.

The cerebrospinal fluid is in command of the metabolism, much of the involuntary operation and the autoprotective mechanism of the system.

Dr. Sutherland calls attention to the fact that secondary osteopathic lesions become less perceptible under the influence of ventricle compression. So it is of value in determining the primary lesion.[1]

There are a number of ways to modify the fast tide in its function in body physiology. Under longitudinal fast tides, there are accelerative, resuscitative, and retardative techniques. Under lateral fluctuation of the fast tide, there are palliative and incitative techniques. There is a combined longitudinal and lateral fluctuation technique. Finally, there are ways to direct the fast tide through a stress area for specific lesion modification.

It will be recalled that cerebrospinal fluid is formed in the area of the ventricles in the central nervous system; it is reabsorbed into the body circulation by venous channels and by perineural channels into the lymphatic system. Thus, many of the ways to modify cerebrospinal fluid fluctuation are applicable through anatomicophysiological mechanisms, which include the lymphatics. The potency available in the primary respiratory mechanism is available in the absorbed cerebrospinal fluid in the lymphatics.

An interesting observation is that it takes about seven minutes to bring the cerebrospinal fluid fluctuation down to and through its stillpoint, in the average patient, using the compression of the fourth ventricle technique. In a case of rheumatoid arthritis, it will take up to 30 minutes to still the tide and bring it through its stillpoint. It feels as though the entire connective tissue framework of the body, with the stasis of fluids within that connective tissue matrix, has to organize itself as a unit from within to bring the whole mechanism down to and through the stillpoint. By repeating this technique once a week over a period of weeks and months, these cases of rheumatoid arthritis will show remarkable changes in physiological vitality as well as general improvement towards health in their clinical problem. The 30-minute time it took in the first visit reduces itself to 15 minutes and then, gradually, to less and less time for each subsequent treatment.

This type of clinical problem illustrates an important point. The total body physiology of midline-bilateral movement is involved as well as the cerebrospinal fluid fluctuation that is being brought down to and through its stillpoint. As indicated by Dr. Lippincott, all involuntary mechanisms change with modifications of tidal functioning. Tissue and fluid tone can be checked before and after such techniques are used. With a trained sense of palpatory skills and a knowledge of the anatomicophysiological mechanisms, the fast tide and the involuntary midline-bilateral mobility within the body unit provide diagnostic data before and after corrective treatment as well as being used in the treatment process itself. "To seek health" in the case of rheumatoid arthritis is for the physician to introduce a compression of the fourth ventricle into the mechanism and allow it to stimulate the health-seeking resources of the patient from within his own self-healing capacities. It is a continuous process, with corrective changes taking place between treatments. In time, the relative health available to this individual with this type of clinical problem will manifest itself. The point is that health is being sought in this patient in his life span, not a cure for his arthritis.

The Slow Tide: 6 times in 10 minutes, it is a physical phenomenon that does occur in body physiology. In some cases, it demonstrates its

122

presence during the application of a corrective treatment procedure, and then again in a similar corrective technique in another case, the slow tide will not manifest itself.

I suspect that it is the type of corrective treatment technique that I use that allowed me to feel the slow tide the first time, several years ago, and many times since. In osteopathy, there are several types of corrective technique, and each of them is guided by specific principles which permit the given technique to be efficient in its use. Articular mobilization, myofascial release, muscle energy, and counterstrain are a few that can be named. In addition, there are the ligamentous articular and fascial techniques developed by Dr. William G. Sutherland, which are applicable throughout body physiology. Some of the corrective techniques listed are conducive to observing the slow tide at work from within the patient, and other corrective techniques make it more difficult to observe this tide.

When I felt the slow tide for the first time, I was using a ligamentous articular technique on a somatic dysfunction in the thoracic area. The technique calls for the physician to use a sensorimotor type of palpation that participates with the area of the strain. He places his hands upon the area involved and, gently but firmly, molds his hands to read the pattern of mobility in the stressed mechanism. He uses a controlled compression and exaggeration, disengagement, modified direct action, or a combination of these directing, palpatory principles to induce the area of strain to seek its own self-correction towards health while the physician monitors, with his sensorimotor skills, the progress the body physiology is using to correct its problem. The physician is also reading the rhythmic fast tide and its concurrent midline-bilateral mobility as it works in the area of the somatic dysfunction. When a corrective change takes place within the stress area and a sense of health functioning comes from within the treatment site to the physician's sensory input, the physician releases his hand contacts. This type of treatment technique permits an opportunity to observe other functioning changes taking place in the body physiology of the patient while awaiting the self-correction to do its work. It was during one such time that the slow tide entered the picture and made itself known to my sensorimotor input.

A general description of the slow tide is as follows: As the self-corrective treatment for the local somatic dysfunction is doing its work, there is a slow pervasive sense of a fluid mechanism spreading throughout the total body physiology of the patient, an expansive feeling of a tidal movement coming in to fill every cell, every space, every fluid channel—a continuous filling sense, not only in the area of stress under treatment but also in all areas of the body including those in relative health. When this tidal wave reaches its maximum filling state, there is a brief pause and it then begins to ebb out. It seems to take as long for it to completely ebb from all the tissues and fluid spaces as it did to fill them. There is another brief pause and it begins to come in again, pause and ebb out 6 times in a 10-minute period.

The quality of the slow tide varies in different patients' problems and in the same patient at different times. An interesting case to illustrate this slow tide at work is one in which the patient had a serious clinical problem that required weekly treatment to give the patient maximum self-treatment input to aid him in his recovery. The slow tide did not show itself for several treatments, but when it did, its first wave was a powerful surging type of body physiological filling with a sense of having to literally force its way against the resistance of the fluids and tissues of the body. It reached its peak, paused, and ebbed out with almost the same type of urgency. There was a brief pause, and the second wave came in with a sense of trying to smooth over the effects of the first wave, a quieting influence. The third wave was practically palliative in its filling and ebbing. That ended the appearance of the slow tide for that treatment session; total time, 6 minutes for the three waves. Meanwhile, the corrective self-treatment was continuing at the site of the local somatic dysfunction but with greater efficiency during and after the three slow tidal cycles. The slow tide did not appear on a regular basis with subsequent weekly treatments. Apparently, the slow tide was meeting a physiological need in that patient for that particular time in his treatment program.

Unlike the fast tide, 8 to 12 times a minute, which can be modified in its functioning by a number of techniques, the slow tide seems to be an inherent entity in itself and in the physiology of the patient, with no need to try to modify it or its work. I find it more efficient simply to continue my efforts to induce self-corrective healing changes at the local sites of strain and incorporate any slow tide effects into the local treatment, even as it is filling and ebbing throughout the total body. The slow tide does seem to improve and shorten the time it takes to carry a ligamentous articular or fascial strain through its stillpoint to a self-correction from within the body.

I have a feeling the slow tide is at work many more times than I am aware of its presence in patients, as I do not make an effort to induce it into action, nor do I consciously alert myself to look for it nor to deliberately plan for its use when it does appear. I accept its presence when it shows itself, and I try to cooperate with it in its work within the patient. It is another self-regulatory mechanism in body physiology.

Structure and Function Are Reciprocally Interrelated

The science of health within body physiology demands the qualities of reciprocal interchange between structure and function to express health. The seeking of health from within is a continuous time, tissue, and tidal effort from conception to the final moments of physiological life. Within every trauma and/or disease entity, there is an effort on the part of body physiology to deliver health mechanisms through the local area of stress to full functioning health capacities. Treatment is more than securing "corrections" in trauma and/or disease problems.

It is true that trauma and/or disease mechanisms are superimposed upon body physiology; that time, tissues, fluids, and tides get organized within these stress areas until they become "closed circuit" patterns that require compensatory adaptations by the body for the patient to function; that chronic patterns of dysfunction, some of them weeks, months, and years old, have to be literally retrained to become a health mechanism again; and, finally, that there is a health mechanism within every trauma and/or disease entity waiting to be awakened to health function again. The physician is in a position to utilize his osteopathic palpatory corrective skills for accurate diagnosis and treatment of acute and chronic trauma, acute and chronic disease conditions. He can recognize the function of health that waits for its delivery from within the problem. In long-standing cases, it may take time and repeated preparatory somatic dysfunction corrective treatment to finally uncover the element of health that should be present. Once this health factor uncovers itself to the palpatory hands of the physician, his effort is directed to working with it rather than the superimposed stress mechanism. In other words, the physician participates with the body physiology of the patient in seeking health from within.

The physician accepts structure and function and its reciprocal interrelationship and develops palpatory skills to use these principles. The body physiology of the patient offers three working tools as guides for the physician to meet physiological needs in the patient: the involuntary, midline-bilateral mobility rhythmically working 8 to 12 times a minute throughout life; the fast tide within the midline-bilateral mobility, a cerebrospinal fluid mechanism with its potency that can be modified to meet physiological needs within the patient; and a slow tide that comes in and ebbs out about 6 times in a 10-minute period of time, a tide that probably has a vitality factor in its functioning within body physiology. As stated at the outset, Dr. A.T. Still said that "to find health should be the object of the physician," and it is also a basic principle in a corrective treatment program.

1. W.G. Sutherland, *Contributions of Thought*, pp. 152-3.

Palpatory Skills

THE ROLE OF PALPATORY DIAGNOSIS IN
THE CRANIOSACRAL MECHANISM
This paper is dated February 1983.

Palpation of the Craniosacral Mechanism

Dr. A.T. Still gave the osteopathic physician the following concepts: The rule of the artery is supreme; the body has the inherent capacity to heal itself; and structure and function are reciprocally interrelated. Dr. William G. Sutherland added another basic concept: The arterial stream is supreme, but the cerebrospinal fluid is in command, and its fluctuation within a natural cavity can be observed by palpation in cranial technique.

Although Dr. Sutherland was speaking about the primary respiratory mechanism—the craniosacral mechanism—we know that body physiology is one unit of anatomicophysiological functioning which includes the primary respiratory mechanism. The craniosacral mechanism is not a separate field unto itself.

To show this rhythmic, involuntary, mobile structure-function interrelationship, consider the following:

Cerebrospinal Fluid: It is formed continuously, presumably from the choroid plexuses, in the lateral, third, and fourth ventricles of the central nervous system. From the fourth ventricle, the cerebrospinal fluid goes into the subarachnoid spaces around the brain and down the spinal canal to the sacrum. It is reabsorbed into the venous system through the pacchionian bodies along the superior sagittal sinus. It also follows the perineural channels or sheaths of the cranial and spinal peripheral nerves and is reabsorbed into the lymphatic fluid system, the third circulation in body physiology. Thus, from a circulation viewpoint, cerebrospinal fluid and body physiological fluids are a common unit of function.

A more important factor views the cerebrospinal fluid as fluctuating, rather than merely circulating, as do other fluids of the body. The cerebrospinal fluid is contained in a natural cavity and its motion, or fluctuation, can be observed by palpation, not only in the cranial cavity but throughout the total lymphatic and body fluid systems. This fluctuation is a tide-like movement, as differentiated from a wave-like motion. This tide is a powerful, rhythmic, constant, involuntary, 8 to 12 cycles per minute of fluid activity, coming in and ebbing out. It is possible, with a sensitive palpatory skill, to control the rhythm of this tide to a degree where all the fluids of the body have a rhythmic balanced interchange.

Dr. Still has said the cerebrospinal fluid is the highest known element in the human body. Dr. Sutherland added that it contains a potency, a Breath of Life factor, which is transmuted as an element into central nervous system physiology. It is for all these reasons that Dr. Sutherland has stated that the fluctuant cerebrospinal fluid is the fundamental principle in the primary respiratory mechanism.

Palpatory clues: The quality of vitality of the patient can be evaluated by palpation. The overall tide within the patient that has a full volume, 8 to 12 cycles per minute, can be compared to a 110-volt pattern of health. The tide that seems to be too slow has less than 110 volts (30 to 90 volts) and feels flat rather than full, indicating many potential problems, including chronic severe stress and others. Such evaluation can monitor the return towards health in a successful treatment program.

Central Nervous System: The central nervous system includes the cerebral hemispheres; the cerebellum; the brain stem with its fourth ventricle, wherein all the physiological centers, including those of respiration, are located; the 12 pairs of cranial nerves; the pituitary and pineal glands; and the spinal cord with its peripheral nervous system. Small movements in the central nervous system have been observed as a result of pulsation in the cerebral arteries, voluntary movements of the head and neck, and inhalation and exhalation during respiratory cycles of the costodiaphragmatic system.

In addition to these movements, there is a rhythmic coiling and uncoiling of the total neural tube, which is the movement associated with the craniosacral mechanism. During the expansive phase, the lateral and third ventricles widen and fill with the incoming tide of the cerebrospinal fluid, and during the opposite phase, the ventricles narrow with the ebbing tide. This constant, involuntary, rhythmic motility of the central nervous system is integrated with the fluctuant cerebrospinal fluid and the reciprocal tension membrane to contribute to adequate venous drainage for the brain, pituitary and pineal glands, and other key functioning.

Palpatory clues: The motility of the central nervous system is difficult to feel, and it is generally not necessary to do so. Expansion of a compressed portion of a cerebral hemisphere can occasionally be palpated during a corrective phase of a membranous articular strain.

Reciprocal Tension Membrane: There are three layers of meninges surrounding the central nervous system—pia mater, arachnoid, and dura mater. The dura mater was named the reciprocal tension membrane by Dr. Sutherland for the way it functions as a unit in its relationship with the craniosacral mechanism.

The dura mater lines the neurocranium as its inner periosteum, passes through the sutures to meld with the outer layer of periosteum of the skull, and merges with the entire connective tissue systems of the body as they hang from the base of the skull. Within the neurocranium, the dura mater has three reduplications: the falx cerebri, the tentorium cerebelli, and the falx cerebelli. An important feature of this arrangement is the junction of the falx cerebri with the tentorium cerebelli at the straight sinus to form a fulcrum where the falx and the two halves of the tentorium become three sickles of mobile functioning. This junction has been named the Sutherland fulcrum.

The three sickles—falx cerebri, right and left tentorium cerebelli—act as a reciprocal tension membrane with their anterior, posterior, lateral, and inferior poles of attachment to the osseous elements of the skull and sacrum. It is a reciprocal tension membrane, not membranes. It is one unit of function.

Relatively, the reciprocal tension membrane moves in an anterior-superior direction during the period of flexion, with widening of the cranial base and lateral sides of the head, and in a posterior-inferior direction during periods of extension, with a narrowing of the cranial base and sides of the head. The Sutherland fulcrum is the fulcrum over or through which the three sickles function physiologically in the maintenance of balance in the cranial membranous articular mechanism. It is an automatic, shifting, suspension, accommodative fulcrum for torsion and sidebending sphenobasilar movements as well as for various malpositions occurring in cranial membranous articular strains.

This constant, involuntary mobility demonstrated by the Sutherland fulcrum and its three sickles is reflected and palpable in all the connective tissues of the body and their enclosed elements—bones, muscles, organs, fluids, cells, etcetera. In addition, all patients live with either a torsion or a sidebending-rotation as a physiologic structural component in their craniosacral mechanism. This component is also reflected throughout the total connective tissues of the body. In the presence of any pattern to be found in the craniosacral mechanism—be it a pattern of health, trauma, or disease—the constant, involuntary rhythmic movement of all parts of the mechanism continues. The reciprocal tension membrane is the working mobile tool through which trained palpatory skills can diagnose and work with these mechanisms within the patient.

Palpatory clues: In working with the reciprocal tension membrane within the neurocranium and the connective tissues of the body, palpation reveals two factors: a constant, mobile flexion/external rotation, extension/internal rotation movement 8 to 12 times per minute and a structural pattern of total body physiology that lives within the individual patient. It is important to diagnose the base pattern of health functioning for the individual as this is the pattern towards which health is to be regained; then diagnose the structure-function of the stress pattern responsible for the patient's complaint. The constantly moving reciprocal tension membrane and connective tissues will reveal these factors to a skilled palpatory touch.

Cranial Articular Mechanisms: There are 29 bones in the skull, but the craniosacral mechanism is only concerned with 22 of them; 8 of them form the neurocranium and the remaining 14 are in the face. There are slightly more than 100 articulations in connection with 22 bones. The sphenoid, occiput, two temporals, two parietals, and frontal(s) form the neurocranium and are directly controlled in their mobility, as to range of motion and pattern of structural integrity, by the Sutherland fulcrum and reciprocal tension membrane. The relative mobility of the sphenoid works with the frontal(s) and facial bones, and the occiput works with the temporals, parietals, and mandible.

The membranous articular patterns within the craniosacral mechanism are described in their relationship with the sphenobasilar synchondrosis. These include torsion (right or left), sidebending-rotation (right or left), and compression. In addition, there are specific membranous articular strains associated with individual suture interrelationships, such as occipitomastoid, frontosphenoidal, frontoparietal, parietal notch, and as many as there are membranous articulations.

The basic patterns named at the sphenobasilar synchondrosis, such as a torsion, will be reflected into all the osseous elements and connective tissues of the total body physiology. This is also true for some severe, specific membranous articular strains, such as an occipitomastoid type of stress.

Palpatory clues: The osseous elements are on the surface of the craniosacral mechanism and are more available for tactile evaluation, but it is important to understand that these osseous elements are a portion of a membranous articular mechanism, and the skill of diagnosis is to palpate the mobile functioning of these elements in health as well as in stress. The bones are primarily going along for a ride on a moving mechanism.

Sacrum: The sacrum plays an important role in body physiology mobility in that it has a complicated side-to-side pattern for voluntary or postural movement of the pelvis and a constant, rhythmic, flexion-extension, involuntary mobility as part of the craniosacral mechanism. The sacrum is at the lower pole of the reciprocal tension membrane and is integrated with the Sutherland fulcrum and the three lever arms or sickles. The sacrum can be locked in its involuntary mobility through trauma and thus can limit movement of the entire reciprocal tension membrane and connective tissues of the body. This constriction can contribute to many problems in total body physiology. A loss of involuntary mobility of the sacrum does not necessarily impose a loss of voluntary or postural mobility of the sacrum, and the loss of involuntary movement is frequently overlooked.

Palpatory clues: A "locked" involuntary sacral mobility can be present for years and can only be found by the trained palpatory skill of the physician. When the sacrum is locked, the whole pelvis—sacrum and both ilia—try to go as a unit into rhythmic flexion and extension with the Sutherland fulcrum. When the sacrum is released to work freely with the Sutherland fulcrum, the sacrum and two ilia are three units of mobility. Palpatory diagnosis of this sacral factor is quite important in determining health patterns for the patient.

This, then, is the primary respiratory mechanism. The unity of the primary respiratory mechanism achieves a basic anatomicophysiological fact: There is a vital, inherent, rhythmic, involuntary movement within the whole body physiology expressing itself as a flexion of all midline structures with external rotation of all bilateral structures alternating with extension of all midline structures with internal rotation of all bilateral structures 8 to 12 times per minute. It is present throughout life. It is a mechanism essential to health in the individual. It is present in both physician and patient and is available for palpatory diagnosis in all parts of the patient's body. Each of the five components is available for palpatory diagnosis, as long as the physician takes into consideration the quality and the type of fluid or tissue involved and its functional relationship to the other components.

134

Palpatory Clues in Clinical Disorders

Many of the clinical problems associated with the craniosacral mechanism will provide palpatory diagnostic clues through one or more of the five components. Examples of these follow.

Headaches: There are headaches in as many ways as there are those who have them. Palpatory clues of suboccipital tensities can support the idea of venous drainage stasis from the neurocranium as a result of reduced rocking of the cranial bowl in flexion and extension. True migraine cases almost invariably demonstrate a sidebending-rotation pattern in the sphenobasilar synchondrosis with the prodromal symptoms starting on the side of the high great wing of the sphenoid and the high occiput. The presence of this pattern is not a cause of the migraine headache but does serve to corroborate the diagnosis.

Hypertension: A common palpatory finding in chronic hypertension is a flattening of the tentorium cerebelli affecting its anatomic functioning. It does not dome upward in extension as much as it should in its rhythmic movement.

Dyslexia: The presence of an intraosseous temporal strain pattern can be found in many of these cases.

Tic douloureux and other trigeminal nerve disturbances: These are commonly associated with dental traumatic strains.

Hormonal disturbances: A limitation in the motility of the pituitary-hypothalamic axis leads to hypo- or hyperactivity of hormonal function. This can be associated with vertical or lateral sphenobasilar membranous articular strains.

Concussion: The reciprocal tension membrane has the feel of a shock-like rigidity in its functioning.

Meningitis and post-meningitis: The reciprocal tension membrane changes in its tonal quality and function from that of "wet tissue paper" in acute stages of the disease to that of "soggy cardboard" in chronic post-meningitis. Chronic venous stasis involving the central nervous system is always present in either acute or chronic cases.

Sphenobasilar patterns: Added trauma can decompensate existing patterns and affect craniosacral and body mechanisms.

135

Specific membranous articular strains: These can be very debilitating, either acutely or chronically, over a period of months and years.

The 12 pairs of cranial nerves: Any of these can be compromised in their functioning relationships. There can be problems in the face involving eye, ear, nose, and throat; in the neurocranium and cranial base creating a vagal syndrome; and down to the sacrum affecting its parasympathetic outflow. An interesting case was one in which the patient lost his sight as a result of a parietal compression, traumatic in origin, forcing the occipital lobe of the central nervous system and its calcarine fissure against the falx cerebri in the area of the straight sinus. The parietal compression, with its loss of membranous and articular mobility, was observed by palpation.

Sacrum: Its freedom to function can be palpated. The presence of a "locked" sacrum following hard falls on the buttocks or inertial injuries (whiplash), a limited return to physiological functioning in postpartum cases, and other contributing factors can be diagnosed by palpation.

Newborns, infants, and children: The role of palpatory diagnosis in the use of the craniosacral mechanism in the newborn, infant, and child cannot be overemphasized. The primary respiratory mechanism at work within the fetus is free to do its rhythmic functioning protected by the fetus' immersion in fluid. Its tide-like movement provides a vitality factor (whatever that may be) and a rhythmic involuntary movement of every cell in the developing fetal body, 8 to 12 times a minute.

The baby is then born and, in the process, molded by its passage through the birth canal. The primary respiratory mechanism continues its tide-like movement within the newborn container of reciprocal tension membrane, connective tissues, and fluids to literally guide the newborn's mechanism towards a total pattern of health, unmolding acquired areas of stress and remolding health back into the function of simple flexion/external rotation, extension/internal rotation motility and mobility. A physiologic pattern of a torsion or a sidebending-rotation will be acquired at this time and will be a part of the total health pattern to be carried by this individual throughout his or her life.

There are no articular gears in the newborn with the exception of the articular contacts of the condylar parts of the occiput in the pits of the atlas. Any bumps, falls, twists, or strains are primarily membranous stresses up to the age of 10 to 13 years, when the bony plates begin to develop their articular status. A diagnostic palpatory skill can examine the craniosacral mechanism of a child in order to find the base pattern of membranous articular health that this individual is developing to carry throughout his life. Any future trauma and/or disease acquired during the life of the patient should be guided towards this health functioning, in addition to correcting the imposed stress.

This is not a time-consuming process. A trained palpatory skill can work with and allow the fluid drive of the tide-like cerebrospinal fluid and the mobile membranous reciprocal tension membrane to demonstrate their basic pattern of functioning within the craniosacral mechanism and, through the connective tissues and fluid matrix of the body, for the total body physiology. Future health or stress patterns for the individual can be better understood if the physician has a palpatory record of his patient's basic, involuntary mobility of life.

In summary, from headaches to the newborn, there is a host of clinical problems that can be diagnosed and treated by trained palpatory skills. In many cases, the palpatory tools are the only way that results can be obtained. In addition, it is also a clinical fact that ligamentous articular strains, fascial drags, and other traumatic or disease-oriented problems can compromise various parts of the primary respiratory mechanism functioning, and conversely, craniosacral mechanism problems can have adverse effects upon the rest of the body. The conclusion that is drawn is that body physiology is one unit of function in health and in trauma and/or disease. Palpatory skills can trace interrelationships of health and clinical problems from the feet to the top of the head and back again.

Palpatory Diagnosis as Art and Science

Diagnosis and treatment are inseparable in the role of palpation in the use of the primary respiratory mechanism and body physiology. Palpation is both an art and a science. From the scientific standpoint, palpation is a quantum leap in sense perception. The moment the physician lays his hands on a patient for palpatory diagnosis and treatment, he is a participator with that patient in a quantum, sharing experience. It is wholly impossible for him to be a neutral or impartial observer as he works with the living tissues of the patient.

The physician is an involuntary primary respiratory mechanism within a living voluntary body physiology. His patient is endowed with the same qualities, an involuntary primary respiratory mechanism within a living voluntary body physiology. Palpation, then, becomes a living interchange between two living bodies. The physician does far more than observe. He is a participator, as his hands, his proprioceptive fiber input, and his sensorimotor areas of the central nervous system record the movements, mobility, and motility of the living body and tissues of the patient. He positions his hands in readiness to receive. His awareness of life within himself desiring to understand the living function within the patient is sufficient stimulus to invoke the primary respiratory mechanism and body physiology of the patient to demonstrate its mechanisms and tissue response to the physician's participatory sense of touch. This is truly a quantum unit of interchange between physician and patient.

An "objective" examination can be made through a more superficial approach if the physician chooses to test the range of motion of an area by passively moving the parts involved. The information he gets is relatively shallow in its content and does not take into consideration how this area functions as a living mechanism.

The physician can choose to make a deeper study of this area. To do this, he must adapt his hand contacts in such a manner as to bring into play an awakened, proprioceptive contact with the flexor digitorum profundus and flexor pollicis longus muscles to record the living movements within the patient and then to allow this mobility and motility to record itself in the sensorimotor areas of the central nervous system of the physician. He is no longer an observer, he is a *participator*. He does not supervise the sensory input he is receiving. He actively, not passively, allows the living function of the area of the patient to report itself to him—its health, its stress, its dynamics of interrelationships with the total body physiology of the patient.

Assessing range of motion by simply observing the motion present is relatively quick in its application and can be objectively analyzed by comparing one area to another. As this palpatory skill is developed and refined by the physician in his daily use, it becomes a valuable tool for diagnosis before and after treatment. It gives some information as to the quality of function for the area involved, although it does not give the physician a full view of the involuntary units of movement, mobility, motility, and finer details of voluntary activity. This requires participation with these units of work from within the patient and the added factor of time to allow the tissues to manifest their functioning. As the physician palpates with his proprioceptive sensory input, he must wait a few moments or even minutes for the awakened primary respiratory mechanism and body physiologic mechanisms to go to work. These mechanisms include all the cells, fluids, connective tissues, and their tide-like movement, mobility, and motility.

An area of health will report this fact to the physician through the tonal quality of the voluntary tissues and the quality of involuntary mobility of the basic rhythm of the primary respiratory mechanism in its flexion/external rotation, extension/internal rotation for the midline and bilateral structures. An area or areas of stress will report these facts to the physician through the change of tonal quality in the voluntary tissues and a limitation or absence of the basic primary respiratory mechanism tide-like movement. The physician should allow the patient's body physiology to report these findings before analyzing them. Function, as shown by living tissues, can be better understood after the work is completed and only to a lesser degree during the time that function is doing its work. After a corrective treatment has been initiated to restore function towards health, it is wise to examine the area of stress to feel for the tide-like rhythm of the primary respiratory mechanism again working its way through the corrected site. The presence of the tide ensures continued, innate self-healing by the patient's living mechanisms; its absent or limited movement indicates a slower phase of local healing function.

Palpation is a self-taught process. This is where the art of palpation becomes a part of palpatory skills. If the physician is using objective, passive motion skills, he learns to read the quality of his movements and those of the patient in the use of these palpatory techniques. If he is a participator and is using the involuntary mechanisms and body physiology of the patient, he learns to read the quality of movement, mobility, and motility from within the patient through his proprioceptive fibers and sensorimotor areas of the central nervous system. To get the maximum sensory insight for diagnosis from the primary respiratory mechanism, the physician needs to become a participator in developing his palpatory skills for the evaluation of health, for the evaluation of trauma and/or disease, and for the guidance of treatment toward health. It is truly an art to learn to use these palpatory skills. All that is required is time, patients, and patience.

DEVELOPING PALPATORY SKILLS
This is an edited transcription of a lecture given in 1986
at a Sutherland Cranial Teaching Foundation basic course
in Philadelphia, Pennsylvania.

WHEN I WAS IN osteopathic college in the 1930's, we were blessed with instructors who gave us the art of treating patients by various manipulative skills, mainly thrusting. What we were taught in school was effective, and when I graduated, I gave a good osteopathic treatment. I had a lot of patients to give them on, and I had to give them a lot of treatments to try to clear up their problems. After eight or ten years of this type of general practice, I discovered I got bored with the fact that these patients were coming back with the same complaints in the same areas that should have been fixed the last time they came in. If I had ten cases of some problem, three or four would make an adequate response within a reasonable period of time, three or four more would make a reasonable response sometime, and the rest wouldn't make any response no matter what I did. What frustrated me was that I wasn't able to differentiate by palpatory skill why one made a response and another one didn't. I finally recognized that you could possess a wide variety of palpatory skills through which you really weren't learning very much, and very obviously mine were like that.

So I went back to the writings of A.T. Still, and literally I decided to give up the practice of "osteopathy" and instead decided to study the practice of A.T. Still. Over a period of time, I realized that in order to understand and use his concept—spelled out in one paragraph in particular[1]—as a goal for development, it would be necessary to drop all my so-called palpatory skills and learn a whole new set-up. I began this by simply putting my hands on various segments of the patients' bodies that related to their complaints, and I learned to listen, listen, listen to the tissues within. I did this because the Old Doctor, Dr. Still,

141

had said every body physiology has a physician within that allows physiologic function to work towards self-correction; all the powers, motive forces, and everything necessary for the treatment of that case are already built into the machine; all that is necessary is to recognize and work with these mechanisms. If the motors, motive forces, and everything else are already in action and in motion, and if even the fundamental principle of the physician within is in motion, capable of whatever is necessary, then I realized I would have to develop a type of palpatory skill whereby I could hear what the body physiology had to say instead of me telling it what to do.

To do this, I put my hands very carefully over the sites of strains, stresses, dysfunctions, or whatever came into the office, and I would sit there a few minutes and quietly try to listen to what those tissues were trying to tell me. I was not just listening to the primary respiratory mechanism, I was listening to the whole body physiology of the patient, including the body physiology of the fascia, the voluntary mechanism, and the involuntary mechanism. I didn't differentiate these in my thinking, I wasn't that smart, I just had my hands on them.

In the early days of this, I felt that when I got through listening, I'd better do something; so I'd go to some other part of the body and give a little correction so the patient would be happy, but I never touched the area I had been working on. After about three to four years, I finally was aware of the fact that I was feeling something happening. Until that time, I was not sure what was happening. In the first year or two, I realized that, although I didn't understand, something must be going on because of the patients' responses. The only encouragement I gained from my patients was, "You haven't done a thing to me yet, doctor, but yesterday, I cleaned the attic for the first time in three months." So I learned to listen to the phrases of the patients as they left the office: "...but I washed seventeen cars and didn't get tired." This told me that something was happening even if I didn't know about it.

Did you ever stop to think how basically lousy our palpatory skills are? Are you feeling anything? Are you actually sensing what's going on? Do you really know what's going on? We have to develop our sense of touch by training our sensory area of the brain; it has never been exposed to this type of feeling. We pick up an orange and an apple, and we can feel that one has a rough surface and the other has a relatively smooth one—big deal. Well, how about the fine motilities and mobilities going on within this body we are feeling? We have to develop palpatory tools commensurate with the complexity and simplicity of this primary respiratory mechanism. We have to learn to feel, but it doesn't happen by being taught. I can't teach you anything about it; you have to learn it yourself on a one-on-one basis. Patients taught it to me from within themselves. I learned it from within them by listening from within myself about how to work with the body physiology. I still don't know everything I'm supposed to feel, I'm still learning.

Five years after I began with my so-called new approach, I moved from Michigan to Texas. When I did, over three hundred people came to me and said, "We like what you do, where do we continue our treatment program?" Believe it or not, that was the first time in the five years of working that way that anybody ever said they liked it; not one single person had ever told me before that it was a good idea. I had only known it was a good idea because it was working.

It is interesting to note that the fact that I could not feel in those early years did not determine the efficiency of the treatment. I could not feel any of the things that I can feel now, but I was working with a body physiology within the patient that could understand that something was going on. It did do something for that patient—not because I could feel it, or give it orders, or tell it to shut up or do anything else, but because I simply did the job of taking hold of the area of the patient that had something to say. It was a job of quietly positioning my hands and then listening through my hands, reading through my hands, feeling through my hands, quietly, for that which the patient was trying to tell me. It was not the patient's ego or intellect but the quietness of their tissue functioning, reporting through to me, that made the necessary changes and allowed the patient to make the physiologic changes toward restoration of health.

The only reason we are talking about developing palpatory skills like these is that this is the only way body physiology works. It does not work according to our plan, it works according to its plan, and it only has one goal—health. We can learn to differentiate, realize, and feel qualities of health. We can learn to read the physiological stresses and strains of dysfunction. We can learn from within. The physician within me is going to be working with the physician within the patient to quietly learn. Why did the patient come to see me? I don't know, but I can go to my physician within and their physician within and learn to shut up and listen. I can listen to their physician within their tissues and get some kind of a report back through my sensory channels. In this way, I can begin to understand. Developing palpatory skill is strictly done on a one-on-one basis. There isn't anybody around except you and the patient. In my book, the patient is the only teacher. The science of osteopathy and the body physiology of the patient are the teachers, and I'm the student. Finally, the sensory areas wake up, and all of a sudden we discover that we can feel.

Now I can give you a few, little clues that will perhaps encourage your capacity to feel more in your palpation. Take my word for it, they have no meaning at all except to aid you in gradually training your palpatory skills. These are just some clues, they are not the exact ways to do it; these are merely suggestions as taught to me by my patients over the decades. The first thing you do, and you're not going to like it, is to give up your egos. You aren't half as smart as your body is or the body of that patient on the table.

Next, it helps to think about four levels of palpatory skills. The first level is a superficial contact. You just casually take ahold of something. You're not listening, you simply register that you are touching something. This contact is using only the touch receptors in your fingers and hands. The next level of palpatory skill is developed by working through the proprioceptive fibers of the flexor pollicis longus and the flexor digitorum profundus, which are the muscles in the forearm that control the motion of the fingers and thumb. You can take ahold of a mechanism with a superficial contact, and then you slightly contract your muscles, and immediately you are aware in a whole different way of the fact that you're feeling an object.

Try it yourself. First just let your hands make a contact somewhere on the body. Then, don't do anything except barely contract your flexor pollicis and flexor digitorum muscles. Do you feel something which you didn't before? Now, go back to not feeling with the proprioceptors. There is a difference in the quality of the feel because with the proprioceptive contact, you are reaching through to a body of fluid and a set of ligaments and muscles, and they are all in motion. With the superficial contact, you are not feeling motion; all you have is ahold of the body. When you use the proprioceptors, you are mechanically listening to the function that's going on in that particular area.

In order to put this proprioceptive contact to work, it helps to create a fulcrum. Place your arms comfortably on the treatment table, and then lean gently on your elbows. This introduces a slight compression into the picture. If you lean too hard into your elbows, you'll lock whatever it is you're trying to feel; you'll be preventing anything from happening. One way to find the right amount of pressure is to lean too hard and then ease up part way on the pressure on the table. Take the pressure off the arms, but do not move the hands, and all of a sudden, you become aware of the fact that something is happening. At this point, you're not locked into the table, nor are you hanging free—you have a floating contact. With this floating contact, anything that happens within that patient is going to reflect back, and you're going to pick it up because your proprioceptors are now in agreement with the exact tensity of that part of the patient's mechanism you have ahold of.

This notion of matching tensities comes up clearly in a patient with an extremely tense and fibrotic lumbar area of stress and strain. When someone comes in with this, get a hand under that psoas, establish a contact or fulcrum point, and then press firmly on your elbow. You might discover that you have to press extremely hard against that table, against that fulcrum point, until you finally match the tensity that's going on in that psoas muscle. Then, as you ease up, you'll find the point at which that muscle goes to work. This is an example of applying a compression through proprioceptive contacts and managing it so as to agree with the pathology felt in the body. This is putting it to work.

In our discussion so far, we've gone from the fingertips to the forearms; now let's go upstairs. Once you've set up your hand contact and engaged your proprioceptive fibers, listen to what is taking place within that body physiology—turn on the sensory area of your brain. This sounds stupid, but how do you talk about something you can't discuss? Think from up there, sense from up there. Sense from upstairs, keep on listening to the body physiology. It's a little bit of a trick, but you finally discover that instead of feeling things happening just down in your arms, you are also recording this information in the sensorimotor area. You can listen and bring the material the body's trying to teach you right up to the sensory and motor areas of your brain. I call this level of palpation, sensorimotor. One side of the central sulcus is sensory and the other side is motor; so they discuss the problem you're feeling down there. Being able to feel from the sensorimotor area is just another tool; it is not a goal to be reached for.

Now, let's take these three layers of palpatory skill—superficial, proprioceptive, and sensorimotor contact—and go one step farther. Knowing that all these tools are working anyway, just listen, listen, listen. You are making a quantum jump, accepting that anything can happen and you don't know why. This is sensing by means of a quantum jump; it is developing palpatory skills you can't define but can guarantee do, in fact, work. The superficial contact gives you one layer of instruction from the body physiology; adding the proprioceptors gives another layer; adding the sensorimotor gives yet a deeper layer of instruction. You can then throw out all three of these and say, "I'm going to Listen, with a capital 'L,'" and you get into a quantum level. I can't explain it, but I get more information at this quantum level than I do with the other three combined.

An analogy I use for this quantum contact is that of a water bug. Do you know what a water bug is? Have you ever seen one running around on a pond? A way to get into quantum mechanics in learning how to palpate is to become a water bug running around on the surface of a body of fluid, which is the body physiology. A water bug never gets wet, drowned, or anything else. He just runs around on the surface of this water, which is living, and he's alive. The water bug moves around on this body of water, finding the areas of stress or strain. Then as the physician, you can focus through and listen through the water bug to what's going on in body physiology. Isn't that nice? The bug does all the work, and you're sitting there listening. As you listen to this little water bug analogy, you can get different impressions of functioning. It gives you just a clue; it's a fun thing you just play with.

When you start examining some patient's problem, quietly think about what's going on and realize you've got a physician's role to play in reading this mechanism. You use your superficial hand contact and get all the input you can. You feel with the proprioceptive and sensorimotor contact and get that input, and then you read with the water bug into the total body physiology of the patient. You consent to be used by the body physiology of that patient as you listen to the messages being given to you through the water bug. With these messages, the patient's physician within is trying to demonstrate how you can help that patient move towards the restoration of health.

Now I would like for you to go to the tables, place your hands somewhere on the body, become a water bug, and listen to anything that could possibly happen–simply observe for ten minutes.

---

1. The paragraph from A.T. Still's autobiography is as follows:
"I am fully convinced that God, of the mind of nature, has proven His ability to plan (if plan be necessary) and to make or furnish laws of self, without patterns, for the myriads of forms of animated beings; and to thoroughly equip them for the duties of life, with their engines and batteries of motor force all in action. Each part is fully armed for duty, empowered to select and appropriate to itself from the great laboratory of nature such forces as are needed to enable it to discharge the duties to its office in the economy of life. In short, that the all-knowing Architect has cut and numbered each part to fit its place and discharge its duties in every building in animal form, while the suns, stars, moons, and comets all obey the one eternal law of life and motion." (p. 148)

LEARNING TO LISTEN

These are excerpts from written notes for various lectures.

COMPARE OUR USE OF palpation to a surgeon in his work. Most surgeons deal with gross motion in working with the body. A microsurgeon deals with small motions in working with the body. He takes months and years to develop his hand-eye coordination and his skills in using small motions. Similarly, we use gross palpatory skills for voluntary mechanisms in body mobility, as would a surgeon. We also find it necessary to take months and years to develop the palpatory skills for the fine movements of the involuntary mechanisms of the body, as would a microsurgeon.

The microsurgeon uses a microscope to magnify his field of work. We magnify our field of work and observation by calling into play our total *living* sensory field. We open all the sensory areas of the brain. We open all the proprioceptive sensory fibers from the head to the feet, not merely the hands and arms. We feel with the whole body in response to the fine mobilities and motilities of the involuntary mechanisms of the body, including the primary respiratory mechanism. We learn to read sensory input from the central nervous system sensory areas to the hand instead of from the hand to the central nervous system sensory areas. Listen through the hands, not with the hands. The patient demonstrates; the physician listens, actively.

We act with our living mechanisms to express life and function. So we learn to act with the living mechanisms of the patient to evaluate his state of health. We become a living pathfinder within the patterns manifesting themselves within the body physiology of the patient. We do this through palpation.

Feeling motion is not enough. One needs to "listen" to what the motion means—listen with the mind, reason with the mind, interpret with the mind, read with the mind. Develop a "mental picture" of what, when, and why the patient's physiological mechanism wants this type of motion.

The physician's role in palpation of the mechanism:
    to watch with sensorimotor input
    to feel with sensorimotor input
    to read with sensorimotor input
    to listen with sensorimotor input
    to allow a water bug to be still while in motion with the mechanism
Consent to be used by the patient's body physiology.
For a discussion of the water bug, see "Developing Palpatory Skills."

A note concerning *listening:* When you listen to the body physiology of the patient, be aware of the level of events happening in the anatomicophysiology of the patient's body as compared to the lack of events when the physician does not listen. The deeper the physician goes within himself to listen to the activity of body physiology of the patient through his palpatory contact, the greater will be the data shown to the physician in his examination.

In this process, stop *thinking* about it and surrender to the total anatomicophysiological output of the patient. Let it be recorded as sensory input to the physician, who receives and accepts this sensory input without making judgement of its content. This permits the patient's anatomicophysiological mechanism to "allow physiological function within to manifest its own unerring potency rather than using blind force from without." The physician consents to be used by the patient's body physiology.

149

Diagnostic Touch

DR. BECKER WROTE A *series of four articles entitled "Diagnostic Touch: Its Principles and Application." They were published by the Academy of Applied Osteopathy in their* Yearbook. *Part I appeared in the 1963 edition, Parts II and III in 1964, and Part IV in 1965, Volume 2.*

For publication in this book, these articles have been extensively edited. The original written version of Part III has been almost wholly replaced with material that had been prepared for a presentation at an Academy meeting. The reader is referred to the original sources for the entire texts. The titles that appear for Parts I-III were given by this editor; the title for Part IV is Dr. Becker's.

The terminology of diagnostic touch, *including the terms* biodynamic and biokinetic energies, *was eventually abandoned by Dr. Becker. In a 1969 letter to Anne Wales, D.O., he explained his decision to stop using the terms. There had been little appreciation expressed for the terminology, he said, and he believed it hindered practicing physicians in their learning to use the concepts. He reiterated to Dr. Wales his belief that the material was valid but stated it would be best to use more familiar terminology when discussing "Still's-Sutherland's basic principles of anatomy and physiology and the palpatory skill it takes to bring these into clinical use."*

DIAGNOSTIC TOUCH: ITS PRINCIPLES AND APPLICATION
Part I: To Feel Living Function

DIAGNOSIS IS BOTH AN art and a science. In the realm of science, we have extended our senses through instrumentation, introducing a battery of tests to diagnose conditions in the human body. The variety and complexity of these tests, and the parameters which they measure, are almost limitless. Diagnosis as a science brings to the physician data that can be learned objectively with a minimum of human error.

The art of diagnosis, however, is that ability applied by the physician himself. Therefore, diagnosis as an art is important; it always has

153

been and always will be. It involves the following factors: the physician's interpretative skill in analyzing the data supplied by scientific tools and the use of the physicians personal skills in evaluating the patient before him. These factors are subjective in nature. They may not bring the finite detail of the instrument, but neither are they limited by the finite detail the instrument is capable of perceiving. There is room for assessing variables: the ability to perceive past and present events and the ability to forecast future changes. A scientific diagnosis is not enough. It is the composite use of both scientific (objective) and personal (subjective) tools that gives the physician a true diagnosis.

Interpretive skills within the physician are a subtle mixture of many years of training, knowledge of scientific tools, experience, and a mind that keeps itself open to any and all approaches that might enhance the physician's abilities. The physician also develops his own personal, subjective tools: the eyes for accurate inspection, the ears for accurate auscultation and percussion, the nose and taste where indicated, and a thinking, feeling, knowing touch. Interpretive skills call for a knowledge of function within the human body—function related to past events, function at the present time, and the ability to project functioning patterns into the near future. This is different from the mere tests for function as recorded by the scientific tools at our command. The latter are transitory findings that reflect the picture of the moment. Assessing true function within the individual patient is the evaluation of what the patient is doing with all of these variables. How is his system coordinating them; how is he adapting to the dysfunctions; where is the potential for the reversibilities of the dysfunctions? In other words, how is this patient functioning as a living being? He is sick. He comes to you for help. Where is he now; where was he when his problems began; what is his potential for a return to normal? It is the intelligent use of the physician's senses that can give knowledgeable answers to these questions.

There are always three factors to consider every time a patient enters your office: the patient's ideas and beliefs of what he considers his problem to be; the physician's concept of what he considers the patient's problem to be; and finally, what the anatomical-physiological wholeness of the patient's body knows the problem to be. The patient may have based his opinion of what is wrong on diagnoses given by other physicians. If you can come up with a picture that will explain his problem to him in a satisfactory way, he is able to cooperate with you. But in the final analysis, he still has his opinion, right or wrong.

The physician's concept of what is wrong with the patient is based on many years of training. He has been taught to create a diagnostic label couched in terminology with which he can communicate his findings. For example, the diagnosis of a peptic ulcer, viral pneumonia or whiplash injury conveys a whole syndrome of findings in the minds of patients and other physicians. While this ability to communicate is necessary, it is also a limiting factor in the true diagnosis. The body does not think of its problem in such a limited sense.

Finally, there is the third factor, the anatomical-physiological mechanism's knowledge of its own case. It has the answer. The anatomical-physiological mechanism and its structure-function carry the total picture for disease and restored health.

To sum up, the patient is guessing as to a diagnosis, and the physician is scientifically guessing as to the diagnosis, while the patient's body knows the problem and is manifesting it in the tissues. It is possible to obtain a more accurate diagnosis, one that is closer to the true pattern, by utilizing the information and know-how of the patient's body to bring this diagnosis into existence. We can train our senses, especially our sense of touch, to lead us into the structure-function of the patient's anatomical-physiological mechanisms and make them give us the information we need. In invoking this process, each physician will have to teach himself the details of the way into and through structure-function. It is a self-taught process. Guidance can be given, but the physician alone is the final arbiter as to methods and results. We have to learn to feel the structure-function messages from within the body of the patient—what is happening now, when did it begin, and how is it going to progress? It is quite a challenge.

Through the sense of touch, we can feel function within the tissues and feel dysfunction when it is present. Motion is not function; function always includes motion, but motion does not represent all the values of function. Witness the patient who complains of a leg ache. We can test the leg for motion and find it working well according to gross motion. Yet, with a touch designed to feel the dysfunction within that, it is possible to say, "I find the source of your disability to be thus and so," though it is difficult to find words to describe function within living tissues.

With regard to the sense of touch, someone said to me one day, "You feel from the heart, don't you?" That is right. You learn to feel into the heart of the patient's problem from a still-leverage point that allows the functions and dysfunctions of the patient to be reflected back into your touch and feel. The first step in developing this depth of feel and touch is to evaluate the patient from the standpoint of the anatomicophysiological mechanism. Just what does the patient's body want to tell you? Take the patient's story and opinion and set it aside, take your opinion and diagnosis and set it aside, then let the patient's body give you its opinion. Place your hands on the patient in the area of his complaint or complaints. Let the feel of the tissues from the inner core of their depths come through your touch, and listen to and read their story.

To get this story, it is necessary to read structure-function in tissues. To do this, we need to know something about potency and something about the fulcrum.

Potency

The knowledge of potency within tissues begins with a statement given to us by Dr. W. G. Sutherland: "Allow the physiological function within to manifest its own unerring potency rather than use blind force from without."[1] These words state the principle upon which we will develop an understanding of what potency is. The diagnostic tool with which we will learn to read and understand this potency is the principle of the use of the fulcrum. We will use the principle of the fulcrum in applying our hands and fingers so as to create a condition in which the principle of the potency may become knowledge for our use in diagnosis and treatment.

The dictionary defines potency as "the state or quality of being potent, or the degree of this; power; strength." It defines potent as "able to control or influence; having authority or power." We have heard for years that the body has within itself all the factors with which to maintain health and to heal itself in case of disease or trauma. This statement is basically true. The body has the capacity to express health through this inherent potency, and it has the capacity to maintain compensatory mechanisms in response to trauma or disease through variant potencies. At the very core of total health, there is a potency within the human body manifesting it in health. At the very core of every traumatic or disease condition within the human body is a potency manifesting its interrelationship with the body in trauma or disease.

It is up to us to learn to feel this potency. It is relatively easy to feel the tensions and stresses of trauma and disease as they are manifesting their patterns. But within these manifesting elements, there is a potency that is "able to control or influence; having authority or power." It centers the disturbance. It can be sensed and read by a feeling touch.

To bring out the idea of what it means to feel potency within a given problem, let us consider something else in nature that demonstrates the power within potency—a hurricane. The principles and manifestations of a hurricane can be shown to be analogous to the principles and manifestations of disease and trauma within the human body.

I have considered potency as a fulcrum point over, around, and through which biodynamic intrinsic forces within human physiology do their work in health and over, around, and through which biokinetic intrinsic forces maintain their disease or traumatic conditions within the body. This potency is very similar to the power or energy field present in the fulcrum point of a moving teeter-totter board or that which can be found in the eye of a hurricane. For example, in large, mature hurricanes, the amount of kinetic energy produced is 100 to 300 times the daily electric power production of the United States. It can be assumed that there is kinetic energy within the still point or the eye of the hurricane over, around, and through which this storm is maintaining itself. It can also be assumed that there is kinetic energy, power and potency in the potencies in the biodynamic and biokinetic intrinsic forces within human physiology in health, disease and trauma.

The eye of the hurricane carries the potency or power for the whole storm, while the spirals of the high winds feeding into the eye manifest the destructiveness of the storm. The eye of the hurricane carries the pattern for the whole storm. Any change in the eye automatically changes the spiraling effects of the winds feeding into the eye and thus the pattern of the storm. If the eye of a hurricane closes, it is no longer a hurricane. So it is the presence of this eye that determines whether it is a hurricane or just an ordinary storm. Within the eye is the potency "having authority or power" to create the manifestations of the spiraling winds making up the storm.

Hurricane Carla struck Texas in 1961, and during that storm, hurricane hunters flying B-29 airplanes flew into the storm and into the eye itself and registered much data concerning her. At the same time, radio and television kept us informed throughout the storm. While those of us who sat on the sidelines were able to watch the growth and progress of Carla's existence, those scientists who flew in the B-29s were able to literally know and experience the high winds in the spirals and the potency of the eye of the hurricane. It was a physical awareness to them. Men trained to understand mechanisms of this type can know the various factors within the storm pattern by the interpretation of their own senses in addition to that information given by the instruments they are watching. They know when they are in the eye or in the periphery of the spirals. They can feel it with their whole being.

Thus, the physician can train his touch to recognize and accept the fact that within every trauma or disease pattern, there is an "eye," within or without the patient, which has within it a potency to manifest this traumatic or disease condition. It is a point of stillness within that focus. It is invisible, to be sure, but it can be perceived by the trained, discerning touch of the physician. How do I know? I have been aware of this potency hundreds of times. I learned by personal experience. It was forced upon me while learning to read structure-function within the patients who brought their problems to me. I became aware of this area of stillness centering the trauma or disease. Slowly, over a long period of time, knowledge and understanding came as to why it existed and its part in the traumatic or disease picture.

If any change had taken place in the eye of Carla before she hit the Texas coastline, her entire pattern of spirals, the intensity of her winds, and other factors would have modified to meet the change in the potency within the eye. Similarly, I am able to observe that when any change takes place in the area of stillness in a patient, there is manifest a whole new change in the trauma or disease pattern, in other words, in potency. This is not something I have discovered. It exists of itself. It merely asks acceptance of its existence and time to develop a sense of touch and awareness with which to perceive it. The problem remains, as always, how to find words to express that which it is and methods whereby it may become part of one's experience. It is a self-taught process.

Fulcrum

To develop this sense of touch, it is necessary to learn the principle of the fulcrum and then to develop a method of using the fulcrum in the diagnostic approach. The dictionary defines a fulcrum as "the support or point of support on which a lever turns in raising or moving something;" hence, a means of exerting influence, pressure, and so forth. Dr. W. G. Sutherland, in describing the fulcrum in relationship to the two halves of the tentorium cerebelli and the falx cerebri, stated, "The Fulcrum (the junction of the falx cerebri and tentorium cerebelli at the straight sinus) is the still-leverage junction over and through which the three sickles function physiologically in the maintenance of balance in the cranial membranous articular mechanism. Like all fulcrums, it may be shifted from point to point, yet remaining still in its leverage functioning." The key to understanding the principle of a fulcrum is to realize that it is a still-leverage junction, yet it may be shifted from point to point while remaining still in its leverage functioning.

On a gross level of functioning, the scientists in the B-29s were relatively still points, riding in a plane that was responding to the storm into which they were flying. Their whole bodies reflected the movements of the storm and the potency or stillness of the eye of the hurricane. This was something they could feel during the flight with their whole bodies, then report and interpret. The physician must use this same principle to a much finer degree. He must set up a still-leverage mechanism with which he can feel the stress and tension in the tissues under his hands and fingers and find the potency or area of stillness within that area of stress. He does this by placing his hand or hands near the area in which the patient is experiencing difficulties and then establishing a fulcrum with his elbow, his forearm, his crossed fingers, or any other part of him that is convenient to his comfort. From this fulcrum, his fingers become the end of a lever that can note the changes taking place within the body. His fulcrum point can be shifted from time to time to adapt to changes within the body, yet remain still in its leverage functioning.

Touch

In placing the hands and fingers on the tissues under examination, do so with the idea that the fingers can mold themselves to the patient's body. It is a gentle contact yet one with firmness and authority. It is necessary to develop, to borrow a descriptive analysis from Dr. Sutherland: "...fingers with brain cells in their tips. Fingers capable of feeling, thinking, seeing. Therefore, first instruct the fingers how to feel, how to think, how to see, and then let them touch."[2] There must be a "finger-feel," a "finger-thought," a "finger-sight" with which to read the functions and dysfunctions of the body. The mechanisms of the body and their potencies are always in action and can be felt with a thinking, feeling, seeing touch, which in time becomes a knowing touch. It is like getting onto a moving train. The train continues in motion and action as I get on it, as I analyze the roughness of the roadbed, the side sway around the curves, the relative speed, and then I get off the train while it continues in action. So it is with the problems of the patient. I move in on a living mechanism that continues to function; I make my diagnosis, administer my treatment, and leave the mechanisms continuing their ever-changing patterns. My touch is think-deep, see-deep, feel-deep and yet does not limit or lock the structure-function of the tissues I am examining.

I can go another step in developing my touch. Through the still point of the fulcrum and the depths of my finger-touch, I can develop knowledgeable awareness of potency and structure-function in tissues within the patient's body. This awareness goes beyond the physical sensations of the physician's five senses. This is not what I feel with my finger-touch; that would be my opinion. Instead this is what the patient's body is reporting through my fulcrum and finger-touch. This is awareness. This is a listening finger-touch. This is the patient's body's opinion and knowledge, not mere information.

I can control the gentle yet firm contact of my hands and fingers by the manner in which I establish a fulcrum. You establish a fulcrum to provide a working point from which to operate and evaluate the case, and yet you must let it be free enough to allow it to shift, while maintaining still-leverage functioning, to adapt to the changing needs from within the mechanisms under examination. Try examining a hyperactive child, and you will see the need for a shifting fulcrum and hand-finger lever, not only within the child's mechanisms but also for the child itself.

You will also find that increasing the amount of pressure at the fulcrum automatically increases the depth of palpatory touch at the end of the lever—the hand and fingers. The reverse is also true. I can modify my touch to meet the various needs of the kinetic energies expressed by the manifesting anatomical-physiological mechanisms and their potencies. Every patient is different, and each patient is different each time he comes in for attention.

Application

Here are examples of these principles in practice. A patient comes in with a low back problem. With the patient supine on the table, it is possible for the physician to sit beside the patient and place his hand under the sacrum with the fingertips extended upward so their contacts are on the lower back. By leaning comfortably on his elbow, the physician establishes a fulcrum from which to read the changes taking place in the back. The patient may flex her knees with her feet on the table, if it is more comfortable for her to do so. The physician's other hand can be brought from the side and placed under the lower back. The fulcrum for this contact can be the edge of the table against the forearm or the elbow on the physician's knee.

By applying a modest increase of pressure at the fulcrum to cause a slight degree of compression through the sacrum towards the head, the physician will initiate the kinetic energy that will allow the structure-function of the stress area to begin to let its pattern be reflected back to his touch. He learns to read these changes from the fulcrum point or points established. He will feel the pull and tug of the tissues deep within them; he will feel the patterns of mobility and motility, and he will become conscious of the fact that there is a quiet point, a still point within the stress pattern. This is the point of potency for that particular strain. This is the point at which the stress pattern is maintaining its focus to be a stress pattern. I am not talking about the anatomical-physiological units of tissues. I am talking about the kinetics of the energy fields that make up this stress pattern. The anatomical-physiological tissue units are manifesting this kinetic energy and are expressing this dysfunction as tissue changes and symptoms. Any change within the kinetics of the energy field of the potency will change the pattern of functioning within the anatomical-physiological units.

Another example would be the case of a liver in hepatitis. With the patient supine, the physician can sit comfortably beside the patient and place one hand under the lower rib cage beneath the sick organ. Then he can place the elbow or forearm of that hand on his own knee, establishing a fulcrum point. The other hand can be placed on the rib cage above the liver and the elbow or forearm placed on some point that is comfortable to maintain its contact. The sick organ is then between his examining hands. By reading from these double fulcrums, the physician will be able to note structure-function changes taking place within the area of the liver. He will be able to sense whether the liver is moving or functioning upon its falciform ligament as it is supposed to do in health, and he will be able to sense whether it responds to the rhythmic, up-and-down movements of the diaphragm during respiratory inhalation and exhalation as it does in health. He will be able to allow the area of stillness, the potency for this particular problem, to come to a focus, and he will learn a great deal about this sick liver with time and repeated examinations. As the anatomical-physiological unit of the liver regains its capacity to respond to respiratory changes of the diaphragm, its normal movements in relationship to the falciform ligament and its venous and lymphatic drainage begin to open and function. The physician then knows that this is a case of hepatitis that has reversed its pathological state and is returning to normal. All these changes are perceptible to the discerning touch.

The application of the principle of the fulcrum is as varied as the list of complaints that walk into the physician's office. Each case calls for its own application, and each physician must develop his or her own approach. The physician must know as much anatomy, physiology, and the structure-function that accompanies anatomical-physiological units as possible. With the development of this type of touch, feeling through fulcrum points into and through the structure-function patterns manifesting their changes under his hands, the physician gains knowledge that increases understanding. This touch opens the door as to why this patient is experiencing the complaints he expresses. Even when laboratory tests fail to reveal the source of the complaints, the physician's trained touch will bring this understanding.

Why is it necessary to establish these fulcrum points? The physician is attempting to feel function within living tissues and to find the still point from which a pattern of stress is manifesting its symptoms. To do this, the physician must feel from the heart of his stillness into the heart of the stillness within the patient.

There is no limit to the application of this type of trained touch. It is a tool that has some use for practically every type of complaint that comes to our attention. It will distinguish the difference between the congestive headache and the vasospastic type of headache. It will locate the specific sinus that is chronically or acutely filled with material. It will localize the specific lobe of the lung that is sick in lobar pneumonia and locate the strains and stresses of the musculoskeletal system. It has uses from the top of the head to the soles of the feet. It is a diagnostic tool that is added to the rest of the available information and will add insight as to the chronicity, present status, and possible prognosis for the case.

Another analogy might be of interest at this point. The electrical engineer is able to apply his art and science because he accepts the fact that electrical energy is present in his machinery. Electricity, too, is invisible but can be measured and felt, both instrument-wise and sense-wise, and its energy can be used to develop functioning mechanisms. The engineer takes his wires, transistors, printed circuits, and vacuum tubes and strings these things together to produce a vast array of electrical products. He knows that the energy for these is electrical in nature and puts it to use. He may not know what electricity is itself, but he can use it to develop functioning mechanisms.

The physician has available to him a form of energy within the living body, which has been called "the potency" in this paper. It is not electricity but a form of energy in the living body and as such can be used by the understanding physician to determine structure-function within the anatomical-physiological units of the body. What is this potency? No one knows. Nor is it necessary to know, anymore than the engineer has to know what electricity is before he puts it to use. At the very core of total health is a potency within the human body manifesting itself in health. At the very core of every traumatic or disease condition is potency manifesting its interrelationship with the body in trauma and disease. Become aware of and use this potency. Within it is the key to reversing the pathology that is present and to allowing the basic potency that is health to manifest itself again.

The principle of the fulcrum can also be used in thrusting techniques to make those applications much more efficient. After introducing the leverage you will be using in the manipulation, pause a moment, establish a fulcrum, pause again and let the thinking, feeling, seeing fingers interpret the degree of leverage and the amount of force you need to use to complete the procedure. You will find you need less application of force from without, and you will be able to control that leverage with much greater precision.

Using the inherent forces is not a time-consuming process. Because we are using mechanisms already in action, it is only necessary to contact them and let them speak for themselves. The patient comes in with a complaint in a specific area. It is possible to go to that area and make an examination that will give the information you need to explain why he is having his difficulties. Of course, this may be only a small portion of the interrelated total picture of his problem, but it is a beginning from which to go to other areas and finally bring the complete diagnosis into focus. Herein is where the physician's knowledge of anatomy and physiology plays an important role. He is able to correlate his knowledge with his sense of touch and to trace the pattern of the disability and dysfunctioning until the whole diagnosis is clarified in his thinking. Subsequent office calls will add more insight, until the physician is able to use his knowledge to understand the past history of the dysfunction, its present status, and to project a prognosis for its eventual outcome. Remember it is possible to utilize that which is already built into the problems we find in our patients. We merely have to contact it and let it do the work for us.

1. W.G. Sutherland, *The Cranial Bowl,* p.8.
2. W.G. Sutherland, *Contributions of Thought,* p.1.

WHAT IS A DIAGNOSTIC touch? It is a form of palpation designed to fulfill the principles expressed in the statement: In the science of health, disease and trauma, allow biodynamic intrinsic force within to manifest its own unerring potency rather than using extrinsic force from without. The physician places his hand or hands upon the tissues and then establishes a fulcrum through which to read the functioning and dysfunctioning from within the living body of the patient. What I feel is my opinion; what the body itself manifests through the fulcrum point to my touch is the body's opinion. It is the latter we are seeking in developing a diagnostic touch.

What are some of the sensations that can be felt from the functioning and dysfunctioning within the body? It is possible to use terminology from all of the natural and physical sciences. A partial list of terms would include compression, decompression, tensity, flaccidity, stress, drag, sag, strain, sprain, shock, contraction, expansion, torque, rotation, twitching, vibration, pulsation, mobility, motility, immobility, agitation, disturbance, oscillation, wobble, restriction, fullness, flatness, swelling, atrophy, dystrophy, irritability, strength, weakness, vigor, force, vitality, tone, power, potency, stillness, balance, fatigue, fluctuation, and many others.

Here are a few questions a physician can ask himself utilizing a diagnostic touch: In a sprained ankle case, can you feel the shock in the tissues in addition to the malposition of the ligaments and articular mechanism? If you have two low back cases come into your office, one with a rotation strain and the other with a hard fall on the buttocks resulting in a compression strain, can you determine this with a diagnostic touch? In a serious psoas muscle problem, can you determine when that muscle is manifesting a better drainage mechanism during the treatment program?

Can you feel the total shock in the thorax that accompanies every moderate to severe postcoronary syndrome? In a case of lobar pneumonia, do you know that there is a relative restriction of temporal bone mobility on the side of the consolidated lobe of the lung? Do you understand the anatomical-physiological connection of the tissues as to why this situation is true? In a case of sinusitis, can you locate the sinus involved and degree of involvement by the use of a diagnostic touch?

In treating a bursitis of the shoulder or a brachial neuritis, can you feel the onset of a better drainage mechanism from these congested areas during a treatment? With severe cases, this is the time to stop treatment for the day in order to avoid fatigue within the sick tissues. Remember, most of the strains of the body make changes at micrometric levels of measurement in structure and function at the core or center of the disturbed area. Can you feel the forces melting out of the strain pattern under examination?

Can you feel the flatness and loss of vitality that accompanies every case of so-called "nervous breakdown" or in all postencephalitic syndromes? Can you feel the upsurge towards the normal vitality during your treatment of that case?

In a recent whiplash injury, can you determine the direction of force in the accident by laying your diagnostic hands on the tissues involved? Can you feel fatigue in tissues, either in the patient as a whole or in specific areas of trauma or disease? This is a most important factor in diagnostic and therapeutic considerations. Can you understand what you are feeling?

These are a few among hundreds of items available to a diagnostic touch. There are qualitative, quantitative, prognostic, diagnostic, and therapeutic considerations for each item listed. In this field of endeavor, diagnostic touch, no one is an expert. That living body lying before you on the examination table is the taskmaster. It is challenging you to find its problem.

There are several steps involved in developing a diagnostic touch.

167

These may be summarized as follows:Position your hand or hands upon or under the tissues you plan to examine. Establish a fulcrum point for each hand contact from which to operate. Let your palpating hand(s) and fulcrum point(s) become one with the tissues involved. Allow tissue functioning and dysfunctioning to come through to your hands and fulcrum points rather than trying to feel something in the tissues; allow biodynamic intrinsic force within to manifest its own unerring potency rather than using extrinsic force from without.

A simple illustration will demonstrate this principle. Take a pail of water, stir it into violent action, and place your hand upon the side of the pail. You will feel the agitation within the pail of water. Next, drop your elbow upon the table, thus establishing a fulcrum point for your hand contact. Now, reading through the fulcrum point, note how much more you are able to feel the agitation of the water within the pail with your diagnostic touch. Note that if you lean with more compression on your fulcrum point, you read deeper into the agitating water, and if you lean with less compression at your fulcrum point, you get a more superficial reading from the agitating water. Within human physiology, the biodynamic intrinsic forces and the biokinetic intrinsic forces and their potencies are already working. It is not necessary to stir them into action, as you did the pail of water.

To see the effect of the fulcrum in the body, try examining a knee and extending the sense of a diagnostic touch through to the thigh and acetabular region. First, sit in front of a patient who is seated on the examination table, and place your hands around one knee with your fingers interlaced in the popliteal fossa. Try to feel what you can, with as much understanding as you can, without having your elbows supported. Then apply a slight degree of compression through the knee towards the acetabulum, and see what you can feel in that area.

Now try this exam using a fulcrum. Let your elbows drop onto your own knees, and read the story the knee is telling you through the fulcrum points you have established. Apply a slight compression through the thigh towards the acetabular region, and again read through the fulcrum points. Feel how the innate natural forces within the thigh and pelvis want to turn the acetabulum either into internal rotation or external rotation. Also, note the quality and quantity of that turning. If you lean lightly on your elbow fulcrum points, you will get a more superficial reading from the tissues, and if you lean more firmly, you will get a deeper and deeper impression. The depth is dependent upon the firmness at the fulcrum contacts, not on the firmness of the examining finger contacts. If there is a problem of stress or strain deep within this area, experience will teach you that it is necessary to make a more firm contact at the fulcrum points in order to read the dysfunctioning manifesting itself within that area. Experience and the nature of the problem you are examining will perfect your understanding.

Let me clarify this point of compression at the fulcrum point and not at the hand contact. In the case of a lever operating across a fulcrum, applying power downward at one end of the lever automatically lifts the other end upwards. This is not the lever mechanism I am describing in applying power or compression at my fulcrum point. My hand contact is not lifted upward into the patient's body. My hand contact is gently but firmly in contact with the patient's body, and I apply compression or power directly downward at my fulcrum point in proportion to the degree of strain or stress I feel in the tissues. The hand contact continues to be firmly but gently in contact with the body physiology of the patient. If a man were to have picked up a 100-pound sack incorrectly, I might be applying considerable pressure downward at my fulcrum point to counterbalance this 100-pound lifting strain, but I would not be pushing my hand contact with the same degree of intensity. To do so would destroy the sense impressions being received from the bioenergy fields within the patient. Try it both ways and learn for yourselves.

This process may require a lot of compression at the fulcrum point of the physician, or it may require very little compression. In the case of the 100-pound lifting strain, the physician will find himself applying considerable compression at his fulcrum point in order to counterbalance the amount of force within the strain pattern. The hand contacts may become more firm, but they will be gentle enough to allow the problem within the patient to go to work. When the physician has approximated the forces within the patient, through his fulcrum points, he will get the maximum response from the tissues under strain in their efforts to position, diagnose, and treat themselves. Interestingly enough, as the physician does approximate the forces within the patient's physiological mechanism, a degree of comfort is manifested for the patient. The patient will frequently remark that the physician is putting little or no pressure on him when in fact, I may have been leaning on my fulcrum point or points with all the weight I could muster.

The physician has to know his anatomy and physiology in order to interpret that which the body is telling him through his fulcrum contacts, and at the same time, he has to divorce himself from doing something to the area under examination, thus letting the story come through to him. This is difficult. As physicians, we are trained to *do*, and here we are told to let something else do the job of *doing*. We have learned to listen to the verbal account of our patient's problem and then *do* something based on that. Now we must learn to listen to a tactile account through our developing sense of a diagnostic touch.

In developing a diagnostic touch, there are no "techniques" involved, in the ordinary use of the word. The physician lets the innate energies within the health, disease, or traumatic condition of the patient tell the story of the problem involved. Thus, the physician has no techniques and is in fact told to get out of the way. How can the body report to you if you keep doing something to it during your examination? Your fulcrum points are your listening posts. Let the tissues tell you their story. Be quiet and listen.

I have said there are no techniques, and yet I have given some instruction. In examining any area of the body, one does position the examining hand(s) upon the body; one does establish a fulcrum(s) through and from which to read the responses from within the body; one does modify the amount of pressure on the fulcrum points to gather various depths of tissue activity and function; and finally, one can add a slight degree of compression or traction through the examining hand(s) to initiate the motive forces from within the tissue under examination. However, this is not actively testing the tissue yourself, such as manually turning the hip into internal or external rotation. Rather, this is activating already existing forces within the patient's body so that they will turn the hip into internal or external rotation with their own built-in power.

Thus, the use of diagnostic touch is more than a passive laying on of hands. It is a form of palpation one might call an alert, observational type of awareness for the functions and dysfunctions from within the patient, utilizing the motive energy deep within the tissues themselves. The patient's tissues within that acetabulum are turning it for you to observe. That acetabular area has a natural tendency to want to go into either internal or external rotation when the forces within it have an opportunity to express themselves. You can feel it happen and are able with your anatomical-physiological knowledge to know whether it is a normal physiological mechanism at work or one that is in a state of dysfunction. If you are not sure, go to the other knee and thigh and test them. They both may be normal, or one will be normal and the other not. That is up to you to determine.

A diagnostic touch is essential because there are subtleties of tissue functioning and dysfunctioning that cannot be explored by any other means than that of a skilled, sensitive, knowing sense of awareness through the use of this type of touch. A case history will serve as an example. A woman comes in with a complaint of violent headaches for the past two years. Her history is taken and various tests are run, and you are able to tell her the type of headache she is experiencing. This is fine as far as it goes. Adding the use of a diagnostic touch, you find the effects of an old concussion in the base of the skull that has limited the mobility there, which interferes with venous drainage from her head and induces an irritability of the intracranial and extracranial tissues through which the nerves pass in connection with her headaches. You ask her, When did she have an accident that produced a concussion or one in which she "saw stars." She then tells you of an accident as a child in which she sat down so hard that she was unconscious for a short time and "saw stars." Now, you not only have located the area of her headaches and determined their type, but you also have found their etiology, both in their early beginning as well as in their present state and disability. This information could not have been gained by any other means than by use of a diagnostic touch, one that told you this was an old injury occurring 40 years ago and manifesting now as headaches, a touch that could literally feel the dysfunctioning within those tissues and tell you specifically which tissues were doing what in their functioning and dysfunctioning. This same touch also gave you prognostic information as to the potential help for this case.

Furthermore, a diagnostic touch is essential because it is a partner with what one might call a therapeutic touch. Taking the case just described, one can give her some symptomatic relief with medication and physiotherapy, but if you were to try to secure a correction for the problem, you would have to do something about removing the etiology, the old concussion that had affected the base of the skull. This calls for the use of a therapeutic touch. A therapeutic touch utilizes the same biodynamic principles and energies from within the tissue as does the diagnostic touch. One of the most important factors in the use of a therapeutic touch is a diagnostic touch to guide and direct you through all the living, corrective processes that take place within that concussion mechanism during its resolution. Therapeutic touch will be discussed later.

Clinical results substantiated the diagnosis made in the woman with the concussion. Within a month after starting a treatment program, she was symptom free and has remained so for the past year. There is still evidence to the diagnostic touch that the concussion mechanism is present, but it has been restored to its compensatory capacity to reciprocate with the physiological balance of the rest of the body. This is another factor in developing a diagnostic touch. In addition to finding the problem area within the patient, one should learn to determine what is happening in its relationship with the total physiology of the patient. Where is the potency or still point or balance point that is maintaining this problem area? What is its potential for restoration to total normalcy or to a compensatory balance in its relationship to the physiological needs of body functioning? In this particular case, a compensatory balance was restored; her symptoms have disappeared for now, but they will recur if and when there is a regression in her body's capacity to maintain physiological functioning within the problem area. Subtleties within subtleties are thus available to the trained diagnostic touch.

There is a particular group of patients diagnostic touch serves well. This is the group who have been told, "I cannot find any reason for your complaints. Your physical examination and tests are all negative. It's all in your mind." These people are frequently called neurotics, psychosomatics, and "crocks." A diagnostic touch defines and confirms the physical evidence to explain the aches and pains these people have. There has to be a somatic component in these psychosomatic problems, and the routine tests are on too gross a level to pick up the dysfunction expressing itself as symptoms. The findings using a diagnostic touch are at a subtler, subclinical level.

This introduces an interesting point. If one's examinations reveal a true physical picture to explain the disabilities that have caused these people to suffer for months or years, can these problems truly be called neurotic or psychosomatic? I don't believe so. The hypochondriac turns out not to be a hypochondriac after all. My reasons for this feeling are based on the fact that if one is able to diagnose the subclinical strains and stresses responsible for the complaints, then one has found the avenue through which these stresses and strains can be corrected, thus bringing back a state of normalcy or recompensation within that individual. A sensitive, highly trained, diagnostic touch can provide the necessary tool to unlock the understanding required in these cases. It is a great help to these people to find a physical basis for their problems.

The body may be considered as basically composed of solids (bones), semisolids (soft tissues), and fluids (body fluids). This solid-semisolid-fluid structure is endowed with the biodynamic living principles of life. It is highly organized and capable of expressing living changes taking place within its own environment. An area that is in strain within this living body can be found because that area of the body is expressing itself as being in strain. What one feels with his diagnostic touch is kinetic energies within that strained area operating as a pattern of dysfunction within a solid-semisolid-fluid mechanism. The physician interprets this kinetic energy manifestation in physiological and clinical language based on anatomical-physiological knowledge of body functioning.

All anatomical-physiological units express and utilize kinetic energy in manifesting their functioning in health, disease, and trauma. The art of learning to use these kinetic energies, with their centering potencies, is diagnostic touch. These energies vary in intensity, quantity, and quality for every situation within patients. In discussing this with an electrical engineer, he made the statement, "It takes a lot of energy to make a transistor or vacuum tube work, but it takes only a small amount of energy to direct that work." Similarly, in human physiology, there is already present a great deal of biodynamic energy at work, but it takes only a minimal amount of energy on the operator's part to learn to read and use that kinetic energy for diagnostic and therapeutic purposes. The physician's minimal energy requirement is applied through the fulcrum point(s) from which he learns to use the biodynamic, intrinsic, kinetic energy already in action within the patient.

The amount of information one can gain as the tissues respond to the use of a diagnostic touch is truly remarkable. The cases that are capable of a good recovery indicate this to a diagnostic touch. The cases that may be slow to respond, or that are making an inadequate response, demonstrate this and give insight as to why they are not responding. This is a big help to the physician, who needs to know how to plan further care for the cases that are giving him difficulty. There is need for a diagnostic test that can give accurate guidance in the care of any case. A diagnostic touch provides this type of guidance.

There is a corollary to the statement: Allow biodynamic intrinsic force within to manifest its own unerring potency rather than using extrinsic force from without. It is: Allow the mind to explore and interpret the biodynamic intrinsic force within as it manifests its own unerring potency rather than using extrinsic force from without. It is necessary to develop a sensitive diagnostic touch capable of palpating this biodynamic force and its unerring potency, and in addition, it is necessary to develop one's mind so as to be able to explore this functioning and to interpret intelligently the changes taking place. Let us set up an example to clarify this thought.

Biokinetic energies or forces are always at work in all physiological and pathological processes. If we were to add an environmental force or kinetic energy to body physiology to produce a strain—such as a blow, a fall, or a twist—we would now have a specific pattern of disability manifest within the body mechanism. It is now a biodynamic energy field plus an environmental energy field—the force it took to produce the strain. We place our hand(s) in this area for examination and establish a fulcrum point for each hand contact through which to initiate and sense the changes taking place within the strained area. Within a few seconds, we will find a change taking place within the tissues as they start manifesting the pattern of disability present within them. It is the biodynamic intrinsic energy within that pattern going to work. To the outside observer watching our work, our hands are apparently lying quietly on the patient, but the motion, mobility, and motility we sense from within the patient is considerable, depending upon the problem. There is a deliberate pattern the tissues go through in demonstrating the strain within them. They work their way through to a point at which all sense of motion or mobility seems to cease. This is the point of stillness. Even though it is still, it is endowed with biodynamic power. This is the area of the potency for this strain pattern. This is a stillpoint within this functioning unit. A change takes place at this time, which the physician records more with a sense of awareness that a change took place rather than actually being able to feel it. Following this point, a new pattern manifests itself as the tissues create a new state of functioning. It is a more normal pattern of functioning as compared to the disability that was present at the beginning of the examination. The amount of correction that takes place may not seem great, but it is a physiological correction commensurate with the tissue pathology that is present and will be all the correction that the tissues are physiologically capable of making for this given treatment.

By following the biodynamic intrinsic forces and their potency and the biokinetic intrinsic forces and their potencies through the potency or stillpoint within the tissue pattern within the patient, I have been able to secure therapeutic benefit for the majority of the pathological conditions encountered within the patient. Needless to say, the irreversible cases, such as those with cancer, eventually expired, but the results of this type of treatment program gave them symptomatic relief during the interim period, more relief than could be obtained by any other therapeutic means.

Other cases wherein there was a potential for reversibility of pathology towards normal health or recompensation responded with maximum capacity on the part of the patient's physiology to return to normal or to recompensation. A physician friend of mine said to me, "Using a diagnostic and therapeutic touch as you are doing, disease states will run through their tidal cycle, but they will do so within the minimum of time for each disease state, and they will do so with the minimum of complications and sequelae. Traumatic cases will have the stress factor that aided in their production washed out of them, and they, too, will permit normal body physiology to reassert itself, or to recompensate itself, with the minimum of complications or sequelae." This has proven itself to be clinically true.

The physician's mind becomes an observing tool, an analytical tool, an exploring tool, and an interpretive tool that accompanies the sense of touch as it follows the changes taking place. One might say that the physician's mind alertly parallels the sense of touch throughout the diagnostic process, just as a trained observer might sit at the sidelines of a visual contest and study the participants of that contest. However, here within this tissue-functioning pattern, the physician's mind must follow deep within the patient's body and go with the sense of touch, as the biodynamic intrinsic energies manifest their own unerring potency in the pattern under examination. The biokinetic and environmental energies within the pattern provide the motive power; the sense of diagnostic touch follows the whole sequence of events from initiation through to what fulfillment is available for this one examination, and the mind observes, evaluates, and interprets the changes taking place. Because the physician has anatomical and physiological knowledge, he is able to interpret his findings in bio-logical, pathological, clinical, anatomical-physiological language. He knows, for example, that it is a psoas muscle strain pattern or a con-solidated lung he has been examining. By his sense of diagnostic touch, he is able to feel this dysfunctioning process as the body manifests it. With time and experience, the physician is able to read some of the past history of that disability, its present status, and prognostic evalu-ations for the future. This is interpretive mental skill. It is highly im-portant to keep the mind alert and, at the same time, wide open to accept that which the tissues have to report rather than that which the physician hopes to find. Here again, let the tissues tell their story. You listen. With experience, an amazing amount of information comes through for interpretation. It is not time-consuming when one has learned the skill of securing the body's cooperation. A lot can be learned within a five- to ten-minute period.

Any fulcrum is the site of the potency—a still-leverage junction over and through which action and reaction takes place. A fulcrum can and does shift from point to point yet remains still in its leverage functioning. You can take a glass of water and by transmitting a fine vibration to it see the water form a pattern centering itself in the middle of the glass. This is a still point around which the pattern of water forms in response to the vibration transmitted to it. It is important to realize that tremendous action takes place in the periphery around a fulcrum center and also that the potency in the fulcrum area is part of this total kinetic energy pattern. Fulcrum points exist in all mediums, in masses of air and liquids as well as in solids.

There is a potency in all the fulcrums of activity within the body's functioning, and like the world of nature in which this body is operating, this functioning provides its own motive power biodynamically. It takes skill, time, and patience to learn to feel this functioning, to learn to sense the motion within tissues as initiated by these living structures, not the voluntary motion of the operator or the patient but that motion which is already present as that patient lies quietly on the table; to learn to follow the patterns being expressed within those patterns; to learn to be aware of the potency within the fulcrum points; to be aware of the moment that a change took place within the potency during the diagnostic or therapeutic examination; to learn to feel the unfolding of the pattern after going through the stillpoint; and to learn to analyze and interpret this material into sound physiological reasoning. Despite the complexity in portraying the development of a diagnostic touch in words, it is a relatively simple procedure in actual practice.

For those without any experience in this field, it is common to have a great deal of skepticism—to believe that a diagnostic touch cannot fulfill all that has been ascribed to its use. A sense of skepticism is a most valuable asset in this work. It serves to keep one's feet on the ground. The physician is seeking information from the living body. If he is totally skeptical about the fact that this information is available to him with the use of a diagnostic touch, he will receive very little information. If he allows his mind to be open to the idea that such information is available, with just enough skepticism to make the body prove that it is providing this information, then he will be in a position to evaluate more accurately that information. Let the body prove itself in demonstrating this functioning and dysfunctioning. It serves a useful purpose to be slightly skeptical.

Diagnostic touch is scientific. A group of physicians who have trained themselves to utilize this form of examination adequately will each come to the same approximate conclusion, upon examining a given patient, concerning that patient's problem. I use the word, "approximate," because successive examinations, one after the other the same day, modify the pattern of disability enough for each physician to get a slightly different picture. However, if the patient has a relatively chronic problem and the examinations are made over a period of time that allows the problem to remanifest itself, each physician's findings will correlate with his colleagues'. A diagnostic touch is scientific because the problem is in the patient, not in the physician's ability or inability to find it.

The development of a diagnostic touch is an added tool for use in understanding a patient's problem. A few minutes additional examination time in every case, learning to use a diagnostic touch, will perfect this form of examination for the physician. In each patient, it will give a depth of anatomical-physiological insight the physician has never experienced before. It will give patients the sense of knowing that the physician is truly seeking the etiology for their particular case and that he understands their problem. The time and effort it takes to perfect the art and science of a diagnostic touch is in keeping with the physician's goal in life—that of serving mankind.

Is it wrong to think of DIAGNOSTIC Touch as providing a fulcrum to a (still point (itself a fulcrum) allowing it to move past its dysfunction?

Part III of "Diagnostic Touch," as originally published by the Academy of Applied Osteopathy, has been largely replaced by material prepared for a presentation at an Academy meeting. All 26 charts Dr. Becker made for that presentation are included here, while only ten photographs appeared in the original article.

A PHYSICIAN HAS TWO jobs to do when a patient comes to him: first, to make a diagnosis of the patient's problems, and second, to administer therapeutic aid for the problems. A diagnostic touch contributes to both of these procedures. The patient and his problem present a challenge to the physician. In this work of using a diagnostic touch, the patient is the taskmaster. His problem is the schoolroom. His biodynamic intrinsic forces and their unerring potency are the teachers. The diagnostic touch of the physician is the pupil. Diagnostic touch involves learning to feel and understand the biodynamic intrinsic forces and learning to be aware of the unerring potency within them. I am asking the biodynamic and biokinetic forces and their potencies within the patient to report their findings to me through my fulcrum points. They do so without failure on their part. When there is a mistake made, it is because of my inability to read and interpret these forces and potencies correctly.

I have learned that these fields of force within the patient are always in action. The tissue elements within their connective tissue envelopes, and the fluid contents, automatically go along for the ride as the bioenergy patterns unfold in their functioning. I have to get out of the way, so to speak, and follow the bioenergy patterns. It is similar to an accompanist in a concert. A good accompanist follows the singer he is playing for and lets the singer take the lead. In using the fulcrum-compression approach, the physician initiates the bioenergy factors within the patient through his fulcrum-compression points and lets the pattern within the patient take him through its cycle of activity.

Diagnostic touch may be defined as a form of palpatory skill wherein the physician invokes the physiological energies and their potencies in the disease, trauma, and health states within the patient for the physician's use in diagnosis and treatment. The physician can learn to feel these physiological energies and their potencies and the associated tissue elements working within the patient's body. It is a self-taught skill. The essence of diagnostic touch is to know, understand, and use the potency in the pause-rest moment of stillness within any given pattern of disease, trauma, or health state.

Clinical application of how to use diagnostic touch in various areas of the body is shown in the pictures which follow this discussion. Briefly, the physician positions his hand upon or under the part of the body he chooses to examine, usually in the area of the patient's complaint. Then he establishes an automatic-shifting-suspension-fulcrum point for each hand contact by dropping his arm or elbow upon the examination table, upon his own person, or upon the patient. His hand contact is gentle, and he is going to control it by the amount of compression he uses at his fulcrum point. When he applies compression or power downward at his fulcrum point (not upward at his hand contacts), biodynamic intrinsic forces and biokinetic intrinsic forces and their potencies within the patient immediately go into action to manifest the degree, intensity, and patterns of the tissue elements in health or disability states.

Biodynamic intrinsic force and its potency may be defined as the physiological energy found in health within the patient. Biokinetic intrinsic forces and their potencies may be defined as the pathological-physiological energies and their potencies found in disease and traumatic states within the patient. It takes added energy from the environment of the patient, in combination with the biodynamic intrinsic force, to produce the condition manifested as a disease or traumatic problem. When a diagnostic touch allows biodynamic and biokinetic forces within to pass *through* their own unerring potencies rather than the use of blind force from without, the physician is securing a corrective process, within the tissue elements of the problem, that leads towards health for that patient.

Potency may be defined as a functioning pause-rest moment of stillness, a fulcrum or fulcrums within biodynamic intrinsic forces and biokinetic intrinsic forces in body physiology over, around, and through which these patterns of activity are manifesting themselves. It can be compared to the power present in the functioning fulcrum point of a teeter-totter board or the eye of a hurricane. A fulcrum has energy and power within it. The physician is aware of this pause-rest period and its potency as he studies these patterns with his diagnostic touch.

After the physician has positioned his hand contacts and established a fulcrum point for each hand contact, the application of compression or power at his fulcrum point initiates activity into the biodynamic intrinsic force and biokinetic intrinsic forces within the patient. The tissue elements and these energies go through three distinct phases of activity at micrometric levels of measurement, and they are read by the physician through his fulcrum points:

(i) It feels as if these energy fields and tissue elements are working their way, within their pattern, towards the point of balance for that pattern.

(ii) A still, pause-rest period, the potency, is reached, at which time all motion apparently ceases. Up to this point, the physician is able to follow these changes through his hand contacts and fulcrum points and thus gain diagnostic insight concerning the patient's problem. When the pattern goes *through* the stillness, a change takes place within the potency. "Something happens" as a result of this change in the potency. This is the corrective phase of the treatment program.

(iii) Motion is again felt within the energy fields and tissue elements. The pattern which unfolds is one that indicates it is a more normal pattern of functioning for the disabled area.

These three phases can take as short a time as one minute to complete their cycle, or they may take several minutes, depending upon the degree and intensity of the pathological physiology involved.

Phase (ii), the physiological pause-rest moment, is the goal the physician is seeking when he uses diagnostic touch. Compression at the physician's fulcrum utilizes the power within the potency in the pause-rest period in body physiology. The physiological energy fields provide the motive power for both diagnostic information for the physician's insight and therapeutic benefit for the patient.

My attention, as a physician using diagnostic touch, is on the potency within this patient because I know if a change takes place within this potency, a whole new pattern will manifest itself towards health for the patient. I know that there is a basic potency that can be found in the patient when he is in a state of health, and I know that when the various energies that are present in traumatic or disease conditions have dissipated, there is a potency and a general feeling of biodynamic intrinsic forces manifesting themselves that tell me this patient is well again.

There seems to be only one way for the physician to learn to use diagnostic touch and that is to go to the problems within the patient and be taught by the problems. In the pictures which follow, the hand contacts and fulcrum points described are merely suggestions. Each physician has to work out his own, for every physician and every patient is different. If you were to watch me doing this work, you would see about as much motion on my part as you observe in the pictures. There is little obvious motion; however, I am in cooperative motion. I am actively following the micrometric levels of motion which are within the patterns I am observing. To my diagnostic touch, there is a considerable amount of movement, mobility, and motility manifesting itself through my fulcrum points. I use a firm but gentle hand contact, which allows the forces within the patient to express their full potential of activity. I vary the amount of compression and power at my fulcrum points to match the forces I am working with in the patient's body during the three-phase cycle of operation. The biodynamic and biokinetic intrinsic forces and their potencies will dictate to my diagnostic touch and interpreting mind the work I am to do for each patient visit.

In summary, biodynamic and biokinetic intrinsic forces are available for use; the potencies which are within these physiological energies are available for use. Diagnostic touch and its partner, therapeutic touch, are available for every physician's use.

In the following pictures, fulcrum points are marked with an arrow. This series was photographed by Dr. Melvin G. Hennigsen, a dental friend of mine from Hayward, California. I have no words to express the depth of my appreciation for the magnificent job he has done in the preparation of these charts.

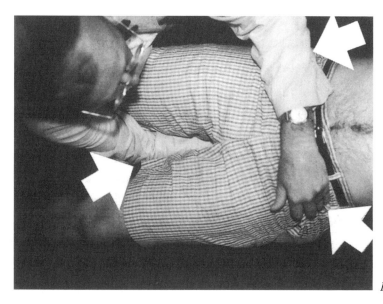

Fig.1

Figure No. 1: Sacrum and Pelvis

The patient is supine and his sacrum is in the palm of the physician's right hand with the fingertips on the spinous process of the fifth lumbar vertebra. The fulcrum point is at the right elbow leaning on the table. The knees of the patient are up, although the legs may be outstretched or one knee up and the other one down. The left arm and hand of the physician are bridging the anterior superior spines of the ilia. Fulcrum points are shown at both ilia because the physician may alternate his use of one or the other anterior superior spine as a fulcrum point in examining the opposite ilium in its functioning relationship with the sacrum.

This position gains understanding from the pelvis as a whole, the sacrum, the ilia, and the interrelationship of the pelvis with the lumbar area above and the acetabular regions below. This is an excellent position to evaluate the functioning of the sacrum in whiplash cases.

Figure No. 2: Sacrum

The sacrum of the patient is lying in the hand of the physician. The fulcrum point is at the elbow leaning on the table.

The sacrum should be considered as functioning as five bones instead of one. There are five segments which make up the sacrum, and all have a degree of flexibility throughout life. At the lower end of the sacrum is the coccyx, which can be sensed with the heel of the hand, and the lower lumbar vertebra can be sensed with the fingertips. Continuity of midline functioning from the sacrum towards the base of the skull can be determined.

The sense of functioning of the five segments of the sacrum can be

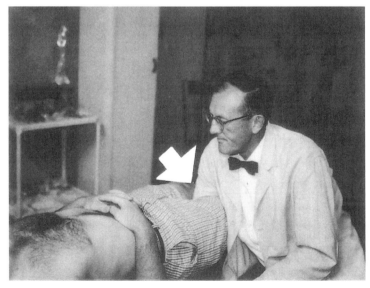

Fig.2

further accentuated by sliding the other hand under the buttock on the same side and placing the fingertips on the five segments so that the fingertips of the one hand are lying between the sacrum and the palm of the other hand that is cupping the sacrum. The fulcrum point for this second hand is at the forearm leaning on the crossed knees of the physician. Through the fulcrum point, this double-hand contact on the sacrum brings a great deal of information to the physician concerning sacral functioning.

Working through the second hand contact and fulcrum to restore the normal flexibility of the sacral segments is good therapy in sciatic nerve irritations.

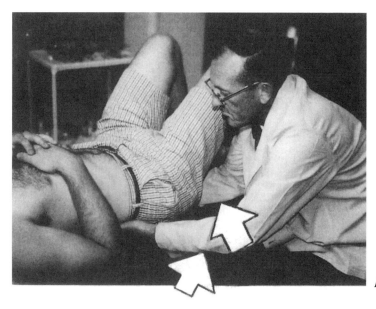

Fig.3

Figure No. 3: Sacrum, Ilio-sacrum, Lower Lumbar

The right hand is under the sacrum, and the fulcrum point is at the elbow on the table. The left hand is under the ilio-sacral articulation, with the fingertips on the lower lumbar spinous processes. The left fulcrum point is on the crossed knee of the physician.

The term "ilio-sacrum" is used rather than sacroiliac because it seems more physiological to me to realize that the direction of lesion production is that of the ilia upon the sacrum rather than that of the sacrum upon the ilium.

Good control for the diagnosis and treatment of the ilio-sacral and lower lumbar strains is afforded by this position.

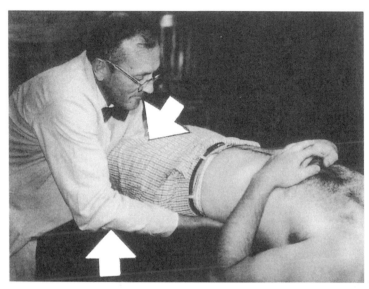

Fig.4

Figure No. 4: Sacrum and Upper Lumbar

The left hand is under the sacrum, and the fulcrum point is at the left elbow leaning on the table. The right fulcrum point is at the forearm on the crossed knees of the physician. The right hand contact is under the upper lumbar area, with the fingertips on the spinous processes of the lumbar vertebra. Various patterns of functioning and dysfunctioning can be analyzed.

Figure No. 5: Upper Lumbar and Psoas Muscle

The examining hand is under the upper lumbar area, and the fulcrum point is on the physician's crossed knees. The other hand and arm are bridging the drawn-up knees.

A lighter compression at the fulcrum point will give an evaluation for lumbar strains because the sacrospinalis group of muscles is more superficial than the deeper-lying psoas muscle. An increase of

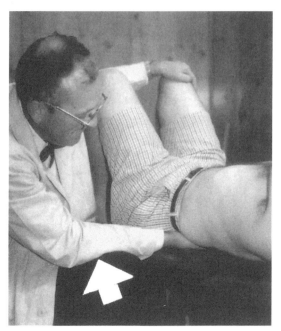

Fig.5

compression at the fulcrum point will reach into the psoas muscle area. The bridged knee contact is meant to compress the acetabular areas with the weight of the arm and hand so as to further activate any psoas muscle disturbance under examination. The sense of diagnostic touch is projected into the lower thoracic area.

Figure No. 6: Lower Thorax

The physician is seated at the head of the table. His hands are placed under the patient at the level of the insertion of the trapezius muscles bilaterally. His fulcrum points are at his elbows on the table.

This position coordinates the impressions received from the lumbar area with those which can be gained from the lower thoracics, lower rib cage, and upwards into the shoulder girdles by way of the diverging trapezius muscles.

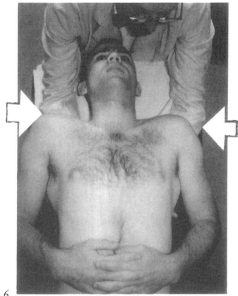

Fig.6

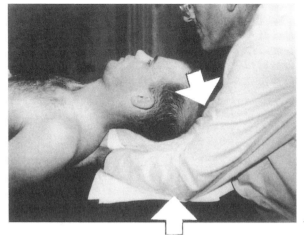

Fig.7

Figure No. 7: Upper Thorax
The fulcrum points are at the forearms, which are resting on the table bilaterally. One hand contact is under the upper thoracic area, and the other hand contact is underneath the first hand. This serves to reinforce the perceptive reading of the biodynamic and biokinetic intrinsic forces and their potencies from within the upper thoracic area. Correlation with the cervical area and lower thoracic area can be analyzed.

Figure No. 8: Upper Thorax
The patient's head is usually on a pillow. The right hand and arm slide under the pillow and contact the upper thoracic spinous

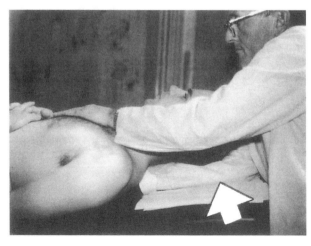

Fig.8

189

processes, with the fingers slightly spread to contact the ribs on each side. The fulcrum point is at the elbow on the table under the head of the patient. The left hand is on the sternum of the patient, and with a pillow under the head of the patient, a fulcrum point at the left elbow can be made by resting on the pillow.

A great deal of valuable information can be gained from this position. Impressions gathered from the lower thorax are correlated here as well as interrelationships between the upper thorax and the cervical area.

Normally, the sternum moves dorsally during inhalation and ventrally during exhalation. It frequently is doing just the opposite when this position for examination is started. By the time the examination is completed, it can be observed that the normal excursion of the sternum during inhalation and exhalation has reasserted itself.

Upper thoracic strains are readily found and easily corrected in this position, using the biodynamic and biokinetic forces and potencies within the patient.

Figure No. 9: Rib Cage

The right hand is under the rib cage, with the fingertips just beyond the spinous processes of the thoracic vertebra for the ribs under examination. The rest of the hand is following the course of the rib or ribs. The fulcrum point is on the physician's crossed knees. The left hand is on the anterior ends of the ribs being examined, and the fulcrum point is at the forearm or elbow that is resting on the anterior superior spine of the ilium on the same side.

The patient's arm on the side of the examination is shown extended over the patient's head. This was done to make the physician's hand contacts and fulcrum points easier to see. I usually have the patient place his arm comfortably on top of my own during this phase of the examination.

Slight compression at the fulcrum point on the crossed knees initiates motion into the heads of the ribs being examined. Rib strains are easily diagnosed and as easily treated, comfortably for the patient

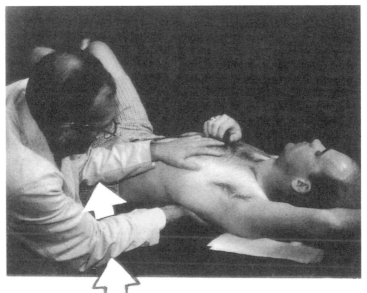

Fig.9

and physician, using intrinsic forces and their potencies within the strain patterns. These hand and fulcrum contacts can be moved up or down the rib cage to find the area of strain and to do the work of diagnosing and treating them.

Figure No. 10: Upper Rib Cage and Shoulders

Fulcrum points are at the thumb contacting the lateral aspect of each scapula. The patient's arms are on the physician's shoulders with

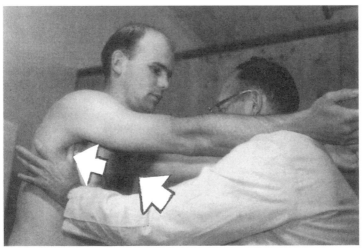

Fig.10

191

the arms externally rotated. When the patient leans forward, the thumb fulcrum points serve to activate each serratus anterior muscle and its origin from the 8 or 9 upper ribs to its insertion into the vertebral border of the scapula. Group strains of the upper rib cage can be analyzed and treated.

I have learned that this procedure is an excellent follow-up after securing correction of any specific rib lesions of the upper thorax. It serves to restore reciprocal tension balance for both sides of the thoracic cage. It is also useful following correction of cervical strains because so many of the cervical muscles find their insertion into the upper ribs.

Figure No. 11: Liver

The left hand is under the lower ribs beneath the liver. The fulcrum point is on the crossed knees of the physician. The upper hand is over the anterior surface of the liver.

This position can be used to examine a sick liver, such as one with hepatitis. The biodynamic and biokinetic disturbed forces and their potencies are readily transmitted through the fulcrum point on the crossed knees to the physician.

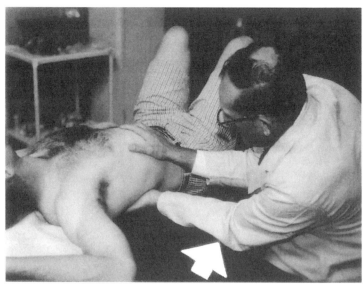

Fig.11

This same type of contact can be used for localizing a consolidated lung in lobar pneumonia by moving the hand contacts, one posterior and one anterior, over the suspected lobe of the lung and setting up a fulcrum point through which to sense the degree of health or pathology that might be present in the lung. A fulcrum point for the right hand can be established on the anterior superior spine of the patient for the examination of the lobes of the lung. This provides two fulcrum points for better evaluation.

Figure No. 12: Cervical Area

The physician's hands are bilaterally bridging the entire cervical area from the base of the skull to the upper thorax. The fulcrum points are at the forearms resting on the table. The arrow points to the one not seen.

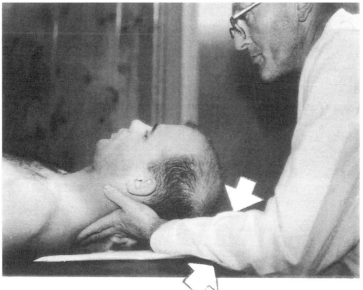

Fig.12

The cervical area as a whole can be quickly evaluated, and then more local finger contacts can be made for the specific cervical vertebra desired, always keeping the forearm fulcrum points on the table. The reason for keeping the forearm fulcrum points on the table is to follow the biodynamic and biokinetic intrinsic forces and their potencies within the area under examination through the fulcrum points of the physicians. The hand and finger contacts can be shifted easily without moving the fulcrum points.

Figure No. 13: Occipitoatlantal Articulation

A finger contact is made against the posterior tubercle of the atlas. The fulcrum is at the forearm on the table. The other hand is on the vertex of the patient's head, maintaining a slight flexion of the head.

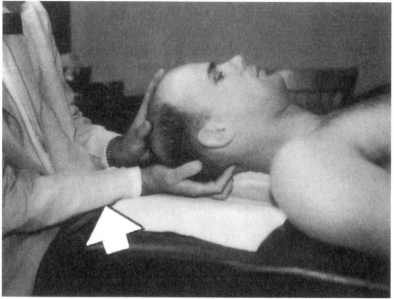

Fig.13

A slight compression at the fulcrum point initiates any pattern of strain in the occipitoatlantal articulations, and the intrinsic forces and their potencies will carry the strain pattern through whatever correction is available for this day's treatment.

Figure No. 14: Specific Cervical Strain

Fulcrum points are at the forearms resting on the table. The fingertips are localizing the specific strain found in the cervical area. Biokinetic forces and their potency provide the motive power for diagnosis and treatment.

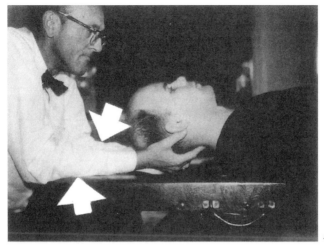

Fig.14

Figure No. 15: Basilar Area of the Skull

The fulcrum points are at the forearms resting on the table. The fingers are lightly interlaced for the physician's comfort and to provide a comfortable sling for the patient's head on the physician's hands. A third fulcrum point is shown at the point of contact between the two third fingers, although any two of the crossed fingers can be used as a fulcrum point for working this area.

This picture merely demonstrates that both the physician and the patient should be comfortable in making an examination or in treating the basilar area of the skull.

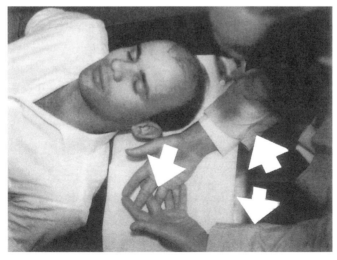

Fig.15

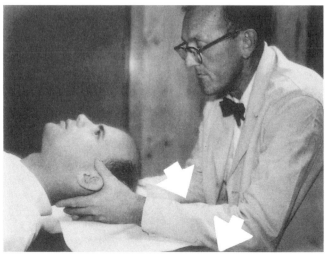

Fig.16

Figure No. 16: Basilar Area of the Skull

The head of the patient is resting comfortably in the lightly inter-laced fingers of the physician, with the thumbs extending above the ears towards the forepart of the head. The fulcrum points are at the forearms on the table.

A very slight compression at the fulcrum points is all that is needed to start an evaluation process that includes the structures of the cranium, those within the cranium, and the cervical areas. An overall sense of continuity of all the midline structures from the base of the skull to the sacrum can be felt.

As indicated in the last sentence, the physician extends his sense of awareness of the continuity of tissue functioning through his fulcrum points and hand contacts. Time and experience will teach him to be aware of much that is going on far beyond his hand and fulcrum points.

Figure No. 17: Basilar Area of the Skull

The head of the patient is resting in the lightly interlaced fingers of the physician with the thumbs along the mastoid portion and process of the temporal bones. The fulcrum points are at the forearms resting on the table.

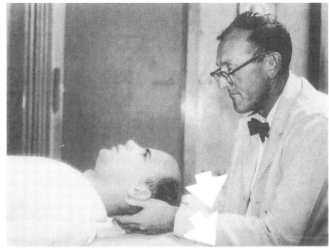

Fig.17

A very slight compression at the fulcrum points starts an evaluation process that includes all the structures of the posterior part of the skull and its contents, the occiput, the temporal bones, the sphenobasilar synchondrosis, the reciprocal tension membrane, the fluctuation of the cerebrospinal fluid, the basilar area of the skull, and the cervical areas.

Figure No. 18: Upper Extremity–Hand to Shoulder
Fulcrum Points: Right elbow against back of chair. Left forearm on crossed knees. Right hand interlaced with thumb and little finger to

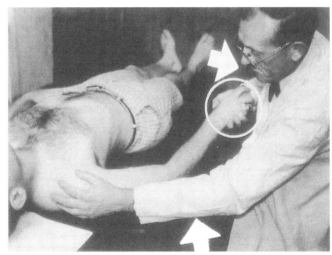

Fig.18

feel through ulna and radius (see circle).

The little fingers as well as the thumbs are interlaced so as to secure a better evaluation between both bones of the forearm. Try this without this interlacing and again with the interlacing. You will observe more when you have interlaced the fingers as indicated.

Figure No. 19: Upper Extremity—Hand to Elbow

Fulcrum points: Right elbow against back of chair. Left forearm on crossed knees. The circle indicates interlaced thumb and little finger hand contact.

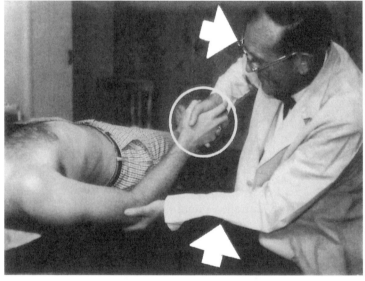

Fig.19

Instead of using the back of the chair, the right arm may be pressed against the physician's own body to act as a fulcrum point.

Figure No. 20: Upper Extremity—Interosseous Membrane Between Radius and Ulna

Fulcrum points: Right elbow on table. Left forearm on crossed knees.

Interosseous membrane strains are frequently present when there is any disturbance in either the wrist or the elbow.

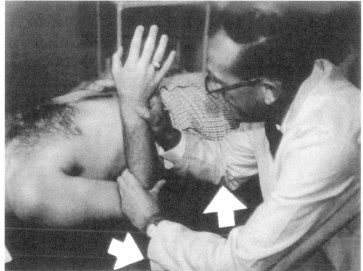

Fig.20

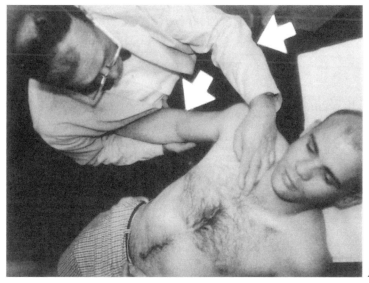

Fig.21

Figure No. 21: Upper Extremity–Elbow to Shoulder and Sternal End of Clavicle

Fulcrum points: Patient's forearm braced against physician's side. Left forearm on crossed knees.

The entire shoulder girdle operates from a fulcrum point at the attachment of the clavicle to the sternum.

199

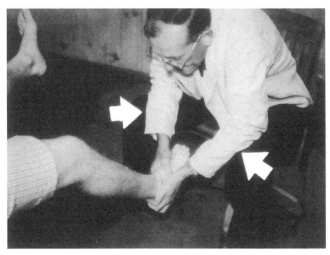

Fig.22

Figure No. 22: Lower Extremity–Foot

Patient supine, leg dropped off edge of table.

The fulcrum points are the physician's forearms against the physician's thighs. Either hand may be behind the heel. Finger contacts can localize specific foot lesions.

Figure No. 23: Lower Extremity–Interosseous Membrane Between Tibia and Fibula

Fulcrum points: Right elbow on table. Left forearm against

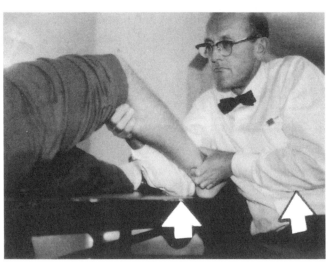

Fig.23

physician's side.

One hand controls the tibia and the other the fibula in evaluating the interosseous membrane between the two. Another approach is to center the upper fingers and lower fingers in towards the interosseous membrane itself. Strains in this membrane usually accompany ankle and knee injuries.

Figure No. 24: Lower Extremity—Knee, Thigh, and Acetabular Region

Fulcrum points: Forearms on knees. Hand contact: Fingers interlaced in popliteal fossa.

A slight compression at the fulcrum points and a slight movement of the physician as a whole towards the acetabulum invokes action into this whole region.

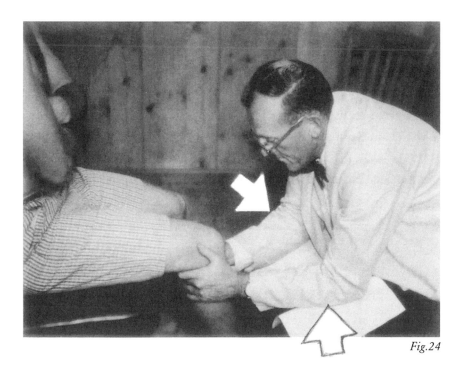

Fig.24

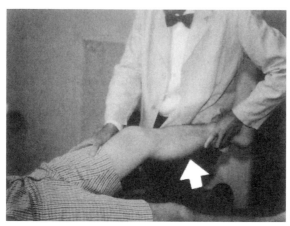

Fig. 25

Figure No. 25: Lower Extremity–Acetabular Region

Fulcrum point: Slightly flexed leg of patient on physician's thigh. Hand contacts slightly compress into acetabular region.

I find this approach useful not only for evaluating the acetabular region but also for following pelvic corrections so as to allow each acetabulum to physiologically reseat itself for the new pelvic balance that has been secured.

Figure No. 26: Lower Extremity–Acetabulum and Ilio-sacral Area

Fulcrum points: Right elbow on table. Left forearm on crossed knees. Hand contacts: Right fingertips in piriformis muscle area. Left hand under ilio-sacral articulation.

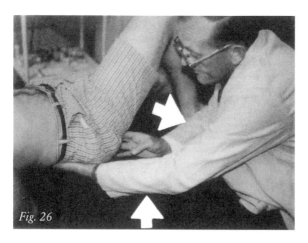

Fig. 26

The fingertips in the piriformis muscle area are directed towards the sacral outflow of the sciatic nerve. I find this approach very valuable in sciatica cases, regardless of what has caused the sciatic nerve irritation.

DIAGNOSTIC TOUCH: ITS PRINCIPLES AND APPLICATION
Part IV: Trauma and Stress

THE PROBLEMS OF TRAUMA and stress in human physiology are complex and wide-reaching. In my patients, it is the effects of trauma and stress upon their specific and general state of health through days, months, and years that brings them to me for attention. That old football injury in college is going to bring the 45-year-old man into my office for back trouble 20 years after the initial injury. The auto accident six months or six years ago has left damaging effects for which the patient is seeking a more accurate diagnosis and a more corrective treatment program. A. T. Still said, "Cause and effect are perpetual. Cause may not be as large in the beginning in some cases as in others, but time adds to the effect until the effect overbalances cause, and the end is death. Death is the end or the sum total of effects. I only ask of the reader to carefully note the different and continued change in effect as additional elements enter the contest and give effect the ascendancy."[1] In light of this understanding, there is no such thing as a "chronic" case. There are only "acute" problems in various stages of compounded effects, whether the injury occurred today, yesterday, or over a long period of time.

Through my use of a diagnostic touch and bioenergy fields, a number of factors have been demonstrated to me from within the anatomical-physiology of my patients. These factors include that there is a bioenergy field of wellness or health within human physiology; in trauma, there are added force factors to the basic bioenergy of health; there are stress factors in trauma; and, finally, a formula can be written to express health and the added force factors in trauma and stress.

Bioenergy Field of Wellness or Health
The bioenergy of wellness is the most powerful force in the

world. It is dynamic. It is rhythmic. It is a force field that begins with the moment of conception and continues to the last moment of death.

The body is a self-contained mechanism, gifted with a state of homeostasis for the stabilization of its internal environment to maintain health and to handle disease, trauma, and stress situations. The body is surrounded by an external environment from which it gets the necessary basic requirements to keep it alive. It is in constant interchange with its external environment physically, mentally, and emotionally. This external environment extends from the person's immediate surroundings to the farthest reaches of the universe. Why, then, separate them, the internal and external environments? Instead of the terminology, man and his environment, these can be joined in one term—biosphere.

The bioenergy field of health is a palpable sensation; it is possible to literally feel the bioenergy of health at work within our patients. It is a quiet, rhythmic feeling of total interchange between the patient's body and the rest of his biosphere. In health, there is a total interchange without any areas of restriction, impaction, trauma, or stress.

There is a bioenergy field of wellness for each individual. It varies continuously from infancy to old age. Every man, woman, and child has their individual pattern. A young woman who has suffered for years with ileitis has a health pattern of normalcy that certainly differs from a woman athlete of the same age. When the physician can sense that the patient and his biosphere are interchanging harmoniously, he can discharge that patient with the assurance that he is healthy again.

Force Factors With Body Physiology

It takes force from without to create trauma within body physiology, and some of this force is left as a part of every traumatic experience. The body absorbs some of these added force factors, which I will call biokinetic energy, and this force becomes part of the physiology within the traumatic area and, in part, throughout the total body. These added force factors can be admitted to the body from injuries that begin before or during birth as well as from trauma in childhood through adulthood to old age. After a trauma is released through treatment or in a case where a trauma leaves no residual, the biokinetic energies totally dissipate back to the external environment, and only the bioenergy of wellness remains.

Since these force factors are not part of the normal bioenergy of health, having come into body physiology from the external environment, it is natural that the body physiology of the patient is constantly attempting to dissipate these biokinetic energies back to the external environment. Compression at the fulcrum points of the physician, with his hands on the injured areas, invokes these biokinetic energies into action along with the basic bioenergy of the patient. The best way to explain how this works in practice is to illustrate with an acute case and then to discuss some of the things that happen in more chronic problems.

Suppose a man lifts an 80-pound sack of fertilizer incorrectly and the next day finds himself with acute low back pain and muscle spasms. He comes into the office, gives his history, and lies down on the examining table in the supine position. I am seated beside him and slide one hand under the area of his lower back where his complaint is most marked, while my other hand and arm are resting on top of his flexed knees. For the arm that has the hand under his lower back, I apply compression at the fulcrum point where my elbow rests on my crossed knees. The weight of my other arm on his flexed knees provides enough compression through his thighs and hips to aid the fulcrum compression point of my other elbow. Since this was an 80-pound sack of fertilizer, I find myself leaning at my fulcrum point on my knees with an approximation of that 80-pound lift. My hand contact under his back remains relatively intact, it is not pushing against his back because of this leverage at my fulcrum point. Instead, it is registering the amount of compression at my fulcrum point, and this in turn is being registered by the tissues in his lower back and its strain area.

The biokinetic energies within the strain pattern are invoked into action and go through a three-phase cycle or pattern of response using their own inherent energy along with the bioenergy of his total

205

body physiology. The pattern of their activity gives me the diagnostic information that I interpret as the fact that he has a rotation compression strain at the level of the fourth and fifth lumbar and that there is considerable muscle spasm in the psoas muscles on each side. The pattern continues to evaluate itself to me by reaching its focus, coming to a stillpoint, going through a point where "something happens" within the potency, and finally unfolding into a corrective normalizing change within all structures involved. The total treatment time varies from five to fifteen minutes. The patient gets off the table considerably relieved and is back to normal in the next few hours or days, if his tissues have not been too seriously damaged.

According to the patient, I did not do much. He may or may not have felt changes within himself during the three-phase cycle of operation. An outside observer might say I did nothing, for he did not see me or the patient in motion. But had they put their hand between my elbow and my fulcrum-compression point on my knee, it would have been a different story. I was applying enough compression to counterbalance the 80-pound sack, enough compression to match the biokinetic force factors added to his body physiology to produce this strain pattern. When I matched this force within the patient, the bioenergy factors within went to work with their maximum level of efficiency to return the biokinetic force factors back to his biosphere, and the pattern that was left was that of the bioenergy of wellness for the patient. I have leaned so hard on my fulcrum-compression points in some cases, I have bruised myself. The patient does not feel it because, in counterbalancing the forces within him, I have voided the sensation of the factors involved within his strain pattern. All he feels is the relief obtained by matching or countering the energies involved. It is far more than a "mere laying on of hands." It is a knowledge of body physiology, bioenergies, biokinetic energies, and the scientific application of many factors for each case each time it is used.

Deeper-seated problems, chronic cases, respond equally well to the use of motive, bioenergy factors. The time interval involved from the onset of the problem until they consult you and the intensity of the pathology has a great deal to do with the progressive corrective results you obtain. The first one, two, or three treatments may "blow off" a number of surface symptoms, and the patient reports he is feeling better, although to your trained touch through your fulcrum points and hands, the tissue strains feel as though very little improvement has taken place. The symptoms return and the patient is sometimes disturbed. In actuality, the tissues had never really made as much change as they indicated to the patient. Sick tissues coming through to make corrective changes do not do so with a sense of relief. They begin their corrective changes by "complaining" that they are now invoked into action and express themselves as symptoms to the patient, not exactly as the patient usually experiences them but as a varied pattern of those symptoms.

Gradually, as the pattern of bioenergy factors and biokinetic energies and tissue elements can come toward the focus for the total pattern, there is an overall sense of "accomplishment" within the patient, felt by him symptomatically and by the physician through his examining hands and fulcrum points. Finally comes the day, usually between office visits and only occasionally during an office visit, when the bioenergy patterns of wellness take the ascendancy within the patient, and he makes a positive change for the better. His biokinetic energies from his traumatic pattern dissipate into his biosphere to the maximum potential for the time he has been under treatment. He may be only in a recompensated stage of recovery, but it is a better recompensated state than he has ever experienced before. If he is dismissed at this time and comes back weeks or months later, his body physiology will show the continued effort of his tissues to restore themselves, as his bioenergy of wellness continues to normalize tissue functioning. He will not show the intensity of his original pathology. He may need more treatment, because he feels the patterns again to some extent, but the physician will be starting at a higher level of functioning in giving him more aid.

Memory Reaction: "Memory reactions" occur within the central nervous system in traumatic cases. An area of the body that has been seriously hurt is going to send thousands of sensory impulses into the spinal cord segments and brain areas that supply that part of the body. If the injury is severe and long-lasting, these messages will be imprinted into the nervous system similar to the imprinting of a message on a tape recorder. After the local injury has finally healed, the nervous system does not necessarily give up its imprinted record. It tends to remember the disturbing message and remain a facilitated area of dysfunction long after the accident.

A man who had a very seriously smashed left leg, which took months to heal, gave the impression at the lumbar area of his spinal cord that it was in a state of shock. The bioenergy field for this area felt abnormal. He was experiencing a considerable sense of chilling in his lower extremities, even though his leg had healed. When the lumbar area renewed its normal bioenergy factor of health through corrective treatment, this sensation disappeared. This type of situation was observed in two other cases. One was a case in which the patient was thoroughly chilled in his lower back and developed a bilateral, psoas muscle strain pattern that resisted treatment until a lumbar enlargement of the cord was brought back into its normal bioenergy pattern. Another case was one in which toxic effects of a series of rabies shots into the rectus muscles of the abdomen had affected the spinal origin of their nerve supply. It pays to consider the segmental origin of any traumatic condition in a treatment program. Any of the cerebrospinal fluid fluctuation techniques can be used to affect the central nervous system and give a normalizing action to wipe out old imprinted messages from disabled areas.

What does an area of the spinal cord segment feel like when it is imprinted with nerve impulses from a disabled area? The only way to find out is to examine a case that comes in with a history of a severe injury. Go to the segmental area of the spinal cord supplying that part, place the hands above and below the area involved with posterior and anterior contacts, establish fulcrum points, apply compression at the fulcrum points, and feel the change in the bioenergy fields within the area being examined. Compare it at each succeeding visit as it normalizes in a treatment program. There will be a distinctive change in tone quality in the tissues at the site of trauma in comparison to adjacent normal areas. Once it is felt and understood, it becomes more easily evaluated in subsequent cases.

I wrote a letter to Dr. W. G. Sutherland in 1954 which will summarize the above brief notes on bioenergy healing as a principle in a treatment program. It reads:

> I have a comment or two to make on explaining so-called "connective tissue reactions" that take place for weeks after treatment to "secure balance in those laws not framed by human hand." At one time I made the statement that a pattern of stress or strain had to go back through its pattern of disability to recover and this proved to be a bright bit of misinformation. It was wrong. I agree.
>
> But here is a new version to explain some of this syndrome of healing. Here in Texas, us ignorant cotton farmers plant cotton until we get no crops because we don't rebuild the soil. So we are told to plant vetch to rebuild the soil during the winter. We do it. The next spring we re-plant cotton, and the crop is a failure. The vetch is given credit for the failure. We don't plant vetch the next winter, and the following spring we again plant cotton. We get a whale of a crop. Our conclusions: Plant vetch, no cotton crop; don't plant, good cotton crop. We are smart. Department of Agriculture conclusions: Plant vetch and the soil is so poor it takes all of the energy of the following year to absorb the vetch and transform the nitrogen into the soil for the next spring when that nitrogen is available for use to grow cotton. Me, cotton farmer, I'm smarter; I know when I got a check.
>
> In cases of severe disabilities, could we use the same simile? As bioenergy levels are restored to living fascias that have been depleted, the first crops of functioning within the fascias express symptoms of

revival towards normalization and use, but they haven't had bioenergy strength for a long time, and an earlier reevaluation of this is expressed as symptoms.

I think you have the idea I have in mind. I have two ladies who have been thoroughly burned out disability-wise for many years. They are experiencing tremendous renewing changes throughout their entire bodies as broad symptom complexes, and yet to my examination, I would say they are fully interchanging their bioenergy field with the environment that surrounds them.

Dr. Sutherland's laconic reply was, "A true bale of cotton."

Stress Factors in Trauma

The general adaptation syndrome enunciated by Dr. Hans Selye accompanies every traumatic experience.[2] "Stress shows itself as a specific syndrome yet it is nonspecifically induced," says Dr. Selye. Trauma as a stressor initiates the general adaptation syndrome mechanism into action. Trauma stimulates the pituitary gland, which in turn stimulates the adrenal glands, which in turn modify a response in the stomach, endothelial systems, and the white blood cells. Selye explains that the whole development of the reaction largely depends on conditioning factors. These can be variables that act upon us from within—our hereditary predispositions and previous experiences (internal conditioning)—as well as variables that influence our body simultaneously with the agent from without (external conditioning). All these are integral elements of the response during stress; they all contribute something to the picture of the general adaptation syndrome.

Furthermore, Selye also refers to tissue-memories as did A.D. Speransky[3]: "The lasting bodily changes (in structure or chemical composition) which underlie effective adaptation or the collapse of it are aftereffects of stress; they represent tissue-memories which affect our future somatic behavior during similar stressful situations. They can be stored."[4]

It was necessary for Selye to develop the fundamental concept of a functional unit of life—the *reaction*—to explain what happens within body physiology and its biosphere. This is a functional unit of energy in body physiology and can be classified as one of the many forms of bioenergy expressed by physiological functioning. He defines a reaction as "the smallest biologic target which can still respond selectively to stimulation."

Trauma is clearly a stressor, and we can discuss a further phase of this concept in relationship to a field in which we, as physicians, have a more direct interest. Selye speaks of "conditioning" through the use of chemicals, drugs, diets, and other things that modify stress reactions. The greatest and most direct conditioners of stress reactions are membranous-articular strains in the craniosacral mechanism that lead to a disturbance of mobility of the cranial articular mechanism, abnormal patterns of mobility of the reciprocal tension membrane, venous retardation, loss of mobility and motility of the pituitary gland within the sella turcica, disturbances of the hypothalamic areas, hyper and hypo irritability of the central innervation of the sympathetic and parasympathetic nervous systems, and hormonal changes that accompany all of this reaction to strain and stress. There are many pituitary hormones involved in the anterior lobe that can be affected, and there can be disturbances between the posterior lobe of the pituitary gland and its nervous connections to the hypothalamic areas through the infundibulum. There are biomechanical answers in the osteopathic concept that explain questions in the general adaptation syndrome.

Knowledge and use of the osteopathic and cranial concepts give the physician direct access to the analysis of stress and its hormone agents. The physician is in a position to analyze the dysfunctioning in terms of mobility and motility of the pituitary and hypothalamic areas and then is able to do something about normalizing it. Birth trauma, head injuries, occipitomastoid lesions, sphenobasilar compressions, condylar compressions, torsions, sidebending-rotations, vertical and lateral strains, sacral concussions, and a host of others are all directly available to our diagnostic insight and treatment programs.

I recall a case in a 16-year-old girl whose growth hormones were disturbed in a most unusual manner. She sustained an occipitomas-toid lesion at the age of 14. As a result, she suffered severe headaches, which were her presenting complaint. Examination revealed that she had developed the left half of her body normally during the interven-ing two years, but the right half of her body still showed the immatu-rity of 14 years of age. This was a cause for alarm for herself and her parents. Correction of the occipitomastoid lesion and its complex not only allowed the headache pattern to disappear but also allowed the right side of her body to normalize its full growth potential over a period of a year, and she was symmetrical by the time she was 17 1/2 years old.

Stress involves the bioenergy factors of body functioning also, and whether they be called reactions or bioenergy, the palpatory skills of the physician are able to localize, analyze, and use these energies in a diagnostic and treatment program for the overall management of the stress pattern induced by trauma. It will differ for each case with each treatment. It is important to study Selye's work so as to be able to define the stress syndrome in traumatic cases, to be able to recognize the symptomatology and concurrent pathology involved, and to know that stress adds a chronological time factor in the recovery of the case. The traumatic condition may make an adequate recovery, but still the patient does not feel he is well again. There is no question in my mind that the stress syndrome is prolonging his total recovery phase, and this factor has to be eliminated to reestablish his bioenergy of wellness. These stress energies can be returned to the biosphere or wherever they go, which allows the bioenergy of health to be the only force left for functioning. Since the cranial concept does include the primary mechanisms for normalizing the mobility and motility of the pituitary gland and hypothalamus, I make sure the bioenergy fields in this area normalize themselves in all traumatic cases. I also check the segmental areas of the thyroid and adrenal glands, the spinal segments of the traumatic areas, and all other areas involved in the general adaptation syndrome. I feel these biokinetic fields of the stress syn-drome are a part of the total traumatic pattern and include them in my overall care of the traumatic case. This contributes to a more rapid recovery of the total problem.

A Bioenergy Formula

As a summary of the discussion thus far, a series of equations can be arbitrarily formulated to explain the reactions of a body physiology to trauma and stress and the body's effort to dissipate these added force factors back to the biosphere.

A few definitions are in order to clarify the equations. In previous papers, I named the bioenergy of wellness or health as "biodynamic energy." So in the equations that follow, the letter "D" will be used for this factor. I have stated that the biodynamic energy of wellness is one of the most powerful forces in the world, beginning from the moment of conception and lasting until the last dying moment. Therefore the first equation can be written: 1. $D = 1$, wherein 1 is the symbol for wellness.

When body physiology is subjected to trauma and stress, force factors are added to the bioenergy systems of the body, and "biokinetic energy" is the term I use to indicate added force factors. The letter "K" will stand for biokinetic energies. The equation will now read: 2. $D+K = DK$.

There is a potency within the body that is constantly working to restore the body to the base pattern of health, $D=1$. Any factors added to body physiology from the biosphere in the form of trauma and stress will find the body attempting to dissipate these factors back to the biosphere. The biodynamic and biokinetic energies and associated tissue elements will automatically wind themselves in towards the focus for that pattern, at which time a change takes place within the potency—the "something happens" phase—and some of the "K" factor is released back to the biosphere. So three new terms are needed for the equations: "Potency," for the inherent power within bioenergy fields in body physiology working towards normalization, "SH" for "something happens" at the point at which the potency comes to a focus in the three-cycle, corrective program, and a small "k" for the force factors left after dissipating some of the "K" factor back to the biosphere. Now the equation can be written: 3. DK→Potency →SH→ (-K) = Dk.

The body continues to normalize itself through the hours, days, or weeks, and the small "k" can be modified to read "$k^{-1,-2,-3,-4,-n}$" to express the descending order of intensity of the "K" factor. The equation will now read: 4. Dk→Potency→SH→(-k) = Dk^n. If the patient makes a complete recovery from his trauma and stress pattern, the equation would read: 5. Dk^n→Potency→SH→(-k^n) = D, wherein only the basic bioenergy of wellness is left.

The patient we see in our practices is the one in equation 4, Dk→ Potency→SH→(-k) = Dk^n, or if he is in an acute state, he would be equation 2, D+K = DK. The physician is going to examine this patient using the bioenergy factors as the motive powers within the body for diagnosis and treatment. He will do this by applying compression through his fulcrum points while his hands are under or on the area of the patient's complaints. This compression at his fulcrum points will invoke the biodynamic and biokinetic energies and the potency within the patient into action, and they will go through the three-phase, treatment cycle operation. It will be necessary then to add the terms "fulcrum," "F," and "compression," "C," to the equation so as to include the role of the physician in the diagnostic and therapeutic program. "FC" will stand for the fulcrum-compression point of the physician in the equation that follows: 6. DK+FC→Potency→SH→ (-K) = D for the case that makes a complete recovery in one treatment. Equation 7. DK+FC→Potency→SH→(-K) = Dk or equation 8. Dk+FC→Potency→SH→(-k) = Dk^n indicates the case that needs many treatments to gradually dissipate the "K" factors to the biosphere. When this more involved type of case finally comes to a focus for the total pattern and is restored to normal, the equation will read: 9. Dk^n +FC→Potency→SH→(-k^n) = D, and the patient is restored to his basic pattern of wellness. D=1 is present again. This is palpable to the physician through his hand contacts and fulcrum points, and he can discharge that patient with full knowledge that the patient is healthy.

Equations one through five represent the body physiology of the patient operating within its own mechanisms to correct its disabilities. Equations six through nine represent the role of the physician in augmenting and aiding the bioenergy factors in body physiology to bring about a more complete resolution of the traumatic and stress experiences.

Why and how this all works is a question, the answer to which is a qualified, "I don't know." I say qualified because I have ideas concerning them that are satisfactory to me in my care of traumatic and stress cases. The bioenergy factors within the patients have given me clues that allow me to follow the progress of each case until I feel the bioenergy of wellness again in the ascendancy within each patient. I can follow the progress of any given case through to normalcy or to the point where I know that a case is irreversible and that certain traumatic and stress factors will continue to be part of that patient's body physiology.

A friend of mine, a space scientist, gives a clue to our use of these bioenergy factors without the total understanding we would like to have in the care of our patients. He told me that it would take 500 mathematicians working for one year to compute the necessary data to plot the flight of the rocket, Ranger IX, to strike the moon as it did in March, 1965. Therefore, the scientists have to rely on data supplied to them by computer machines. They feed their information into the computer and then take the results of the machine with less than total understanding, accepting it as the answer to that phase of the problem, and add this information to the next phase of the problem involved. Finally, the Ranger IX is sent into space and corrective procedures are invoked based on material given to them by the computers. The point is that they do not understand all the steps between each new calculation but accept the machines' analysis from early measurements until the final crash landing on the moon's surface. They have confidence that the computer is correct, and in this case, the successful launch and termination of this particular flight within four miles of their target is proof of their accepted understanding. If this is true in nonliving systems, how many more variables do we, as physicians, have to accept with partial understanding when we work with the phenomena of life?

Bioenergy factors are present within the body physiology and biosphere of each patient. They are available for the physician's diagnostic insight and therapeutic care of that patient. The bioenergy approach has been tested and retested in case after case within my own practice, and the validity of its approach is beyond question. A continued search to explain the in-between steps will bring answers to the physician to many of the problems involved. But meanwhile, the patients continue to benefit with resolutions of many disabilities, although the physician does not have total understanding. I believe the key lies in analyzing what occurs during the stillpoint of the three-phase cycle when "something happens." I am certain that when this door is opened to understanding, it will reveal many more doors for which more keys will be needed to further deepen our knowledge of the phenomena of life.

1. A.T. Still, *Autobiography*, p. 202.
2. Hans Selye, *The Stress of Life*, revised edition (New York: McGraw Hill, 1976).
3. A.D. Speransky, *A Basis for the Theory of Medicine*, ed. and trans. C.P. Dutt (New York: International Publishers, 1943).
4. Source of quotation unknown.

Principles And Methods Of Treatment

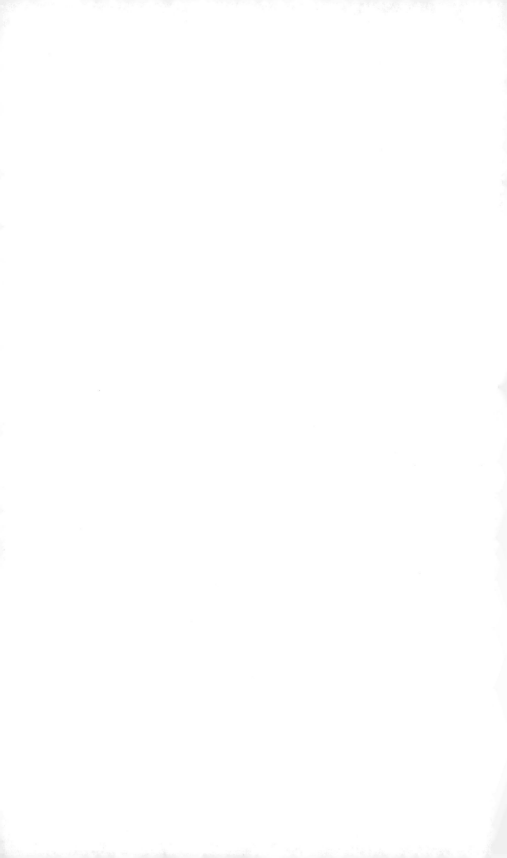

TREATMENT PHILOSOPHY AND METHODS

This is an edited transcription of a lecture given in 1983 at a
Sutherland Cranial Teaching Foundation basic course in
Colorado Springs, Colorado.

THIS TALK ON TREATMENT philosophy and methods is simply a resume and reminder of the things you have already been experiencing in this course. In the first few days of the course, you have been working to feel function and make a diagnosis, but in reality you haven't quit treating since you arrived in this room. Diagnosis and treatment are inseparable.

It is extremely difficult to find words to express health. Health is a word with an unknown meaning. We think of health simply as "health;" we don't have any definitions for it. We can't prove that we're healthy; we can't prove that we register health. However, health in the broadest sense, "Health" with a capital "H," is a something. It's the very reason we're all here–I don't mean in this class, I mean here on earth. We're here because we have Health. So as physicians, we would like to know and experience this quality of health in the living body physiology of our patients. Using our palpatory skills to read this living body physiology, we're allowing this patient's body physiology to show its patterns of health as well as its patterns of stress and/or disease. That is why diagnosis and treatment are inseparable.

Learning the science of osteopathy doesn't come with specific directions; it's a road of experiences, a road of development. I have been up every blind alley you can name in developing my principles of osteopathy for the way I practice. I have fought my way back to the main road many times, only to discover myself in another blind alley. I have made all the known mistakes you can possibly make, and I will probably make more before I'm through. Even Dr. Sutherland, clear up to the last week of his life, was learning the science of osteopathy and developing better ways to accommodate to it. It's an enjoyable trip.

Learning from Body Physiology: One thing that has unlocked doors for me is a willingness to observe and let the body physiology teach me. It's frequently very difficult to realize you are in a blind alley. A simple clue as to how to recognize it is to keep observing. In my practice, when a patient comes in with a problem or stress in their body physiology, I work out an approach to that case and gradually work it out until we secure the necessary "corrections" for the given problem. It might take three minutes, several weeks or several months, but eventually the patient goes away happy. Then the next time that patient comes back to me (and they do return, perhaps for some other problem), I go to the areas of the original stress and carefully test that area as to its quality of being. It may have modified itself so it is not creating symptoms, but maybe it has merely compensated to a point of somewhat better function, and underneath, there is still a sense of gravel—as if it is saying, "Just give me a few years, old buddy, and I'll be right back there and let you have it."

If I feel that, then I realize the principle I devised for that particular type of approach is not on the mark, and I need to start over again. We then use this second go-round as an excuse to finish up the other job, and the next time the patient comes back, if there is no sense of gravel, then great, that principle has worked—I can use that one again. The body physiology *is* the principles of treatment, it *is* the methods of treatment. The body physiology of every patient *is* the laboratory to teach *it* to seek health. We are there merely as guides, as teachers, as active philosophers. Philosophy to me isn't worth a thing unless it works, unless I can *make* it work. So, yes, I've gone down many blind alleys and have managed to wander back again.

You have the right to self-test your skill as long as you obey the laws of the body's physiology. You have a simple mechanism that allows you to test for these rules—a simple flexion/external rotation, extension/internal rotation—not the gross motion in bones and ligaments but a tide, a fluid tide that is literally doing these things, creating flexion/external rotation and extension/internal rotation. It's a guide. It's restricted in areas where there is stress. It also gives you a clue as to what the patient is capable of contributing towards securing health. It is a clue to look for when you reexamine a patient. Does it feel better? If it does, good, but then six months later, when the patient comes back, if you feel that it has gotten tied up again, it's a clue that perhaps you should reevaluate your thinking, let go a little more, listen a little harder, learn a little more, and work for that patient again.

We are talking about principles of treatment. I'm not trying to teach you anything, nobody can teach this work; only the individual can learn it. Dr. Irvin Korr, one of our famous physiologists, was a speaker at our conference years ago, and he said it's impossible to teach palpatory skills because only one person can put a finger on one spot at a time. This is true. Palpation is literally a self-taught art. You can teach the ideas and principles and some of the things that perhaps you're going to find, but then it's up to you to figure out how you can translate it into your body physiology and use it to understand the patient's body physiology.

Seeking Health: Here is another point in the philosophy of treatment which I have learned only in the last few years. When a patient walks into the office, he wants to have that left sacroiliac fixed so that it will quit hurting him. He wants something done for that sciatic pain, or he wants that rib cage unwound so that it ceases to be a problem. This is fine. But my idea is that when a patient walks into the office with a particular problem, I want to deliver the health pattern within that strain, not merely stop with diagnosing it and attempting to treat the anatomicophysiological process that represents the iliac strain or the sciatica.

As an example, I'll tell you about one patient I had. (This is not a hero story; I don't know any. I haven't been a hero in 49 years of practice. The patient is the hero.) This man fell from a 20-foot skylight and shattered his leg, drove the tibia right up into the femur.

Afterwards, the problem was that his legs stayed ice-cold 24 hours a day; on a 105-degree day in Texas, he wore wool underwear. How many tens of millions of messages were going from that shattered limb to the lumbar enlargement of the cord, for "x" number of days, weeks and months? Think of it. That lumbar enlargement of the cord was in a state of total shock from the hour of the accident to the time I saw him. I laid my hands under him with one hand up under the enlargement of the cord, and it felt as if he had an icicle in there. Don't ask me what an icicle feels like three inches deep, but that's what it felt like.

So I treated merely to change the quality of arterial circulation to and in and around the lumbar enlargement of the cord. In this case, I did not use the principle of seeking health. I was not seeking health at that time—we're talking about 20 years ago. I was seeking a good, adequate correction; that's all I was interested in. So we tried to improve the arterial supply, the venous drainage, the lymphatic drainage, the autonomic control, and to push every button the man owned. I used compression of the fourth ventricle and balanced the sacrum—anything that would influence the circulatory pattern to and from the lumbar enlargement of the cord. To make a long story short, during one treatment, we were working, and all of a sudden, it felt as if someone put a hot poker into that thing and it melted. It warmed up and his legs were warmed; the physiology came back to normal health. What took place? A correction of a shocked lumbar enlargement of the cord? No. It was a restoration of health. Literally. Now the cerebrospinal fluid tide could go into flexion and extension through that lumbar enlargement of the cord. Until that time, it couldn't.

This approach of my seeking health is not a new idea. It is an extension of the notion of what I would like to see accomplished within the patient. In this approach, I'm not confining myself to the tunnel vision of, "I'm going to correct this spot." It's a little bit different—I'm letting go to see that health is the thing that comes through rather than a correction of a lesion. This is truly a treatment philosophy. And it works.

Chronic Patterns and Closed Loops: Of course not every problem is just going to melt away. The physiology of tissue that is functioning with some old scar tissue that's been lying around for twenty years is not about to wake up and be healthy; it's got to be trained back into health. Chronically involved tissues have to be trained. Chronic strain patterns tend to form a closed loop. My experience with one particular unwinding technique I was shown was that after all the movement, the patient felt better—the treatment got the thing well-oiled. But then the very next week, when the patient came back, he had the same strain, same place, same everything. A closed loop—once you initiated it, the thing never came to an end, round and round you'd go. The body literally set up a neuromuscular, biofeedback closed loop.

This means you've got to tune through that strain pattern. You are seeking, What is the health for this area? And once you've gotten through to that strain pattern, bore a hole in it so it has to dissipate, have it do something besides staying a closed loop. You can then begin to get a correction in that problem. If it's been there for years, ligaments have to soften, musculoskeletal tensions have to change, autonomic systems have to modify their functioning, lymphatics have to wake up and find out they have got a job to do, and the Breath of Life has to literally flow into those tissues and become as strong as it is in the rest of the body. Lots of things have to change, and they will slowly. You can feel that thing gradually heading towards, not a correction, but towards literally dissolving itself, with the health pattern becoming the dominant pattern.

Naming Pathologies: One other thought along these lines. When you learn to palpate through to it, the pathology in living tissues does not have textbook titles. You're feeling body physiology functioning as it is designed without a label on it. You do not just treat a bursitis or a shoulder problem for instance. You find things are happening below, above, around and through that all contribute to that shoulder complaint. (I'm doing everything I can to avoid the cranial-sacral mechanism in my examples; I want you to realize there's more to life. We're using the primary respiratory mechanism in everything we're talking about; we're just not using the words each time.) When someone trips and falls down on their shoulder, there are other things involved. As you are working with a patient, there are many things happening during the tissue change that you can't call by a pathologic name. It's a new picture that you're seeing unfolding within those tissues. It's a moving pathology, it's a pathology coming alive, and it is correcting itself. We need to realize that when we say, "This is a torsion left, this is a frozen shoulder," these are just the labels we put on things. The function within is a moving picture during corrective cycles. Labels have their use, and you can make up your own labels. I've got a long list of labels I choose for various things I recognize are relatively the same type of pattern. But it's only just a name so I can recall what it was that I theoretically had been working on. The label is not the pathology involved.

Evaluation of the Patient: When a patient comes into my office, the first thing I like to do after I listen to their complaint and try to get a little history, is to go to that patient's body physiology and place my hands under their area of primary complaint (because this is the thing they are going to want something done about). But that's strictly to introduce myself to the patient. I then go to some other part of the patient, to their craniosacral mechanism or to whatever else seems to be indicated, to give me an evaluation of what should be the health for that patient as a whole.

With new patients who come into the office, I also try to find out what type of pattern they are living in. What is their base pattern? We've already been finding out in this course that no two of us are alike, and no two of us have the same pattern. In other words, if you get your hands on me, please try to discover I have a torsion pattern and that I want to be left in it when I get fired from your services. I try to find a total body physiological pattern that represents how this person gets about. That then gives me a guide towards understanding what is the base pattern the patient has been living with and how his base pattern functions in flexion/external rotation and extension/internal rotation. I can then go back to the area of trouble and see how this patient relates to his type of pattern.

In this evaluation, I also note the quality of that patient's mechanism. For this, I use the idea of the mechanism registering 110 volts in health. I note whether it feels like the patient's mechanism has 110 volts coming in and 110 volts going out. If it comes in and goes out at 50 volts, that gives me a clue. A 110-volt battery in a living patient suggests good quality in those tissues for ligamentous or membranous articular strains to be corrected. In this case, you've got adequate juice to work with; the battery is full of vim and vigor. If he's only got 50 volts, his local tissues, especially in the area of the stress, are going to fatigue much faster, and you've got to be a little bit more careful about what you are introducing to that body, what you are attempting to accomplish that day. That body may only tolerate a few minutes of treatment before it fatigues.

There's a very cute story that relates to this about a guy who had an acute psoasitis that you would not believe. I got my hands under that psoas muscle, and after exactly 30 seconds, I was told to get the hell out of there. "I've heard you, now shut up," his mechanism said. Two days later, he came back and we got to stay almost two minutes this time, until another little, tiny change took place. The local batteries were shot. He was then supposed to come back in a few more days, but he got called out of town. However, orders had gone to his primary respiratory mechanism, orders had gone to his body physiology, and on his way down to a meeting in East Texas, all hell broke loose. It almost threw him out of the car as it made a self-correction. When he came in on the next visit, he said, "I went home the first day and my wife asked, 'What did he do?' and I told her, 'He just examined me, he's going to see me in two days.' Then after my next appointment she asked me again, and I said, 'He didn't do anything. He just examined me again and said I'll be alright.' Well, Doc, at first I had my doubts about your approach, but now I realize you were doing something and I feel great. I'll be back for another 'examination' next week."

The point is that you need to read the quality in that tissue, read the ability of that tissue to respond, assess the quality of the battery, and assess how much it can respond in a given treatment. That's a principle. Next, choose the stress pattern that you are going to work on. Start off with a diagnostic phase on the stress area that you choose. Then somewhere along the line, while you are attempting the diagnosis—listening to the body physiology explain it to you in great detail—you'll suddenly discover you're in a treatment mode. It is a step, it's almost an invisible step. You think you're diagnosing, and then, all of a sudden, you say, "Hey, by golly, now's the time to perhaps see if we could just give it a little coaxing and maybe something will happen." So we put just a little more compression or some other contact in, and all of a sudden, we're in the treatment mode for that given day. This is not a time-consuming process, believe me. Most of the work can take place in a relatively few minutes.

Principle of Permitted Motion: There are five different patterns of permitted motion that we use as potentials for treatment procedures. Exaggeration is probably the most common—carrying the tissue strains toward the direction they went into when they got strained. Exaggeration can also be used in testing. If I were testing the cranial base for a torsion right pattern, I would deliberately initiate that pattern and then allow the tide to carry it into a torsion right and then come back to neutral. Then I would initiate a torsion left. This principle applies for general patterns, specific patterns, local patterns, voluntary strains, etcetera.

Another pattern of permitted motion is direct action, in which you literally guide the parts right back towards the position of neutral or health or whatever. Direct action is sometimes specifically used in a very acute type of strain, where if you attempt to exaggerate it, the intensity of the patient's discomfort increases. But if you attempt instead to guide it back, allowing physiologic function to help you do it, the patient feels more comfortable. Direct action is the name for this. (Again, I don't like labels, including these.)

Disengagement is what its name implies. In a frontosphenoidal lesion, there can be an impaction, with all those prongs interdigitated, and you've got to disengage it. That is one of the treatment methods.

For the pattern of opposing physiologic motion, an occipitomastoid lesion is what comes to mind as an example. With trauma, the temporal bone can be driven into a traumatic internal rotation pattern extending through the membranes, while the occiput is driven towards a flexion attitude or mode. If we have an old chronic occipitomastoid lesion that has been lying around in the closet for years, we perhaps would want to use opposing physiologic motion. We would guide the temporal bone or attempt to have the temporal bone go towards external rotation while guiding the occiput towards extension, being extremely careful to read with great delicacy the quality of the tissue changes taking place in the membranous articular pattern. I'm not giving you an occipitomastoid technique, I'm describing opposing physiologic movements.

Finally, there is molding technique. Actually, these are *not* techniques; these are literally the principles that the primary respiratory mechanism, the reciprocal tension membrane, and the body physiology of the patient uses to self-correct its own problems.

For those of you who are taking the course for the first time, these are valuable ways with which to manually take ahold of a patient and guide those tissues back, using exaggeration, direct action, or disengagement, to find a point in membranous balance where the patient's body physiology will go to work for you, and then you can ease off. You can manually exaggerate a certain pattern and find a point at which all the tension is ready to do something for you. The battery is in there; you support it and let it happen. These patterns of permitted motion are principles of treatment which are used as guiding principles to treat body physiology and the primary respiratory mechanism.

For those of you who have been in the game a little longer, you may use these principles accidently. We'll take the example of a relatively severe type of strain somewhere in the area of the pelvis or in the neurocranium. You may choose any one of the patterns of motion, and you kind of imply to that mechanism that you're going to do it; yet you may find yourself cooperating with a body physiology that's trying to take it away from you. It says, "Well, look, doc, that's fine, you're smart and intelligent, but let's go this way." You turn on all your listening aides for this mechanism within the patient, and you discover that it is going through these motions. You will feel this particularly if it's a severe strain or old chronic strain. You will find that the body itself exaggerates, directs action, disengages, etcetera. It uses those very principles deep within its own unlabeled pathology and physiologic system of self-treatment. During the treatment, it can go through all these things, and then all of a sudden it makes some kind of shift or change; it clicks and tells you to get out—leave me alone. What have you done? You've experienced the mechanism doing the same thing you were doing manually.

There is another point I want to make. You've only given the orders for the treatment; what you did was not the treatment. The patient does the treatment. You've given the orders to the body physiology. You have told it: "We recognize your problem. We have told you where the potential for health is. Now go to work."

Why do these principles work? Well, we're just lucky they do. That's really the only answer I can give, but I'll tell you another one. The innate physiological mechanisms of a fluctuant cerebrospinal fluid, a motile central nervous system, and a mobile reciprocal tension membrane are moving the cranial articular mechanism and the involuntary mobility of the sacrum between the ilium. In addition, the total fascial envelopes of the whole body and their fluid content are in reciprocal interrelationship with the primary respiratory mechanism. The initiation of function in any of these elements initiates physiologic action in all the elements. That's the reason it works. It's only words. Palpatory experience verifies it.

Response to Treatment: How often do I treat? I like a minimum time of at least a week between treatments, unless we have a patient with acute psoasitis who will kill you if you don't get to him quicker. When the patient comes back for the next visit, get your hands on that case and start a diagnostic program to determine how things have matured or not matured. See if it feels like, "Well, yes, I tried to do some work last week, but I'm not too sure I understood you." So you discover you have to give it another whatever. When he comes back the week after that, the same routine. Then he comes back the next week and this time his mechanism says, "Look, Doc, I'm finally beginning to hear you, but I'm not quite through with those other things; I'm still working on those last three." So you taper him to every other week, then you taper him to once a month. I try to treat them just often enough to keep directing them back to whatever I'm working on, back towards the patterns that are healthy for that particular individual.

In the course of treatment, it is possible to create some magnificent reactions. I have managed to create some wonderful reactions, as opposed to responses, in some of the cases I've worked on. This was especially true in my early days. There were reactions where they had to lie on the table for two and a half hours before they could get up after I had tried to make a correction somewhere in the area of the temporal bone. These can be brought under control. We can cool off reactions by certain skills we'll discuss later, including compression of the fourth ventricle.

These kinds of reactions aside, most of the time when a patient feels something after they leave your office, it has to do with the work going on for their particular problem. For the next two to three days or a week, they can actually feel worse because you have given orders to the tissues, the fascias, the connective tissues, which like to do the loudest screaming. You woke them up. An unhealthy tissue does not wake up and say, "Oh, joy, peace in the world!" It wakes up and says, "Who the hell told you to disturb me?" Sometimes they come back at you and they complain very bitterly.

As a rule, if I sense a person will perhaps respond that way, I very quietly warn the patient that she can either feel ten times worse or better, and I don't know which it will be. I tell her that if she needs to, call me, and I will explain it to her because I have observed what took place in those tissues after I finally quit listening to them, and I have a pretty good idea where they are going to end up complaining and what they are going to complain about. In this way, I can encourage the patient to just wait it out for the rest of the week, and the patient will. And the funny thing is that while some area is complaining louder than it did, the patient has the strange feeling that maybe it is alright. You've spoken to her private physician, and that private physician is "in" and has good ears, and it tells that patient that this is not a reaction, this is a response. Often the patient will say something like, "I never hurt so bad in my life, but I got six rooms of furniture cleaned for the first time in a month." So always listen for a "but I...." It helps you to understand where you are.

In closing, we thank all of you in this room. Whether you know it or not (this is a simple statement of fact, you don't have to believe me), we have all become one body physiology since the day we started putting our hands on each other. So thank you. It's one unit.

FLEXIBILITY IN OSTEOPATHY

This paper was written in the 1980's.

THE ROLE OF THE physician is to serve man. The science of osteopathy offers a direct, one-on-one, clinical approach in this service to mankind. The purpose of this paper is to demonstrate the use of the science of osteopathy in a wide variety of clinical syndromes, with some evaluation and anatomicophysiological interpretation as to diagnostic and treatment results in the cases selected.

To clarify this discussion, it will be assumed that the physician is using the science of osteopathy as enunciated by A.T. Still and W.G. Sutherland; that the structure-function of the body physiology of the patient will be manifesting its innate, involuntary primary respiratory mechanism and its anatomicophysiological integrated mobility, motility, and fluid drive; that the physician can use these elements of manifesting life from within the body physiology of the patient for diagnostic and treatment service to mankind.

In my personal experience, I have learned that each patient visit brings with it three factors in the restoration towards health: 1) the patient's opinion as to his/her diagnosis and/or treatment program; 2) the physician's knowledge in his diagnostic and treatment program; 3) and the patient's body physiology in a direct, one-on-one relationship with its specific, manifesting patterns of function and dysfunction.

To insure greater accuracy in diagnosis and treatment, it is helpful to get the patient's opinion of his/her condition. It is also helpful, as a physician, to have some input into a diagnostic and treatment approach. But most importantly, the physician can use a trained palpatory skill to read, listen, and feel the dynamics of the patient's body physiology manifesting its health functioning and the dysfunctioning that brought the patient in for evaluation and treatment. In other words, the patient's opinion is interesting, and my skill as a physician gives me deeper insight into the problems presented, but neither are as informative or as productive as desired. When my attention is drawn away from the patient's opinion and away from my professional physician's input, I can go directly to the body physiology of the patient and become a student again, a student who uses palpatory skills to feel, to listen, and to read the anatomicophysiological changes within the body physiology of the patient as they express health and/or dysfunction. I become a student and the patient's body physiology is my teacher. The science of osteopathy provides the tools for evaluating both diagnostic and treatment programs directly from the inborn health mechanisms and the areas of dysfunction and their mechanisms.

As one learns to work with the teacher (body physiology of the patient), one leans less and less on the opinion of the patient or the evaluating input of the physician. One realizes, more and more, that the teacher-student relationship, using trained palpatory skills, is providing basic, clinical, diagnostic and therapeutic interchange with the body physiology of the patient. The flexibility in the science of osteopathy is expressing mobility, motility, and fluid drive mechanisms. Palpating the elements of function from within the patient through these mechanisms can give the student (physician) the available factors that represent health for that individual as well as those factors that are expressing dysfunction.

Again, there are three factors presented with each patient: 1) the opinion of the patient, which is inconclusive; 2) the input from the physician, which is frequently inconclusive; 3) and lastly, the accuracy of the output from the body physiology of the patient, which is wholly conclusive in production and information. Thus, the physician must learn to trust the teacher (the mobility, motility, and fluid drive of the body physiology) and become a student using his palpatory skills through which to listen, to read, and to feel the instruction from the teacher.

How is body physiology manifesting its living functioning as tools in the science of osteopathy? It is an involuntary mechanism that is a simple, mobile, motile, fluid drive, with flexion of all midline structures and external rotation of all bilateral structures alternating with extension and internal rotation. This rhythmic, balanced, involuntary interchange occurs 8 to 12 times per minute. As a total unit in body physiology, it is essential to life and health. The secondary mobile, motile, fluid drive in body physiology is the voluntary mechanism in use by the individual in his/her daily activities. Both involuntary and voluntary mechanisms within the individual can be observed and worked with by the physician through his trained sense of palpatory skills.

In clinical application of these principles (involuntary and voluntary mobility, motility, and fluid drive), they are one unit in operation. Consider a young woman who was sleeping in the back seat of a car when it was involved in an accident, struck an abutment, and stopped abruptly. After she recovered from the emergency care of her case, she came into the office with a complaint of swelling of her right lower extremity. It would be fairly normal in the morning but would become more involved by the end of the day.

Palpatory examination of the involuntary and voluntary units of her body physiology revealed that on the left, healthy, lower extremity, her fascial envelopes would alternate into external and internal rotation patterns freely with the rest of her body physiology, while on the right lower extremity, the fascial envelopes would only go into internal rotation while the external rotation was relatively locked in its pattern so as to retard venous and lymphatic drainage. It turned out that her right lower extremity had been in an internal rotation pattern while she was sleeping in the back seat of the car at the time of impact. Corrective treatment to release the fascial drag of internal rotation towards the health mechanism of functioning restored adequate venous and lymphatic drainage.

Another interesting case was a man, age 46 years, who came in with a complaint of chronic backache over a period of several years. His history included an auto accident with a front-end collision sixteen years earlier. Palpatory findings revealed two major deficits in body physiological functioning. One was a glass-like feel to all the muscles and fascia in the thoracic and cervical areas. The second deficit was a "locked" sacrum with total loss of involuntary mobility. The whole pelvic girdle—the sacrum, the two ilia, the lumbosacral area, and the two acetabula—was not being rocked individually 8 to 12 times per minute by the rhythmic mobility, motility, and the fluid drive unit of motion. This basic fluid drive has an important task of providing an adequate trophic interchange between all the cells of the body and the entire connective tissue or fascial framework. In this man, for 16 years, this fluid drive and vital mobility and motility had been impeded in their activity, leading towards a withering field in function in all the tissues involved.

The voluntary mechanisms in his body were relatively free of symptoms and not too much impaired on palpatory evaluation. Palpatory examination of his involuntary mechanisms, however, found disturbances of function from the top of his head to his feet, including all the fascial envelopes. It took three or four offices visits to get a clearer insight into the total patterns presented. At the time of the accident, he had been lifted out of his seat and slammed back into it so as to freeze the involuntary mobility of the sacrum between the ilia. As this immobilization continued, the sacrum even lost its tonal quality of living bone. It had the feel of a unit of concrete between the two ilia. It is difficult to read this loss of involuntary mobility and motility, but it can be learned with practice. After several office visits, this man's sacrum was saying, "You probably can't feel me easily, and I am more or less like concrete in my functioning, but I am here for you to work with and to help me to get well."

Treatment once a week was given, using the resources of this patient's body physiology, and in about five months, the "concrete" sacrum had changed towards a "dense oak" with some improvement in tonal quality. At the end of nine months, he walked into the office with a total recovery of the normal tonality of an osseous sacrum and a total health mechanism of a rhythmic, involuntary, mobile, motile, fluid drive unit of function. He was dismissed. Five years later, he came in for a minor complaint, and palpatory examination indicated that all musculoskeletal and fascial units in his thoracocervical areas had made a complete healing. He is now in his early seventies and continues to be in good health. What would have been the story if the original withering field had continued its pattern?

This last case cited is an example of a whiplash or inertial type of strain associated with loss of involuntary sacral mobility. The palpatory evidence of this type of injury is a frequent finding. Over the past 30 years, my records show that every seventh new patient showed palpatory evidence of this type of strain pattern, with a relative loss of involuntary mobility of the sacrum between the ilia, even though this was not a part of the presenting complaint. When the patient was asked, "When did you have an auto accident?", the reply was frequently negative until the next question was asked: "When did you have such an accident and not get hurt?" The answer would then be positive, as he or she would recall such an inertial strain in a time ranging from a few months to a period of several years ago.

In most cases, this is not the reason for their seeking care from the physician, but during the physician's palpatory examination, there is found a unilateral or bilateral limitation of involuntary sacral mobility. The mobile, motile, fluid-drive, 8-to-12-times-per-minute, rhythmic cycle is not delivering its full trophic potential in the patient's body physiology. Since the patient came in for other problems than that of the locked sacrum, a treatment program can be developed for whatever the patient presented with, but during the treatment phase, one can allow a short time to go to the sacral dysfunction and work with the body physiology to release the sacrum into its involuntary freedom to function. This release process coordinates with all other treatment corrections towards health. There are many forms and types of inertial injuries and each one of them requires specific evaluation, diagnosis, and treatment. The whiplash sacral syndrome is used as an example because of the frequency with which it can be observed, diagnosed, and corrected towards health.

Working with body physiology and its innate involuntary and

voluntary mobility, motility, and fluid drive will allow palpatory patterns to show themselves during a physician's examination. Three cases of a "shocked" lumbar enlargement of the spinal cord are examples. Case one was in a colleague of mine who fell from a skylight and drove his left tibia into his left femur. Five months later, he came for treatment to restore body physiological functioning in his leg. He came wearing wool underwear in Texas, 100-degree weather because of a loss of autonomic nervous system control to his lower extremities. Since the time of the accident, think of the millions of messages of impairment being relayed between the shattered leg and the lumbar enlargement of the spinal cord. The potential for giving him help required his body physiology to reawaken and make a corrective release of his spinal cord vitality in the area of the lumbar enlargement. The tool for this restoration was the mobility, motility, and fluid drive of his involuntary mechanisms. Weekly treatment in the area of the cord was given to encourage his body physiology to influence its self to release the "shock" that the spinal cord was experiencing. After about 12 treatments, there was a sudden release or corrective change from within in the area of the lumbar enlargement. There was a sense of heat radiating from the spinal cord segment, and his lower extremities became warm with resumption of autonomic nervous system control. He returned home with continuing self-healing changes.

Case two was less dramatic and of shorter duration, but again, it showed a direct involvement with the lumbar enlargement of the spinal cord. The patient came in with a history of getting thoroughly chilled after sitting in a cold draft for two hours. Within 12 hours, he developed a bilateral psoas muscular contracture that would not release its effects within the area involved. Reasoning from the relationship of the origin of the psoas muscles and the source of the nerve supply to these muscles, it seems probable that the external chilling of the patient had bombarded the lumbar enlargement and created a dysfunction in the spinal cord at that segmental level. Attention was therefore taken away from the contractures of the muscles and directed towards working with the body physiology and its mechanisms of involuntary activity in the area of the lumbar enlargement. During the third treatment, there was a sudden radiation of heat from the spinal cord segment, and the patient made an uneventful recovery.

For the physician, it is an interesting palpatory experience to be present when such a release takes place, but the same type of correction can and usually does take place between treatments when the patient is at home. The patient reports this change at his next office visit and the palpatory evaluation by the physician can verify the result. It is a fact, in working with the body physiology within the patient, that during the office treatment, the body physiology is initiating its corrective changes towards health, and the actual treatment results take place between office visits. The next office treatment confirms the changes made and provides data for what the continued needs are to further the treatment program. As a teacher, body physiology is most accurate in its diagnostic and treatment results.

The third case showed a similar type of impairment in the lumbar enlargement of the spinal cord but for an entirely different reason. A man, in his fifties, came in with chronic circulatory disturbances in the lower half of his body. This had been going on over a period of several years. He had made the rounds of several physicians without success. His history revealed that he had received a series of 28 rabies shots 20 years earlier into the abdominal muscles supplied by the lumbar enlargement of the spinal cord. With passing time, the toxic effects of these shots had compromised the quality and the functioning of the spinal cord in that segment. The tonal quality was very poor in the muscles and the lumbar enlargement. This tentative diagnosis was suggested to him, but he did not wish to follow through.

Findings reported with disturbances of functioning of the lumbar enlargement of the spinal cord are not uncommon. The three cases presented describe varying types of effect mechanisms to initiate a response in the spinal cord. The nature of that response was an overload or a shock to specific sensory, motor, and autonomic nervous system segments. With persistence of inflowing sensory input from the initiated trauma, the shocked spinal cord in the lumbar enlargement

237

establishes a closed-loop type of phenomenon. It can be compared to a closed-loop tape recorder message. Incoming messages from the injury report trauma, and the feedback becomes a repetitive event even after the site of injury is stabilized. It can persist for weeks, months, and years.

The basic activity of body physiology is a rhythmic, involuntary, flexion and extension of midline structures with external and internal rotation of bilateral structures 8 to 12 times per minute and a fluid drive for trophic interchange throughout the body. Why this basic activity fails to neutralize or cancel its closed-loop circuit between the injury and the spinal cord is difficult to explain, but the fact remains that there is a shock in the lumbar enlargement that will lead to withering fields in cellular and fluid functioning with the passage of time. However, there is also an opportunity to work with the basic body physiology to cancel this closed-loop circuit. Two of the cases described demonstrated this release towards health.

The lumbar enlargement of the spinal cord is not the only area that can experience this type of response. It can be found in any part of the spinal cord supplying a portion of the body subjected to a severe injury. Anatomicophysiological reasoning can work with body physiology to localize and define the areas that need attention.

If such a problem should present itself—for example, a patient has had a major accident and the case has apparently stabilized but still has problems—check with the body physiology of the patient to evaluate the presence or absence of a closed-loop circuit in the spinal cord segment for that accident. This is done by comparing the quality of the basic body physiology in an area of relative health for that individual and in the area of the closed-loop or accident site. The health area will report adequate quality in fluid drive interchange with the whole of the body, while the tissues involved in the accident will show impaired quality at a local or segmental area. Work with body physiology in the area of the traumatic mechanism and in the potential closed-loop circuit to promote health. Allow the impaired quality of living function to more closely resume the relative health tested in the initial examination.

238

Thus, the physician has a working tool for diagnostic and treatment insight before, during, and after each treatment session. If the patient's traumatic sites make some type of healing change in the treatment for that day, the physician can assure himself that the patient's body physiology had done its work for that visit and will continue its effort between treatments until the next office visit. If some type of correction takes place, but there is no indication that the body physiology of the patient has up-graded its quality in the traumatic sites, the so-called corrections do not meet physiological needs. The before and after tests for quality of health in the areas of relative health and in the closed-loop circuits will provide insight in working with the patient's own living mechanisms. The day will come when the patient walks into the office, and his mechanism announces, "I'm well." Testing his basic body physiology tools of mobility, motility, and fluid-drive units of function verify his statement. His closed-loop circuits have disappeared, and all traumatic units are working their way towards health.

Another palpatory finding available to the physician who is developing his sense of touch to work with the body physiology of the patient is that in the presence of a myocardial infarction, there is an implosion in the thoracic cavity that occurs at the time of the attack. The first time this was observed was in the case of a woman in her sixties who was taking treatment for a relatively minor ailment when she had a major myocardial infarction. She survived the event and returned to the office for further treatment. In evaluating the quality of function in the thoracic area, it felt as if the whole chest wall was in a state of fascial restriction. This factor was noted as a definite change from the type of thoracic tone felt in the chest before she had the myocardial infarction. It was as though there was a modified shock or implosion affecting the chest, an implosion that could be found and treated to cancel itself towards further restoration to health.

Through the years, this implosion has been observed in several patients who developed this phenomenon as part of a thoracic fascial response to the shock of a myocardial infarction. Whatever other complaints the patient may be seeking service for, treatment to cancel the implosion can be added to supplement further healing from the heart attack. This is an example of one of those silent physiological events that shows itself to the physician's palpatory skills from within the body physiology of the patient. Any release from the fascial drag of the implosion can only be beneficial in the overall care of the patient's health needs.

Body physiology is the silent partner and the foundation for health within the total human being. There are two basic principles expressing this health. There is the involuntary flexibility for all movements, mobility, motility, and fluid drive with which to express life. Every cell and all fluids in every organ, viscera, musculoskeletal mechanism, circulatory network, lymphatic system, central and peripheral nervous system, fascial framework, and cerebrospinal fluid fluctuation are rhythmically expressing a simple flexion and extension of all midline tissues and fluids accompanied by external and internal rotation of all bilateral tissues and fluids. This movement can be compared to a tide, similar to that in an ocean, except that in body physiology, it occurs approximately 10 times per minute rather than twice a day. Like the ocean tide, there is power in this rhythmic pump with every fluctuation, power that the physician can feel, read, listen to and palpate in all of the tissues and fluids. This is the involuntary activity of living motion expressing health. Think of the resources within the body physiology of the patient, and accept their livingness for use. Motion is not life, but motion expresses life. The fluid drive, as it fluctuates in body physiology, is one of these elements. All tissues and fluids express this involuntary movement as one unit in health and as one unit in stress. The second basic principle is the patient expressing voluntary activity with which to live his daily life, even as his silent partner continues a living tide-like movement centered within to maintain his health functioning.

The patient is subject to developing trauma and/or disease, which will be found in specific areas of his body and organized being. His silent partner continues its rhythmic balanced interchange in relative

240

health for the whole body while it becomes impeded or modified in the presence of trauma and/or disease. The quality of health can be measured anywhere in the whole body to serve as a guide for measuring the quality of restricted tidal movement in the stress area. Flexibility is also reduced in the problem area. The science of osteopathy is deep but simple, if you understand the mechanism. As treatment is administered to restore health, the quality of involuntary mobility, motility, and fluid drive in the stress area begins its progressive release towards health functioning. The effects manifesting in the area of trauma and/or disease do more than make a mere correction; they literally melt, leaving health recentered in physiologic functioning. Whatever corrective measures the physician may be using, the rhythmic tidal units are working about 10 times per minute to act as penetrating oil with other trophic factors to cancel the stress area and to return to health. The physician can develop his touch to feel, to read, and to experience these healing changes within the body physiology of the patient. Flexibility is restored as part of the healing process.

The role that body physiology plays in service to mankind and within each individual is very real and very attainable in a one-on-one relationship between physician and patient. The point is not what the physician can do for the patient, but what the physician can do to open the doors to allow the patient to heal him or herself. In each of the cases described earlier, all that underwent treatment made restorations towards health by using the basic principles of body physiology, involuntary mobility, motility, and fluid drive functioning, and voluntary mobility as used by the patient in his day-to-day living.

The physician accepts the livingness of these principles from within the patient and develops the palpatory skills of feeling, listening, reading, and knowing the relative qualities of health being demonstrated in the patient and the relative qualities found in trauma and/or disease expressed in the stress areas. The physician's sense of touch can find these local specific dysfunctions and can work with the innate restorative basic principles to allow the patient to return to health. It is an accepted fact, at least in words, that the body physiology of any individual is constantly seeking health, whether he or she is aware of it or not. But to translate these words into a one-on-one experience on a day-to-day basis in a patient-to-patient context is a real challenge.

GUIDED BY THE MECHANISM
This is an edited transcription of a lecture given in 1988 at a
Sutherland Cranial Teaching Foundation course in Tulsa, Oklahoma.

OVER A PERIOD OF many years I have worked towards the establish-
ment of a one-on-one relationship between the Life within me and
the Life within the patient during treatment. If you take away your
personality completely, take away your name, take away everything
you own in life, then you are simply a body physiology at work.

If I can work on a one-on-one basis to understand what their mechanism is trying to tell me, then I will be guided by the type of pattern
and the type of function that is within that patient. The patient's
mechanism is literally in charge of things, in charge of that patient.
When treating, I am not looking for a pattern within that mechanism;
I listen to the mechanism functioning and let it inform me.

Here is a clinical case to illustrate this point. A patient comes into
the office, and he's been having brachial neuritis for over 18 months.
He's a tough, young man who has also been having a lot of headaches, and he generally feels miserable. He has all kinds of complaints
focused around the brachial plexus region. When a patient comes in
with so many complaints, I remind myself that these patients are going to be living for a long time, and I don't have to solve all their
problems the day they come into the office.

We then begin a treatment program, and after two or three treatments, I am aware of the fact that he is not improving. He hasn't
made any changes at all. Normally, the body physiology is constantly
making changes, and this fact is used to make an assessment at the
follow-up visit: Did they or did they not make any changes since the
last treatment? The body physiology of the patient gives you something to make a comparison with from treatment to treatment. I am
aware of the fact that the potential for change is actively there for

every single treatment on a one-on-one basis.

So, after about the third treatment, this guy is still having the same pain in the same area, and he isn't particularly happy with it. Then I realize that I must be sitting at the wrong end of the lever. All the noise is coming from the upper body, but nothing is having an effect there. He gets no relief. Then I go down and get my hands underneath the sacrum, and the thing is so completely locked that it is impossible for it to go into flexion and extension. To test for motion down there, I get one hand under the sacrum and the other forearm across the ilia. Then as he flexes and extends his feet, I feel the whole pelvis dip as one unit. This means that his sacrum is totally locked down in that pelvis; otherwise, when he moves his feet, the sacrum and ilia would feel like three units that can function independently.

So, the sacrum was locked in his pelvis, but where were all the symptoms? Up at the other end. They were complaining up there because they literally had to function against the totally locked pelvis. There was pain, there was neuralgia, there was a pull on the fascia. His symptoms were coming out of a totally locked pelvis that had to be the result of something, so I got to questioning him. It turned out that he owned a sports car, and he'd had the engine out on blocks to work on it, but the engine weighed 250 pounds and he weighed 150 pounds. He had lifted that heavy engine over and put it on the blocks. In the process of doing that, in that awkward position, he locked the sacrum right down between his two ilia. It had no other place to go. To treat this, I applied a hold across the pelvis, across the involved tissues, and worked with it utilizing the tidal mechanism coming down through there 10 times a minute.

When you get ahold of a strain pattern, you put it to work. You grab ahold of the tissues in and around that area and add a little compression. You tease the mechanism, which is automatically going into flexion, extension, internal and external rotation, and follow the strain patterns within that area. I place my hands in the involved area and apply enough compression through my arms, or otherwise, to make some type of change. In this case, compression on the ilia acts in such a way as to tease them, to say, "Hey, wake-up; we're working on you."

In the case of this young man, after another couple of treatments, I was able to read in those tissues that there was something beginning to function in that 18-month-old problem. The next time he came back, all of a sudden, the pelvis shook, the sacrum went back to work, and he lost all of the symptomatology.

The point that I'm trying to make is that we are guided by the living physiology of the patient to go looking for the places we need to work–not where they are having symptoms, but where there is something that can be done to allow their body to train itself to let go of its problems.

By constantly reading the situation, we can realize what the tissues did, what we think they might do, and then we can patiently help them to do what is needed. There is a constantly-shifting source of information available within the patient. What does that body have that it wants to tell me? How can I tease it to make it speak louder? How can I feel something that's going to happen, and then all of a sudden, I'm aware that it did happen, so I'd better let go and let it go home and get well? It's an organized approach for allowing a human mechanism to make a human change in a living body by a living physician. A lot of things can get done on a one-on-one basis.

THOUGHTS ON TREATMENT

These are excerpts from written lecture notes
with dates ranging from 1969 to 1986.

THERE IS A CONSCIOUS and unconscious tendency to separate cranial osteopathy from body osteopathy in our thinking. We need to eliminate this notion of separation from our thinking, consciously and unconsciously. It is essential that we eliminate this dichotomy in our thinking and *know* the body as a whole in the science of osteopathy. It is one unit of functioning from the top of the head to the soles of the feet. When it comes to managing a clinical problem, consider it always as a problem involving the total science of osteopathy.

♦ Technique versus principle: Doing something to a problem is technique; working with an inherent mechanism within the problem is an application of a principle, not a technique.

♦ Healing: an individual manifestation of a universal principle.
♦ Health: harmonious, effectual living.

♦ Treatment: Treat people, not clinical problems in people.

♦ Can you listen and observe the inherent effort of the anatomicophysiology of the patient to self-correct? Can you allow the living needs of the patient to manifest themselves and to cooperate with their program for return to health?

♦ Once you open the door—when you first make contact with the patient's mechanism—it may take 30 seconds or a minute for it to recognize that the door has been opened.

♦ Health is being restored when flexion/external rotation, extension/ internal rotation of the involuntary mechanisms of the body manifest themselves.

♦ The treatment phase is knowing when to take your hands off–knowing when the treatment is through. Up until then, it is *all* diagnostic phase.

♦ Patients and their problems do not retrace steps to return to health: Health is NOW.

Frequency of Treatment: What does the patient's physician-within report? What does the innate vitality of the tissues tell you? How long does it take between office visits for the initiating treatment to absorb into the patient's tissues? Remember that treatment takes place between office visits, not in the office on the table. Shorter times are needed for acute cases, longer times for more chronic cases. Some cases require time to "prepare the ground to receive the seed" of a successful program of treatment.

Space treatments so as to allow the *initiated* changes at the treatment site to continue their correction at the problem site and to work their way throughout the whole of body physiology. The whole patient is under treatment, not just the local area which brought the patient to the physician.

Over-treatment: If you get a patient who has a feeble quality to their tide, you can over-treat them. I've done this many a time; I'm an authority on it. They come in with a rate of 6, and you think you're heading them back to 10 or 12, but you end up beating them down to 3 or 4. If you find a patient who is rundown with a rate of 6, that's all you've got to work with, so stay within its tolerance, and that will allow the patient to recharge to a higher level. Don't force the patient down into another level or up to a level they can't reach.

Asymmetry: If you lay your hands on a patient's chest and have them take a big breath, you will observe that no one is bilaterally symmetrical. As a person breathes in, one side of the body is going to rotate out a lot, while little happens on the other side of the body; but then with exhalation, the side that didn't move much will internally rotate a lot more than the other side. Similarly, as the fluctuation of the cerebrospinal fluid expands in its tidal movement, you're going to feel the body go into external rotation on one side more easily than it does on the other, with the opposite moving more freely during the extension/internal rotation phase.

Father Dura

At a 1986 Sutherland Cranial Teaching Foundation Faculty Meeting, Dr. Becker described a technique called "Father Dura," which was taught to him by Dr. Sutherland.

Dr. Sutherland states that you can actually feel a difference in the direction of movement between the inner and outer table of the vault bones. If you observe carefully, the inner table is moving slightly differently from the outer table. To work with this is a matter of quietly sitting there and gently increasing the pressure on that ossification center until you find the point of balance, then quietly holding that point of balance, reading the point of balance, and allowing a shift between the inner and outer table of each vault bone.

Patterns of the Cranial Base

The experience of learning to go through the patterns of the cranial base with our minds and our hands, and to appreciate the living reciprocal tension membrane's capacity to shift the sphenobasilar mechanism into various patterns, is useful because these patterns definitely have clinical significance in certain types of problems. It is also important to understand these patterns in a broader sense. When we go through these sphenobasilar synchondrosis patterns, we're finding out for ourselves the pattern in which this patient lives. There's more to it than just finding out that the reciprocal tension membrane is able to do all this wiggle waggle in each of our heads.

It is important to know whether a patient has a basic torsion, sidebending-rotation, or vertical or lateral strain pattern underneath a specific membranous articular strain involving two bones—that is, to know what their pattern of physiologic function was before they got a superimposed strain. It is good to know when we get through with the corrective procedure of the specific membranous articular strain that a normal cranial base pattern has been reestablished for that particular patient.

We do not name a torsion lesion, for example, and then try to make the mechanism fit the picture; we go to the mechanism and discover these structures are in a particular relationship—so what do we call it? If we think in terms of the function of these areas, then we can put a name on the lesion for the way it works. Dr. Sutherland struggled for many years to find names to fasten onto things. He felt these things function, and then he had to come up with a name to fit that which the body was teaching him as he listened to it.

What health patterns do we seek in our patients?

1. Determine the base pattern or patterns the patient has lived with all his life. Observe the normal to-and-fro movement of flexion/external rotation and extension/internal rotation of the primary

respiratory mechanism and body physiology, *and* the presence of a torsion, sidebending-rotation, or whatever other pattern is the patient's life mechanism.

2. Note the quality of function of these base patterns. Is there good vitality or poor vitality? What is the quality of the battery? 110 volts or 50 volts? Are there round and full excursions during rhythmic cycles of function or flat and indistinct ones? Ask yourself, How can this body physiology respond to a treatment?

3. What added stress patterns are present that brought this patient to you for diagnosis and treatment?

4. Choose the area you are going to work on. Choose a stress pattern which seems to be the area that switches the physician's intent from a diagnosis to a treatment mode—in other words, you find that while you are diagnosing the area, it moves into a treatment mode.

CAUSE AND EFFECT
This paper was written in the 1960's.

Cause and effect are perpetual. Cause may not be as large in the beginning in some cases as in others, but time adds to the effect until the effect overbalances cause, and the end is death. Death is the end or the sum total of effects.

I only ask of the reader to carefully note the different and continued change in effect as additional elements enter the contest and give effect the ascendancy.[1] *—A.T. Still*

LET US UTILIZE THE thinking of Dr. A.T. Still and discuss, briefly, the role of the osteopathic lesion in cause and effect. How many times a day do we manipulate or mobilize the osteopathic lesion or lesions in our patients and feel that we are doing all we can for those cases in this area of our treatment program? If we were to think deep with Dr. Still as we analyze a lesion problem, we would discover we are dealing with effects and not cause in our handling of a case.

We know in our medical care that a high percentage of the medications we prescribe are designed to modify the effects or symptoms of a problem with little or no design to change the cause. This is also true with mere manipulation or mobilization of osteopathic lesions we find, if we confine our efforts and thinking to them alone. We modify their pattern of motion and the result is a modification of the symptom pattern for the time being. The next time that case comes to us, we find the lesion pattern has returned to approximately the same condition as before. As Dr. Still says, "I only ask of the reader to carefully note the different and continued change in effect...."

In the early days of osteopathic research, Dr. Louisa Burns applied traumatic force and produced osteopathic lesions in animals and then studied the subsequent phenomena that followed this lesioning process. She and other research workers since that time have been able to develop a very complete picture of all the stages of tissue changes that follow such a lesioning mechanism. We are all acquainted with the details of these changes, so we do not need to discuss them at this time. In Dr. Burns' work, after the lesion phenomenon was permitted to exist for several weeks or months, she applied a corrective force to normalize the lesion mechanics, to bring back into those areas the capacity to function normally, and again she studied the changes that took place in the tissues as they returned to their former health. Thus, she was able to prove the validity of the osteopathic lesion.

Editor's note: The current terminology for the osteopathic lesion is "somatic dysfunction." For a description of its pathophysiology, the reader is referred to Foundations For Osteopathic Medicine, *ed. Robert C. Ward, (Baltimore: Williams & Wilkins, 1997).*

We, as members of the osteopathic profession, have learned to focus our attention on looking for the osteopathic lesion. We find it. We fix it. We leave it alone. That is not enough. We have not included the traumatic force it took to produce that osteopathic lesion. The osteopathic lesion is an effect which in turn is leading to other effects "as additional elements enter the contest and give effect the ascendancy." Note carefully, Dr. Burns applied a traumatic force to produce a lesion. If we are to reason with Dr. Still, we should think through this lesion pattern to the traumatic force it took to produce it and include this traumatic force in our effort to correct the lesion mechanism. It is possible to do this with a trained palpatory touch that can think deep, feel deep, see deep, and know deep.

What kind of traumatic forces do we look for? There is the whiplash injury case wherein the patient may weigh as much as 15 tons at the moment of the impact upon the bumper of the car six feet away from the patient's body. Every molecule of his body is hurled forcewise towards the point of impact. This total impact of force must be included in the correction program for his case. Then there are the literally hundreds of thousands of little environmental traumatic forces that produce various strains in body mechanics: picking up a hundred-pound bag of fertilizer the wrong way, twisting and reaching too far to make a bed, reaching overhead to bring a heavy box off a shelf, a sudden cough or sneeze in an awkward position, stepping off a curb we didn't see, carrying a load of fireplace wood away from our bodies so as not to get our clothes dirty, and as many more ways as you care to investigate or discover for yourself or learn from the histories of the patients who come to you. Each of these force factors is individualized, and each has been added to the body physiology of the patient who is seeking your help. Each of them must be evaluated and added to the diagnostic survey you are making in this patient before you. Some of this detail can be learned by a careful history as to the exact type of strain, the direction of its impact, the amount in quantity and quality of the load involved, the movements of the body of the patient, the time element since the accident occurred, and all other information pertinent to the case. The trained palpatory touch can read the tissues involved and gain as much or more information as the history can.

What about the osteopathic lesions we find associated with disease rather than that of known traumatic forces? These, too, are forces but are more subtle in their beginnings as causes for osteopathic lesions. These are forces at the molecular levels of germ and virus particles that are truly as environmental as that heavy load of logs we attempted to carry into the house.

In either case, trauma or disease, the osteopathic lesion or lesions we have found are effects and not causes. To find them and treat them as a unit in themselves is to neglect one half the reason our patient came to us. We are only giving her symptomatic relief if this is as far as our reasoning extends in her care. We must learn to read through the osteopathic lesion pattern and to pick up the beginnings of it as a traumatic or disease process and to include the energies that it took to produce it in our diagnostic and therapeutic procedures. This is, in part, the osteopathy that Dr. A.T. Still would have us practice in our daily work. As a mental exercise, review the problems you saw yesterday. In how many cases did you or I attempt to reach back to the cause and thus to produce a corrective change towards total health for that patient?

1. A.T. Still, *Autobiography*, pp. 202-203.

DOMINION OF HEALTH

This is excerpted material from lecture notes dated May 23, 1973.

"Health holds dominion over the body by laws as immutable as the laws of gravitation, and so long as we obey the laws that make for health, one need have no fear of disease." —*A.T. Still*

Cause and Effects—Section I: Case Histories

1. Woman, age 26. Severe headaches and pain since 18 years old. Portion of parietal-temporal bone removed on right side for cerebral decompression at age 19. Cerebral edema, multiple central nervous system and peripheral nerve disturbances, vagal syndromes, and somatic problems. In last year, had five major diagnostic surveys with pneumoencephalogram at each survey. No diagnosis established. Difficult labor at 18 years with second child.

2. Woman, age 44. Severe, intractable headaches and pain for four years. Multiple medical evaluations. No relief. Severe fall on sacrum on a rock when ten years old; in bed for a week.

3. Young woman delivered triplets, the three weighing 21 pounds. Nine months after delivery, she came in walking and functioning as though pelvic mechanism was still carrying triplets.

4. Woman who had pneumonia in her twenties with "good recovery." 15 years later, had secondarily induced hepatitis with three years of disability, cortisone, etcetera. Developed cirrhosis of liver.

5. Man with an auto accident in his teens, with loss of normal involuntary mobility. 20 years later had developed symptoms of glass-like rigidity and trophic changes in the cervical and thoracic areas.

6. Several cases of men with severe falls on the sacrum, completely locking its respiratory movement and distorting the sacrum. This alteration in low back function persistent for 20, 30, 40, 55 years. This

situation is difficult to diagnose due to total lack of sacral respiratory motion with chronic fibrotic changes. They present with gradual musculoskeletal problems through the entire spine with increasing age. They have vague and not-so-vague symptoms, which bring the patient to you year after year.

7. 30-year-old man with constant pain in cervical and thoracic areas for ten years. Saw many specialists, with no diagnosis or relief. He had bulbar-meningeal polio at age of nine years. Intensive care in hospital for one month. Physiotherapy for a year. Good athlete.

8. Man with rheumatoid arthritis who required bilateral hip protheses.

There are multiple short-term diseases and traumas that need adequate diagnosis and treatment to prevent future problems. Most of the above could have experienced short-term problems if they had received adequate physiological diagnosis and treatment in the beginning. All the above are effects, powered by a potency for every clinical problem.

Cause and Effects—Section II: Health Patterns

Primary respiratory mechanism

Muscular-skeletal-fascial systems
Peripheral nervous system

Visceral systems
Autonomic nervous system

All health patterns are functioning *effects*.

All are integrated, all are intermeshed, all are intrameshed for health with the capacity to work, to play, to think, to emote, to pray, to shift in functioning to meet every need, to interchange within and without the environment and the universe in which they exist.

This is the pattern in which "Health holds dominion over the body by laws as immutable as the laws of gravitation."

This is a *dominant* pattern of *functioning* health specific for each individual, and it is powered by a potency.

Cause and Effects—Section III: Diagnosis and Treatment

When a patient comes to you and me, they come with a complaint or multiple complaints and a history of trauma and/or disease. We take a history, we make an examination, do laboratory studies, etcetera, and with our skilled hands, we feel for a possible physiological and pathological reason for the patient's problem. We diagnose the problem as a problem of disrupted health.

Our number-one task should be to seek and be aware of the dominant functioning pattern of health that dwells in each individual, to *feel* it in its functioning, and to understand that which is specifically health for that individual at the time of the initial examination. Our second task should be to recognize the existing patterns of dysfunction as an overlay on this *dominant* pattern of health. Understand the specific, fundamental health pattern we are seeking for this individual, this office visit, this diagnostic and treatment time, and plan to bring it through for full functioning. All the cases described in Section I are effects, traumatic or disease effects leading to more disabling effects with the passage of time.

The dominant health patterns described in Section II are *effects*.

The traumatic and disease patterns are powered by a potency specific for each effect and specific for each tissue involved in the traumatic or disease condition in order for it to exist, but these are *not* dominant potencies as long as there is reversibility left in the tissues with which to return to health. If they become irreversible, these potencies become dominant for the specific trauma or disease. Some cancers would be an example.

The dominant health pattern in man and woman is powered by a potency to *be* health. It is the power source the physician should seek and work with in determining the dominant, functioning health pattern he is seeking in each patient with each treatment session.

It is not enough to be able to diagnose the key strains or disease patterns manifesting as complaints that bring the patient to you. Whatever diagnosis or treatment program you set up for that patient, let your mind, consciousness, awareness, and hands go *through* the tissue-oriented trauma or disease entity and determine the dominant pattern of health and functioning that should be and is present for that area of physiology and pathology. Utilize the greater potency of the health pattern to deliver a change towards health functioning in the traumatic or diseased tissue while you examine and treat the patient. Do not be satisfied with just a diagnosis and treatment of a trauma or disease entity in itself.

Take dominion over the health pattern that is present in that individual and deliver it into action. Be conscious and aware that you have aroused the dominant health pattern and can feel it in action with your trained sense of touch within the patient in your treatment program. Do this daily with every patient, every visit.

EMOTIONAL FACTORS

This is an edited excerpt from the article, "An Osteopathic Concept and its Relationship to the Osteopathic Lesion," which was published in the 1952 Yearbook of the Academy of Applied Osteopathy (currently named the American Academy of Osteopathy).

WE HAVE BEEN TAUGHT that the differential diagnosis between a neurosis and a psychosomatic illness is that a neurotic develops a consciously motivated resistance to some factor in their environment while a psychosomatic illness is characterized by unconsciously motivated resistances to environmental factors, and "these resistances constitute objective phenomena that serve to indicate the dynamic biologic significance of the total illness."[1] These patients rarely know what is bothering them and will protest that there is nothing wrong with them when the possibility of a hidden tension is brought to their attention.

Osteopathic treatment for both classes of patients is one of the finest therapeutic measures available. As the recognized osteopathic lesions present are normalized, the hidden tensions tend to be brought to the surface and resolved. The osteopathic treatment, when "scientifically prescribed, accurately dosed, and skillfully administered," as Dr. Arthur D. Becker used to say, tends to normalize the free flow of blood, fluids, energy and other vital forces to the lesioned areas and, what is equally important, normalizes the free flow of blood, fluids, energy and other vital forces away from the lesioned areas. A true normal ebb and flow towards health.

We can carry our reasoning one step further. In addition to recognizing the therapeutic value of treating the osteopathic lesion in these complex cases, we can also see the osteopathic lesion as a powerful diagnostic aid in the analysis of neurosis and psychosomatic illness. In the differential diagnosis of somatic ailments from the neurosis and psychosomatic cases, it is noted that there is an added resistance factor in the latter two that exists in addition to the resistance of disordered physiology in somatic illness. This added resistance can be recognized and, in part, interpreted by the thoroughly trained, alert, and aware osteopathic touch. In other words, if the osteopathic physician will consciously realize, as he examines every case that comes to him, that environmental factors may be adding their resistances to the osteopathic lesions in the somatic problem that is so apparent to him, he will gather a greater insight into the true cause of the disturbance before him. This can be and is clinically demonstrable; it is an aid to use in diagnosis, and definitely contributes a valuable asset to one's practice habits.

Adding this diagnosis of environmental factors to the diagnosis of somatic factors does not necessarily mean every case will be dramatized with great discoveries. However, the added service of knowing as to when, where, and how the lesion occurred is a tremendous help to the patient and provides a more lasting, therapeutic relief when the disordered physiology is brought under control. Occasionally, the physician will be able to recognize a more serious, long-standing, hidden resistance, which may be an environmental problem or a fear of cancer, tuberculosis, or some other equally disabling phenomenon in the patient's way of thinking. Then, as this resistance is gradually resolved in the subsequent examinations, discussions, and treatment, the doctor has a friend for life as well as a thoroughly satisfied patient.

1. Hart, Andrew D., M.D., "Psychosomatic Diagnosis," *JAMA.*, Jan.17, 1948, 136:147-149.

BALANCED MEMBRANOUS TENSION

This is an edited transcription of a lecture given in 1976 at a Sutherland Cranial Teaching Foundation basic course in Milwaukee, Wisconsin.

WHEN A STRAIN OCCURS, the membranes carry this pattern of strain, which has the effect of shifting the "normal" fulcrum over towards the point of strain, the point at which the area went into strain. Within this strain, there is a point of balanced membranous tension. There is a fulcrum point, a relative point of stillness around which all the forces are gathered. When you bring all of these forces into focus, the mechanism goes through a stillpoint, a fulcrum point, a moment of stillness. And when it goes through that stillpoint, the fulcrum shifts back towards the so-called normal pattern for that individual—towards the Sutherland fulcrum—and you have a correction for that particular day. Through this process, you are shifting the fulcrums within the cerebrospinal fluid and reciprocal tension membrane. The stillpoint is often obvious, although many times you'll go through the thing without ever realizing it. In these cases, you will notice that instead of a lot of arguments going on inside the head, it feels as if it's smooth, it feels comfortable, and maybe the head gets hot; then you know you have gone through it.

How do you use the principle of balanced membranous tension? Say you decide for that day that your treatment is to be directed at a torsion right lesion; you initiate it into that torsion pattern, you allow it to go to the full excursion, and then you gently hold it in that area and do not allow it to come back to neutral again. As you hold it there, it goes through its cycle of argument, goes through a stillpoint, and then you allow it to drift back to whatever new neutral it has discovered.

In doing this, you have not only worked on a torsion membranous articular strain pattern, you have induced a change through the fascial structure of the thirty-four muscles attached to the base of the skull and through all the fascias of the system. You have corrected a torsion pattern for the entire system of the body. Therefore, if you run into one that has a lot of arguments and takes forever, be glad; it is not that the local cranial problem is holding you up, it's that there are torsion factors in the fascia, clear down through the pelvis to the feet, that also have to get quieted down and shift gears so these forces can come and go through a stillpoint. Also, you will find that somebody with a sick body is going to respond slower than somebody with healthy fascia.

When you focus your treatment on a local strain, a specific membranous articular pattern, you're shrinking the mass of stuff that's being worked on to the small area of the membranous articular strain. But even then, you not only have all the local membranous articular strain factors but also the fluids, the dynamic forces, and the associated fascias as part of the traumatic pattern. When you are working on a local cranial membranous strain, the stillpoint may seem smaller, but it is the same. The membranous articular shifting is at a smaller level—you're dealing with a wristwatch, not an alarm clock. There is little motion in the skull in comparison to the rest of the body anyway, and we're going to shrink it even more to get at the specific membranous articular strain. No matter the size or location of the strain, the principles are the same.

This balanced membranous tension is not a static thing. I may find that I'm using exaggeration to kick off the pattern, and as my hands are working with this area, it may need disengagement, and I may even introduce a little bit of opposing physiologic mobility, but I'm not necessarily doing it consciously. I may discover after I have gone through the cycle that I have induced all those factors because I was consciously following a membranous articular pattern that told me I should introduce those factors during the treatment program.

These principles we give you are principles of treatment, true, but they are also principles we apply as we train our palpatory skills. A famous conductor once said that a conductor commands a sound image of the author's symphony to manifest itself and expects the musicians in the orchestra to bring this living sound image forward in response to the command. I wonder—what is the difference between that and laying your hands on a patient, contacting a flowing, living mechanism, and commanding a response from the tissue? The musicians are the multiple tissues involved, and they are going to respond in return to your command and cooperate with you to manifest the perfection you're trying to bring through for the body's health. Beautiful.

CHILDREN: DIAGNOSIS AND TREATMENT
This paper was dated September 1984.

THE ROLE THAT OSTEOPATHY in the cranial field plays in infants and children is one of the great contributions in the science of health care. Health care in today's science has shown a phenomenal growth of technological skills, from microsurgery to biologic tests and treatment procedures. The cranial concept is as much a part of this technology as are all the other units of health care. All units of health care are dependent on the same innate vitality in the patient and rely on it for the results the physician desires to obtain. The cranial concept's role in diagnosis and treatment is a one-on-one active use of the innate vitality of the infant, child, or adult. This concept, together with trained palpation tools, provides the technology for understanding the details of health in body physiology. In diagnosis and treatment, it is one unit of life in motion in the individual, whatever the age.

The adult is a relatively stable body physiology, functioning as a basic mobile mechanism. He is not a bilaterally symmetric structure-function unit. His mechanism includes an element of torsion or sidebending-rotation as well as other potential patterns that are his anatomicophysiology in health. There are as many superimposed variations in the structure-function of body units as there are individuals, but all of them carry a specific pattern within that says, "This is this individual's health functioning." And this is the health pattern within that the physician is seeking in his care for the patient. These variations begin in the prenatal, natal, and postnatal periods and on up through the early years of life. In this time, there are few articular gears, and those which have developed have been modified by external forces.

In early life, the cranium, as a structure, is still developing. The frontals and parietals are membranous plates and have a membranous interlacing. Those bones at the base of the skull are developing in cartilage. There are 11 small pieces of cartilaginous bones in the cranial base at birth—four for the occiput, three for the sphenoid, and two each for the temporal bones—held together by intercartilaginous unions and by the reciprocal tension membrane with its three sickles and its inferior pole of attachment at the sacrum. These eleven pieces become four—sphenoid, occiput, and two temporals—as time permits ossification centers to mature and unite. Consider all the fascial and connective tissue elements that fasten to the base of the skull and form the framework for the body. Consider the rhythmic fluctuation of the cerebrospinal fluid and the midline and bilateral 8-to-10-times-per-minute mobility taking place in all these developing tissues. If the cranial base were totally free in its development, what would be the structure-function of the body? Then consider the reality, where there are at least minimal and often more severe modifications of the cranial base from external forces that occur in the prenatal, natal, or postnatal period, or later. What would be, and are, the patterns of structure and functioning in the infant, child, or adult?

The only articular gear operating at birth in the cranium is at the junction of the condylar parts of the occiput with the pits of the atlas. The adult occiput is one bone, while the occiput, through the first seven to nine years, is in four parts—a basilar portion at the anterior end of the foramen magnum, two condylar parts forming the lateral borders, and posteriorly, the occipital squama with a cartilaginous union between it and the condylar parts. The condyles converge anteriorly and inferiorly and diverge posteriorly. With the fetal head resting in the pelvis, a compressive force through the amniotic fluid from a labor contraction can drive these condyles into the facets of the atlas, a fulcrum point and the only bony contact at that age. Depending on the direction of force, the condyles can be modified in their cartilaginous contacts with the squama or the basilar process of the occiput to produce a structural pattern a tiny bit different from that which a freely functioning cranial base should be. This will be reflected into the total body structural mechanism as the body matures.

It may be a simple torsion or sidebending-rotation, or it can be the onset of a scoliosis that will appear during the teenage period. Condylar parts dysfunctions are responsive to palpation for diagnosis and treatment.

In this way, compression of the condyles can act as pincers on the basiocciput by approximation of the anterior ends of the condylar parts, resulting in any of a number of possible lesion positions of the sphenobasilar synchondrosis and the reciprocal tension membrane. These are flexion, extension, torsion, sidebending-rotation, vertical strains, lateral strains, and compression. These are lifetime, structural, mobile mechanisms in body physiology. Torsion and sidebending-rotation are considered basically physiological whereas some or all of the others can create unphysiological patterns of disturbance later in life as various maturing elements show some type of dysfunction. An example is a boy, age ten, whose speech was so poor, it could not be understood. His intelligence was normal. He had a lateral strain pattern, sphenoid right. His problem did not appear until two, three, or four years of age, when a child is supposed to start speaking clearly. His lateral strain was gradually corrected over a period of six months, and he became free of his disability. Needless to say, his parents and teachers were grateful.

More serious strains of the cranial base can contribute to cerebral palsy or to any abnormal color, actions, crying, feeding, growth, etcetera. One of the most unusual cases I ever saw was an infant, nine months old, who cried continuously and whose skin from the top of the head to the soles of the feet was covered with open skin lesions, so that it was difficult to find one spot of clear skin on which to put a finger. The history was that this condition existed practically from birth. Not knowing what else to do, I used a fluctuant cerebrospinal fluid technique in the area of the condylar parts of the occiput, quieting the existent, fluctuant pattern until it went through a stillpoint. That was the treatment for that day. Believe it or not, within twelve hours, the infant grew new skin from head to foot without one single blemish, and it slept all night for the first time in its life. True

266

evidence of innate vitality. The infant was brought back for further treatment over a period of several months, and it did have a few areas of skin irritation but never like its original pattern. In thinking about this now, I reflect on the fact that the central nervous system and the skin both develop from ectoderm, and both were involved in this particular case.

Trained palpation skills with knowledge of the anatomic mechanisms can evaluate total body patterns as well as more specific problems at local sites. Some of these are fascial or ligamentous articular strains which can be found anywhere in the body as a result of the child's activities in his/her day to day living. Allowing the proprioceptive touch to diagnose and work with the treatment of restoring health in lesioned tissues is a one-on-one relationship between the physician and the innate vitality of the infant or child. A case in point was a boy, nine years old, who had a fall the year before and developed a persistent limp. Examination revealed a ligamentous articular strain in the left acetabular area. Palpation testing for the rhythmic external-internal rotation in the right hip showed it was in health, but on the lesioned side, this external-internal rotation was limited or inactive. Corrective treatment of the ligamentous articular strain was made, and reevaluation of the alternating external-internal rotation was checked in both hips and found to be equal. This indicated a restoration towards health was achieved in the left hip.

The craniosacral mechanism of the infant or child has a number of specific sites for lesion production. Some of the most common membranous articular strains found in older children are occipitomastoid, frontosphenoidal, and temporal strains. In these early years, the emphasis should be on the membranous. The time between production of the strain and symptomatology can be weeks, months, or years. In one patient, a blow on the occiput at age four, compressing it inward at the mastoid portion of the temporal and right tentorium cerebelli, gave no symptoms until age 24. A girl's fall on her sacrum at age ten, locking its involuntary mobility, showed itself as severe head pain at age 42. A whiplash type of locked sacral dysfunction showed itself as trophic disturbance in the upper thoracic area 20 years later. Any of these strain patterns can be diagnosed by training one's palpation skills and using them to also effect a corrective treatment program towards health.

There are two diagnostic and treatment aids that I have found useful in working with the patient's mechanisms, and they also save time for the physician using them. The first is the use of testing the inherent, alternate, rhythmic fluctuant cerebrospinal fluid and midline and bilateral mobility at the site of lesion and some other portion of the body that is in health. Testing before and after treatment is valuable evidence for checking the results desired. The second is that in the child's skull, the articular gears take until 10 to 13 years to begin to develop the stability of the adult. Therefore, the reciprocal tension membrane is the dominant factor for the craniosacral structure, and the fascia is dominant in body structure. I have found it easier and more efficient to work through and with one or both of these units in the care of infants and children. Any diagnostic information and treatment change reports itself to me through these units of function.

In closing, I once heard Dr. Sutherland make a statement, "If you understand the mechanism, your technique is simple." How true! No infant is too young or a child too old that he or she cannot be examined and treated using the basic principles of the science of osteopathy. Any corrective work done at this early age is preventive care for later years, and you get better health in the process.

The Nature
Of Trauma

FORCE FACTORS WITH BODY PHYSIOLOGY

This article has been extensively edited from the original, which was published in the 1959 Yearbook *of the Academy of Applied Osteopathy (currently named the American Academy of Osteopathy).*

THE LITERATURE OF THE day is filled with discussion of the effects of force *upon* body physiology. All traumatic experiences call for an analysis of what has happened to body physiology and what course of action is to be undertaken to treat the problems that have arisen as a result. It is also important to view this traumatic experience in another light, that of recognizing the role that the traumatic force plays in its relationship *with* body physiology. To clarify this picture, it is necessary to have a concise picture of body physiology itself, and this can be found, in part, in a discussion of homeostasis. The first part of this paper will be a short discussion of homeostasis, and the last part will discuss some of the principles involved in understanding the role of force with body physiology.

Homeostasis

In 1932 in his book, *The Wisdom of the Body*, Walter B. Cannon perfected the theory and the work of Claude Bernard concerning the processes of self-regulation within the body and gave it the name "homeostasis." Cannon has defined homeostasis as "a tendency to uniformity or stability in the normal body states of the organism." The theory of homeostasis can be compared with the principles of A.T. Still's osteopathic concept; the similarity is evident.

Cannon starts from a recognition of instability and sets his task as that of understanding how the body remains stable at all. Homeostasis is that principle of the body that indicates the automatic stability that the body is forever seeking—the capacity of the body to operate on a functional basis within an inherent, normal range of activity.

The stability of the body has its origin in its "natural instability," as Cannon calls it. It is a cyclic biochemical, physiological, mechanical, electrical mechanism beginning its work for a specific task, performing its work to a conclusion, and automatically returning the body condition to its given level again in preparation for a new task. Such a viewpoint clarifies the automatic feature of the body, which is "set in motion at the very beginning of a disturbance," according to Cannon.

All the physiological processes of the body exhibit this principle of natural instability: the pulse wave, the electrocardiographic tracing, the electroencephalographic reading, the blood sugar curve, the acid-base equilibrium of the blood stream, the CO_2 concentration of the blood, and a host of others. Within each process, there are dynamic pivotal points that initiate the stability of the body system; all functioning starts from these points and returns to them in readiness for their next cycle of change. William G. Sutherland once referred to this pivotal point in the respiratory cycle as "...the midway point between inhalation and exhalation, not at the end of inhalation or exhalation but at the balance point between inhalation and exhalation."

The capacity to be forever ready for action in response to any stimulus can be more readily understood if the body is visualized as starting from a dynamic, natural instability factor rather than from a static stability factor. The term homeostasis can be very misleading for "stasis" indicates stagnation, a status quite different from the biodynamic vitality of the physiological processes involved. Homeostatic controls are ones that work automatically, in a compelling way, to bring a given entity back to a discernible baseline of maximum operating efficiency; they are genetically determined in the biologic world. It is rather overwhelming to consider the composition of subatomic particles, atoms, molecules, cells, fluids, gases, solids, organs, and systems that make up the whole body—all in reciprocal balanced interchange. Even when the body is at total rest in deepest sleep, there is an integrated wholeness of purposeful activity operating constantly.

Today's world of the science of health and disease has produced a multitude of tests to measure the end products of physiological functioning but practically none that indicate the processes themselves during their active phase of production. A urine test or a blood analysis only indicate the state of the body at the time the sample was taken. When the tests are run a few hours later, the body has developed a whole new set of quantitative and qualitative values. The fault lies in the instruments themselves. An instrument, to be accurate, necessarily has to be limited in its adaptation in order to have validity, and in that limitation, it can only cover a small field of reaction, while a multitude of factors that contribute to that reaction are left untouched.

The problem is not insurmountable, however. The physician who is willing to learn the many parts of the body, both as to their positional location and their functional aspect as they operate within the integrated body, has made a great stride towards this understanding. He must know where each part is in the scheme of the framework and know what is its maximum operating efficiency in its functioning status within the framework, using the total physiological functioning of the body itself as a point of reference. This is more than merely testing for the end products of its capacities. For example, such a physician does not just test the passive range of motion of the acetabulum by external and internal rotation of the thigh upon the pelvis; he seeks to know the capacity of the body to externally and internally rotate the acetabulum as demonstrated by the body itself with its own self-regulatory, reciprocally balanced mechanisms. This is what Dr. Still was referring to when he made the statement, "Anatomy [and physiology] understood."

By developing perceptual skills in his touch, the physician should be able to sense these self-regulatory mechanisms within the biodynamic framework of the body. He should be able to reinforce, aid in the restoration, direct and control the processes that are already working within the body to attain the maximum baseline of equilibrium. To do so, he must know the body as it operates in health. If he understands it in health, he will recognize dysfunction when it manifests. The body carries templates of normal functioning within every phase of its self-regulatory mechanisms. The physician can learn to use the forces already present in these templates to guide his corrections from states of dysfunction towards normal functioning. The body does its own work automatically in maintaining health and will do its own work, to a large extent, in assisting the physician to restore it to health when treating disease or injury.

The body is in dynamic reciprocal balanced interchange between all of its components–mechanically, biochemically, and electrically. The body is forever seeking to restore the perfect balance in the wholeness of its activities, and it is necessary to work with it, if the maximum baseline of efficiency is to be obtained. Rather than the application of force from without, the physician listens to the living body itself for the *modus operandi* for its own restoration of health.

The energies involved to produce and maintain this integration of a homeostatic mechanism are poorly understood. Andrew Taylor Still, Arthur D. Becker, William G. Sutherland, Carl P. McConnell, and others have indicated that these energies exist and can be studied and used in diagnosis and treatment. There is a great deal of work to be done to create a better understanding of these energies. Such studies should include more than biological information. They must include all the forces of physics, chemistry, and other allied sciences as well as all the known laws for gases, liquids, and solids, and laws that have yet to be discovered. In addition, there is a deeper layer of activity that has been barely touched upon. This deeper layer has to do with the energies that integrate the animated, living, homeostatic body. The day will come when they, too, will be catalogued and their laws understood. Until then, the physician reasons with the physiological functioning that is apparent and works with it as he develops a better understanding. This, then, is a brief analysis of homeostasis and is the foundation on which a discussion of trauma or force with body physiology will continue.

Force With Body Physiology

It is the purpose of this portion of the paper to fuse force with body physiology. Victor F. Lenzen, in his monograph, "Causality in

Natural Science," makes an important interpretation of force on a given body, not as an activity or mere symbol but as a characteristic of the external bodies in the environment of a given body. He says that force is not merely something that has occurred *to* the body but is one of the factors of environment that functions *with* the body.

Body physiology is never at rest. The "still" body is never still. Its internal environment is essentially fluid and is in constant motion. So any external force is being added to an internally moving mechanism. Body physiology is a collection of living cells bathed in moving fluids, whose biodynamic structure is modified when force is fused with body physiology. Cellular systems take on new patterns of functioning with the addition of the force factors. Subjective and objective symptomatology become the order of the day with limitation of motion, pain, neuralgias, myositis, fibrositis, ligamentous and membranous articular strains, and other disturbances. As long as the force factors are present, the body physiology must compensate for this new addition to its normal physiological functioning. The patient must include force factors in every move he makes, in every voluntary activity he undergoes, in every involuntary activity of his internal environment. It has become written into his cellular structure and function, into his homeostatic mechanism.

My current thinking is that these force factors driving into the body physiology carry a wave-like motion into every cell and into the fluid matrix. This in turn is recorded by the peripheral nervous system, and this nerve imprint becomes part of the central nervous system pattern. If there has been a strong enough impression made upon the central nervous system, it includes this data within its makeup of orders that are fed out through the motor system, the trophic system, and the autonomic nervous system. The whole organism has created a new pattern for functioning in keeping with the body physiology plus force factors. This is in addition to the local injuries that have been endured by the body, which are usually the only thing treated by the physician.

Cell intelligence is a recognized quality of all biologic tissues, and in circumstances of trauma, thousands of cells have had their inertial patterns suddenly disturbed from their normal patterns of functioning into new patterns that include force factors thrusting them in specific directions for action and motion. The sensory nervous system records these new sensations. If the impression has been great enough, such sensory nerve messages are continued for hours or days, depending upon the injury. They will be continued as long as there is shock in the tissues, and that is long enough to establish a definite change within the central nervous system data. Thereafter, the central nervous system must include this new data in every voluntary and involuntary use of the local areas involved and in varying degrees throughout the entire body physiology.

This is why we often find it is comfortable for the patient to voluntarily move his body in the direction in which the force factors were introduced into his body, but if that given motion is in any direction at variance with the introduced force factors, it is disturbing to the patient. He is cooperating with the data that has been written into his nervous system in one case and is going "against the grain" in his other movements.

As time goes by, this basic imprint into his body physiology becomes part of his new mechanism, with a subsequent loss of baseline efficiency as compared to a body physiology without the additional force factors. Local tissues under direct orders from all these stimuli become more susceptible to further injury and strains by the lowered resistance.

The trained perceptual touch and examination by the skillful operator provide the first clues to this syndrome in the majority of cases because it is through the physician's perceptual knowledge that he reads the tissue functioning and tone quality and recognizes that it is different from the normal. He then makes inquiry of the patient as to recent or old injuries that might account for his findings. The patient frequently does not remember any accident that might explain the findings but on subsequent visits will tell the operator of an accident, after his memory has been refreshed. Thus, it is important for the operator to train his perceptual touch to be able to find these areas of disturbed functioning. Here is where his knowledge of what is the normal baseline of equilibrium for every area of the body is the keystone to his understanding. Every accident writes its own story into every type of body physiology that is presented to the operator.

In the diagnostic process, instead of testing the area under stress for the positions that are limited in functioning capacity and are distressing to the patient, the physician should reverse this process. The area is positioned, anatomically and physiologically, towards the point of maximum comfort. Also, since the vast majority of these accidents involve force that has been put upon and is within the patient, a moderate amount of compression is induced by the operator as he seeks the focus of maximum efficiency—not enough compression to interfere with the physiological action of the area but just enough to cooperate with the tissues as they seek their new baseline of equilibrium. This is part of that tone quality mentioned in the last paragraph. The important point is to go towards the focus of comfort, not to try to see how limited the area is but to read the tone quality of maximum efficiency. The tissues will tell the story.

For example, in a woman who had her leg curled under her in a car wreck, when she was positioned according to her accident story, the tone quality and physiological functioning of her injured leg was almost as good as the other leg, especially when a moderate amount of compression was added to the picture to represent the driving force of the sudden stop. The same holds true for all such cases. Each pattern has to be individualized for each patient and each added force factor. There is a perceptible dissipation of these added force factors when the injured areas have been accurately focused in their anatomical and physiological positioning. It is part of the treatment program to so position them that the physiological functioning patterns are brought to the point at which this force factor dissipation can take place. The primary point of treatment is to leave only basic body physiology innate within the injured areas. A more complete healing can then take place, and residual complications are minimized.

Editor's note: Dr. Becker did not always grossly position the patient; instead, with his hands, attention, and small movements of the body, he focused many of these force factors.

Frequently, the tone quality of the tissues is such that it is impossible to secure good, corrective results until the vitality of the areas has been brought up. Correcting the structural abnormalities may appear easy and may take place while the patient is on the table, but the tissue tone and nervous imprinted patterns may be such that the patient has already undone his treatment before he has walked to his car to return home. These imprinted tissue patterns are easily fatigued, and a treatment program must stay within this fatigue factor for each case with each treatment. When the tone quality has come up to something more normal, the basic corrective measures will continue to aid body physiology in restoring itself to its normal baseline of equilibrium. A well-developed perceptual touch will confirm the patient's subjective knowledge that he has resolved his problem.

A treatment program should include all the factors present in each case: a careful history and a perceptual examination; knowledge of the local areas as to their normal baseline of equilibrium and the new baselines of functioning; local mechanical, chemical, circulatory, electrical, and fluid matrix tone qualities; the imprint of the functioning pattern upon the central nervous system through its sensory, motor, trophic, and autonomic factors; and the synthesizing of the whole picture for total evaluation and treatment.

Force affecting body physiology may be imposed from without or created by the individual in his application of his body to his environment. Being hit by a flying object is an example of the former, while a lifting strain illustrates the latter. Force or energy in any form has an influence upon the internal homeostatic mechanisms of the body.

Case Histories

For purposes of illustration, several brief case histories will be given. They serve to illustrate the different applications of energy forms upon each problem and the resulting picture and outcome of each case.

Their purpose is also to bring to your attention that force plus body physiology is an entirely different physiological picture than mere body physiology alone.

Case 1: A man in his middle thirties came in with a complaint of shoulder pains, brachial neuralgia, and recurrent stiff neck over a period of 18 months. The usual local lesions for each of the complaints were present and treated three or four times, with some relief each time, but problems recurred within a few hours after each treatment. Finally, he gave the history that he was a sports car enthusiast, and shortly before all this trouble began, he had taken the engine out of his car to work on it. When it came time to replace it, his helper was not present and he lifted it back into the frame. He thought it only weighed 150 pounds but subsequently learned it weighed 250 pounds. With this history, his chief sustaining problem was found and resolved in two more treatments. There has been no recurrence of any of his symptoms in over three years.

In this case, the force of the lifting strain had locked the sacrum between the ilia at the area of the second sacral segment, although there was no disturbance of the movements of the sacrum upon the ilia at the sacroiliac joints. With a loss of free motion and integrated function of the sacrum between the ilia, the paravertebral muscles and ligaments, including those to both shoulder girdles, were limited in their integrated functioning, and his voluntary use of those structures imposed stress, which was recurrent. Resolving the force factor of the lifting strain and integrating the normal functioning of the sacrum released the problem.

Case 2: A lady in her twenties was in a car accident in which her left ankle sustained a compound fracture. When the problem was supposedly healed, she was left with generalized swelling of the left limb from the pelvis to the foot during the day, with subsidence of the swelling at night. She had experienced this disturbance for one year since the accident. Physical examination revealed ligamentous articular strains in the right iliosacral area, acetabular socket, knee, ankle, and foot, all in internal rotation strains. Eight osteopathic

279

treatments to correct these various internal rotation strains resulted in some reduction of the patterns and some relief of the symptoms and swelling, but the satisfactory progress that seemed to be needed was not made. At the ninth visit, she told me that, at the time of impact, she had been asleep in the back seat. I asked her to assume the position on the treatment table, and she curled herself up on her right side in such a manner as to produce the total pattern of internal rotation for all the structures involved in the symptom complex. The forceful impact of hitting a bridge abutment at 30 miles per hour had created a total pathological, physiological pattern for the limb in question. Treatment to correct the force field maintaining the internal rotation patterns permitted complete normalization of physiological functioning in two visits. In nine years, the symptoms have not recurred.

Case 3: The next case describes another kind of inertial force. A lady in her middle fifties was riding near the rear of a commercial airliner. During the flight, the plane suddenly dropped a few thousand feet without warning, tossing many of the other passengers out of their seats. Many passengers required first aid, although she was not one of them.

Subsequently, she developed tension pains in her shoulders and neck, which radiated into the suboccipital areas. These persisted for three months until she received a treatment that resolved the problem. When there was a sudden change in the direction and speed of the flight, the fluid matrix of the body suffered a new force factor to be added to her body physiology. As long as this force factor was present, her body physiology plus force created a new pattern of functioning. When the force factor was resolved, normal body physiology reasserted itself. One treatment was sufficient to do the job.

Case 4: The next case was that of a young man who was driving 55 miles per hour down the road when another car pulled out in front of him. There was barely time for him to get his foot on the brakes, and he hit the other car. He was not seriously hurt, although his car was severely damaged. He did have some contusions and a sprained ankle. The next day, examination showed local strains as well as the typical lesion found in most whiplash injuries, a loss of motion at the second sacral segment. In addition, the patient complained, "I don't feel as if I am in one piece."

Again, there was a sudden change of inertial motion affecting body physiology. It should be remembered that the body is essentially fluid, and if this man had been a pail of water sitting on the car seat at the time of impact, the water in the pail would have been splashed all over the scene. Treatment to resolve the force factors involved permitting the normal templates of body physiology to reassert themselves, and he left the office feeling in one piece. His various aches and pains also cleared themselves rapidly in the next two days.

Case 5: A similar case was that of a 15-year-old boy who was in a motorcycle accident in which he suffered a compound fracture of the right thigh and twelfth thoracic vertebra and a severe concussion. While he was in the hospital, it took treatment twice a week to resolve the shock in the tissues and in his body physiology. It took until the end of the first month before there was evidence to the perceptual touch of the operator that the normal reparative mechanisms of the body were fully able to do their job without the added insult of the force factors that had been added to his problem.

Case 6: The final case in this series was a 39-year-old man who, two years prior to his initial office visit, had lifted some 100-pound sacks and suffered a disabling low back injury. He had been continuously disabled and was scheduled to go to surgery for a low back fusion operation. His radiographic summary was as follows: 1. grade one spondylolisthesis; 2. extensive spondylosis and arthrosis involving the lumbosacral segments, associated with a nearly complete fusion between the anterior margins of the fifth lumbar body and first sacral segment; 3. marked degeneration of the disk at the fifth interspace suggested by the extensive narrowing involving this interspace.

He had 28 treatments over five months and then was seen monthly for five more months. In that time, there was complete resolution of his disability. He could ride horseback, outrun his son in 100-yard races, and lift buckets of sand from a well on his ranch. After these results were obtained, he was sent to another radiologist for a survey of his problem. The radiologist's report was a duplicate of the first report, yet there has been no recurrence of his symptoms in the past six years. The man still carries all the potentials of a congenitally unstable back with degenerative changes, but his primary problem in this case was that he had added force factors to his body physiology. When these were resolved, his normal compensatory mechanisms had reasserted themselves for his normal functioning.

Included here are two additional case histories taken from other articles.

Case A: A man came to me with a vagal syndrome of severe intensity. He had episodes of violent paroxysmal peristaltic contractions, diarrhea, and other vagal symptoms lasting two to three days. This had recurred one to two times a month for six years. He had been a pilot in World War II and had flown in many missions, making many a multiple, G-force pullout from steep dives. When he was finally shot down in the Burma jungle, he suffered a fractured skull, among other injuries.

It took several office visits to determine the dysfunction: There were many ligamentous articular strains through the spinal areas from the sacrum to the skull, a complex pelvic imbalance, a basilar compression strain pattern, and an occipitomastoid cranial lesion on the left side. Careful resolution of these strains over a period of nine months, with a reevaluation of the predominant role or roles for the functioning that needed corrective care for each treatment, resulted in a good recovery. He is now a professor and occasionally reports to me by mail that he has one or two very minor episodes per year. One can assume that the skull fracture and left occipitomastoid lesion were the primary factors in the vagal syndrome, but it took treatment for the whole body, which had been involved in a whiplash type of strain pattern, in order to restore normal, balanced, autonomic nervous system functioning that would carry him through day-to-day living.

An interesting note can be made about fighter pilots in general. I have examined a few from World War II, the Korean War, and some present-day jet pilots. During steep dives and while pulling out of them, pilots subject themselves to a sustained, whiplash type of movement that crowds them into their pelvises. This pattern can be found on examination. Maybe this is what is meant by the statement, "He flies by the seat of his pants." It is a factor to consider in some of their disabilities.

Case B: In this case, I am going to include four 20 year olds and a 55-year-old female as a group. The young people were each in severe auto accidents, were each unconscious for six months after the accident, and came to me years later. The lady was in an auto accident in which her head was buffeted by the windshield visor and the side of the car. All of these cases had severe cerebral hemisphere damage. All of them were manifesting severe stress syndromes. All of them still had a great deal of "shock" in their whole bodies as well as in the multiple lesion areas.

The initial treatment program was to give physiological care to correct the stress syndrome and shock because then the available physiological functioning in the more normal areas of the body could reassert itself towards the maximum potential healing possible. Irreversible pathology will not correct itself, but a great deal can be done for this type of problem in restoring reversible areas to function again.

What follows is a letter written by Dr. Becker to a colleague, dated September 4, 1981.

Re: Force Factors *with* Body Physiology
Dear Doctor:

In response to your question, I have reread the article after 20 years, and it is too wordy and repetitious, but its basic premise, force factors *with* body physiology, is as valid today as it was when it was written. A brief story as to why it was written is indicated.

The first part of the paper on "homeostasis" can be summarized as the fact that structure-function and function-structure are inter- and intradependent in body physiology. Furthermore, there are the voluntary mechanisms of the body and the rhythmic involuntary mechanisms that work to create flexion with external rotation and extension with internal rotation from the top of the head to the soles of the feet in every cell of the body.

With this background, let me make a point concerning palpation. I used the palpatory skills associated with articulatory-mobilizing techniques for ten years and had such palpatory skills as were adequate for that type of approach. When I realized that structure-function, voluntary and involuntary mechanisms were a reality in body physiology, I had to change my total approach to palpatory skills philosophically and physically. This changeover and retraining period to learn to read basic homeostasis factors in action in body physiology took me three to five years to develop. By now it was 1949.

Over the next ten years, the body physiology of patients demonstrated structure-function, function-structure, voluntary and involuntary mechanisms in health, trauma and/or disease. Surprisingly, a large number of the patients also demonstrated force factors *with* body physiology in their mechanisms. Thus, the paper was written.

The section of the paper with the case histories is still valid after 20 years because there were no recurrences of disability in any of the cases offered as examples. I can also report that every seventh new patient that comes through my office brings with them force factors *with* body physiology in their systems. This is picked up by palpation primarily and then verified by history secondarily. In addition, every air pilot, retired or still working, demonstrates a locked involuntary mechanism from the top of his head to his feet, and all of them show force factor patterns.

The middle part of the paper is an attempt to find an explanation for the phenomena of force factors with body physiology, and I am not satisfied with the idea or ideas offered. A book, *Sensitive Chaos*, by Theodor Schwenk (published in Great Britain, Garden City Press, 1965:1976, 3rd printing), gives alternative solutions to the problem. Read it. I trust it will be of help to you.

X............WHIPLASH INJURY
This article has been extensively edited from the original, which was published in the 1961 Yearbook *of the Academy of Applied Osteopathy (currently named the American Academy of Osteopathy).*

THIS ARTICLE'S TITLE EXPRESSES the beginnings of the whiplash injury: the point of impact "X" which causes the whiplash. It will be the purpose of this paper to discuss these beginnings and some of their effects upon the patient. Three of these effects will be emphasized: the mental and emotional changes induced, the trophic influences within the involved tissues, and the effects of time or chronicity in these patients.

Forces Involved

An analysis of a whiplash problem begins at the point of impact. This point of impact is typically not within the physiology of the patient but is on the vehicle in which the patient is riding at the time of the impact. This force, emanating from the point of impact on the vehicle, comes to involve the whole patient. The whole patient is either in motion, and is brought to a sudden stop, or the direction of his inertial motion is radically changed, or he is in a stopped position and his car is struck by a moving car. In either case, from an inertia at rest to sudden motion or from motion to sudden, relative rest, there is profound physiological shock and change of direction within the whole individual.

Add to this picture, the individual physiological units in active contact with the vehicle. When struck from the rear, the point of contact is the back of the seat in which the patient is sitting. The neck and upper parts of the shoulders are relatively free and are whipped at the time of impact. If the blow strikes the front end of the car, the patient is thrown forward and strikes some part of his body against the dash, steering wheel, or seat belt. In addition, the driver usually has his foot on the accelerator, brake, or clutch pedal, and the force involved is transmitted through the involved extremity. Then, too, the speed of the moving car is always a factor. An experiment done a few years ago shows that objects placed in the rear of a parked car were driven forward at the same speed as the car which struck it.

Given these factors, knowing the details of the accident can be helpful, but it is difficult to get a true picture in most cases. Unless the accident was of recent date, the patient doesn't usually remember much. I have found evidence of these accidents 10 to 30 years after their occurrence.

The physician must understand that the patient has been exposed to a unidirectional arc of force throughout his entire being. The physician, therefore, should try to visualize the patient within that arc in developing an understanding of the physiological changes that have taken place. Add to this picture the specific points of active contact against the patient's body and try to extend these forces into the physiological mechanisms involved. To begin at the patient's body is to adopt a too-near approach to the problem. The direction from which this force came is one of the factors that leads to better understanding of the whiplash injury.

Physiological Body Types

The next factor for consideration is the different types of people and their anatomicophysiological patterns involved in whiplash injuries. Some of these people will be the slender type (ectomorphs) and some the round build (endomorphs). Each of these anatomicophysiological mechanisms will have a different response to the added force from the whiplash injury.

But this is only the beginning. Among individuals, there will be anatomicophysiological variations, such as alterations in the lordotic-kyphotic pattern—the individual with the straight lumbar area and an anterior thoracic spinal mechanism. There will be scoliotic patterns of varying degrees for each individual. It is obvious that each of the variations is going to respond to the whiplash force in an individual manner. Even the simple mechanics of the difference between the female and male type of body calls for a different response. In some types of build, the force will carry the pattern in the same direction as the pattern involved, while in others, it will be the opposite. The kyphotic pattern may have the force driven into the kyphotic area opposite to the direction in which the kyphosis is present, while the anterior thoracic area may have its anterior direction exaggerated. This is a simple illustration and can be compounded by the detailed analysis of each type involved.

It is also necessary to add other factors that are always present in these cases. These are the accommodative mechanisms that have come to accompany each of our basic physiological patterns in response to earlier strains. These accommodative patterns have also been subjected to the arc of force generated by the whiplash injury and must be considered. It has been my observation that these accommodative patterns become disrupted as a result of the whiplash injury and, like sleeping tigers, come to life to add their share of symptoms to the induced, whiplash injury symptoms. It sometimes takes a bit of doing to unravel the various factors operating in these patients as the weeks, months, and years go by. Are they hangovers from the whiplash injury directly or are they accommodative strains that have been aroused and need to be corrected to a quiescent state to bring the patient back to comfort? This calls for accuracy in diagnosis in the recalcitrant case. As long as there is a definite degree of force acting within the body from the whiplash injury, that force is one of the factors tending to maintain the awakened "tiger," and it is a diagnostic tool to measure the healing response the patient is making by observing how rapidly the accommodative mechanisms can return to a quiescent state again. The ones that do not return indicate that there is still something preventing the reversibility of pathology, and this "something" is usually some of the force factor that was put into the body at the time of the whiplash injury. From personal experience, when this factor is resolved, these accommodative mechanisms tend to restore themselves to more normal physiological functioning.

Pathological Physiology

Next, let us try to give a brief picture of the whiplash injury itself upon body physiological mechanisms. Let's take the case in which the patient was struck from behind while in a parked car. The moment of impact was upon the rear bumper and the arc of force involved the whole individual in the sitting position. A direct point of contact would have been the top of the seat over which the head, neck and shoulders were thrown backward before they recoiled forward. There may be tearing or stretching of the anterior longitudinal ligaments and annulus fibrosus, possibly associated with hemorrhage and edema, as well as damage to the intervertebral disk or the apophysial articulations and narrowing of the intervertebral foramina with consequent nerve root damage. There will be alteration of the physiological curves of the spine from the sacrum through the cervical areas. There will be paravertebral tissue changes—from ligamentous, articular and visceral effects. There will be modification of the fascial envelopes that surround every involved muscle, nerve, artery, vein and viscera at the cellular and multi-cellular level. This point is important because every one of these fascial envelopes has been subjected to the entire arc of force emanating from the point of contact at the rear of the car.

Now, let us consider the role of the sacrum in this syndrome. As the patient was thrown backward, his entire spine, including the sacrum, was lifted from the pelvic bowl, and as he was thrown forward, he was forcefully reseated into his pelvic bowl. As a result, the sacrum tends to become locked at its respiratory axis of involuntary motion. (Normally, the sacrum rocks between the ilia; during the inhalation phase, the sacral base rocks posteriorly, and during the exhalation phase, the sacral base rocks anteriorly.) This involuntary motion is frozen after the whiplash injury so the sacrum no longer rocks independently in rhythm to the respiratory cycle. Instead of the sacrum rocking between the ilia, we now find the sacrum and ilia moving as one unit during the respiratory cycle, posteriorly and anteriorly. This loss of the normal respiratory movement of the sacrum is usually bilateral in blows from the front or rear of the car and unilateral in blows from one side or the other. It has profound, maintaining effects in whiplash injuries.

In this situation, the long paravertebral muscles and ligaments that reach from the crests of the ilia to the shoulder girdle become limited in their capacity to function, not only during the respiratory cycle but also during voluntary movements of the shoulders and neck. There is a palpatory sense when palpating in the upper areas of a fixed base at the pelvic bowl instead of a normally floating base. Every movement the patient makes with his shoulders, arms or neck is operating with resistance from the locked pelvic mechanism. This is one reason why the shoulders and neck stay sore, fatigue easily, and maintain some of their disabilities in these cases.

Fastening to the sacrum is the anterior longitudinal ligament, which has been injured at a higher level and which carries limitation of function clear down to the level of the sacrum. The dura mater surrounding the spinal cord hangs freely from the level of the upper cervical vertebrae and foramen magnum and then fastens firmly again at the level of the second sacral segment. With loss of the respiratory motion of the sacrum, the spinal dura as well as the dura of the cranial cavity suffer a limitation of normal respiratory motion during inhalation and exhalation. Also, the filum terminale of the pia mater, which finds its attachment in the coccygeal area, is restricted. There will be limitation of the normal upward movement of the spinal cord and its peripheral nerve structures during inhalation and limitation of the downward descent during exhalation. Physiological disturbance of the spinal cord and the central nervous system yields a continuing level of dysfunction that contributes to chronicity and trophic changes in whiplash injuries.

The other postural movements of the ilia upon the sacrum have not been disturbed as a general rule, so we do not often find so-called sacroiliac strains accompanying the whiplash injury, unless, of course, accommodative mechanisms have been disrupted. The sacrum is not the key in all whiplash problems, but in many cases, it does play a very real role in maintaining the whiplash and accommodative mechanism strain syndrome.

There is another bit of anatomical detail that I think is of clinical importance in whiplash injuries. This is a ligamentous band, firmly attached to the anterior longitudinal ligament over the fourth and fifth thoracic vertebrae and extending downward and anteriorly to blend with the fascia, which covers the esophagus, trachea and aorta. This ligament is shown in *Bassett's Stereoscopic Atlas of Human Anatomy*, Section IV, The Thorax, slides No. 128-1 and 132-3. I have not been able to find reference to it in other works of anatomy, but it is a strong ligamentous band.

Why is it important? Any ligamentous restriction is an initiating factor in dysfunction, and here we have a suspension ligament involving the mediastinal fascias. Superiorly, the mediastinal fascia is continuous with the deep cervical fascias through to the base of the skull. Inferiorly the mediastinal fascia blends with the pericardium, the diaphragm, the right and left crura of the diaphragm, and the psoas fascias, which pass through the pelvic bowl to fasten to the lesser trochanters of the femurs. Our knowledge of applied anatomy tells us that ligamentous strains in the mid-thoracic area that also involve this described ligamentous band could extend the difficulties we find in whiplash injuries into the structures of the mediastinum, posterior abdominal wall, pelvis and acetabulae, and superiorly into the anterior cervical areas.

Again, as with the spinal cord and central nervous system, this may be only a minimal stress in terms of gross dysfunction, but it is a continuous stress that will serve to limit the free mobility of these areas during the respiratory cycle. It is freedom of function in all parts of the body during the respiratory cycle that contributes a major share to the adequate drainage through the minute veins and lymphatics. Again, too, we must realize that whiplash patients have had an arc of force imposed upon their total mechanism—fascial envelopes, spinal and cranial mechanisms, sacrum, and viscera.

Psychological Complications

A quotation from the September, 1960 *World-Wide Abstracts of General Medicine* will bring this aspect of the problem into focus:

Whiplash...injuries are accompanied by psychic complications characterized by anxiety, depression, irritability and especially bewilderment. Patients require an unusual amount of explanation, reassurance, personal attention and sympathetic handling. Prompt treatment is essential.

In 47 consecutive cases (23 in men and 24 in women), the severity of the psychologic symptoms could not be correlated with the severity of the injury. Nearly all the accidents occurred when an automobile was stationary or moving slowly, and its occupants felt quite secure. The violent assault from the rear came without warning, rendering a comfortable situation perilous and painful.

Most of the patients deny all knowledge of the collision. This mechanism is believed to come into action because the accident is so sudden that in many people, the ego cannot mobilize the usual defenses and so invokes the more drastic mechanism of denial. This makes it impossible to work through the meaning and the discomfort of the accident emotionally.

It is as if the ego unconsciously perceives that to accept the injury means to accept the possibility that the control—the head and neck, which have been injured—can be severed from the body. In this respect, the whiplash injury of the neck is psychologically unique. Both its suddenness and its unconscious meaning tend to mobilize greater anxiety in ordinarily well-integrated and stable people than do injuries to other parts of the body.

In this view, the emotional aspects are an integral part of the whiplash injury; they are not dependent on the accompanying circumstances and are not significantly related to pre-existing psychiatric disease.

This concise report covers the situation very clearly and serves to emphasize some of the points already made in this paper: the wholeness of the problem, the difficulty in getting a clear history, the intensity of the application of a sudden force, and the nervous system's reaction. There is also a physical, anatomicophysiological component that sheds additional light on why these people express some of the symptoms they manifest. This component makes it easier to evaluate the situation.

The brain and spinal cord are covered by the three layers of the meninges: pia mater, arachnoid and dura mater. All three layers, with their visceral contents, are whipped in an automobile accident. Between the inner and outer walls of the cranial dura mater are the venous sinuses of the skull. The blood stream enters the skull through arteries that pass through protected channels, while the venous drainage is dependent upon the venous sinuses within the dura mater. The venous drainage of the eyes empty into the cavernous sinus, that of the vein of Galen into the straight sinus, and that of the superior cerebral veins into the superior sagittal sinus. Interestingly enough, the superior cerebral veins empty into the superior sagittal sinus at an angle that faces anteriorly while the blood in the sinus is flowing posteriorly. However, it is only during the exhalation phase of the respiratory cycle that the veins point forward, counter to the flow. During the inspiratory phase, with expansion of the parietals and the slight widening of the sagittal suture, these veins empty at right angles into the sagittal sinus.

Within the viscera of the central nervous system are the reticular areas of the medulla and pons, with ascending nerve pathways to the thalamus and cerebrum and descending nerve pathways from the cerebrum to the spinal cord and peripheral and cranial nerves, all giving off association fibers. Just above this area are the emotional centers of the hypothalamus and thalamus. Within the floor of the fourth ventricle are all the physiological centers, including that of respiration.

This whole mechanism is shocked by the whiplash injury. The dura mater, as a membranous envelope, tends to lock down like air brakes on a train when it is shocked. Normally, it has a most important role in rocking to and fro in a rhythmic pattern during the respiratory cycle of inhalation and exhalation in order to initiate and maintain adequate venous drainage within the venous sinuses of the skull. This becomes limited after a whiplash injury in varying degrees of dysfunction with membranous articular strains of the craniosacral mechanism. These can be diagnosed by a skilled tactile touch and an understanding of the mechanisms involved. What is happening to the venous drainage from all these important nerve centers? What is happening to the venous drainage from the eye sockets? The nervous system is normally motile in a rhythmic motility of its own. With the filum terminale and the pia mater restricted at the sacrococcygeal area, there is further limitation of functioning within the central nervous system.

Is it any wonder that these patients are anxious, depressed, irritable and bewildered? Some of them will tell you that they feel as if their eyes are being pulled out of their sockets or pushed into the sockets. With a locked dural membrane and inadequate venous drainage, is it not easy to see why?

Another of these limitations is a disturbance of the normal fluctuation pattern of the cerebrospinal fluid, which is a serious pathological process leading to dysfunction, equally as important as the venous stasis. This fluctuant fluid contributes an important nutritional factor in the interchange between the central nervous system, the arterial system and venous system. Therefore, the cerebrospinal fluid helps in normalizing the patient when it is permitted to do its job of fluctuation within the craniosacral mechanism. A trained touch can learn to recognize changes from the normal in the fluctuation pattern and dural membrane tone quality and can learn to nontraumatically correct the membranous articular strains always found in whiplash injuries.

Yes, psychological factors play a big role in these whiplash injuries. They are effects of the physical factors, and the physical factors contribute to maintaining the psychological impact. Diagnosis and treatment of the physical factors offer a major breakthrough in the resolution of not only the psychologic effects but also the pathological physiology. It has been my personal experience to see these symptoms clear rapidly with the restoration of the normal physiological motility of the central nervous system, the normal mobility of the investing membranes, and the fluctuation of the cerebrospinal fluid.

Trophic Changes

Trophic disturbances in the body mechanisms begin from the moment of impact in the whiplash injury and involve the whole individual. To understand these changes it is necessary to understand the role that the fascia plays in the economy of body health and disease. A few words from Dr. A.T. Still will give us some foundation stones on which to build:

> The fascia gives one of, if not the greatest problems to solve as to the part it takes in life and death. It belts each muscle, vein, nerve, and all organs of the body. It is almost a network of nerves, cells and tubes, running to and from it; it is crossed and filled with, no doubt, millions of nerve centers and fibers to carry on the work of secreting and excreting fluid vital and destructive. By its action we live, and by its failure we shrink, or swell, and die. Each muscle plays its part in active life. Each fiber of all muscles owes its pliability to that yielding septum-washer that gives all muscles help to glide over and around all adjacent muscles and ligaments, without friction or jar. It not only lubricates the fibers but [also] gives nourishment to all parts of the body. Its nerves are so abundant that no atom of flesh fails to get nerve and fluid supply therefrom....
>
> ...When you deal with the fascia, you deal and do business with the branch offices of the brain, and under the general corporation law, the same as the brain itself, and why not treat it with the same degree of respect? [1]

It is the vitality, the tone quality, the capacity for functioning of this tremendous fascial system that Dr. Still refers to when he says, "By its action we live, and by its failure we shrink, or swell, and die." The patient who has suffered a severe whiplash injury, who has been exposed to an arc of force throughout his entire body, is going to find

that his fascial envelopes have had air brakes applied to them in varying degrees of intensity from the head to the toes. Cellular nerve supply is disturbed, venous and lymphatic drainage is curtailed, arteriole
and capillary blood supply is less efficient, interstitial fluid interchange
is impaired, hormonal and enzyme mechanisms are under stress, and
many other changes have taken place. Some of the chronic pain and
illness cases we see are in reality post-whiplash syndromes.

The importance of the fascial pumps can be simplistically understood when we realize that we have a heart that is pumping 7,000
liters of fluid a day out to the tissues, but we do not have a peripheral
heart to return all of that juice for recirculation. We depend, primarily, on the tone quality of the fascial pumps and the muscular agencies of the body to bring the fluids back through the veins and lymphatics. Impair these pumps and we have a chronic stasis, minimal in
degree but persistent in dysfunction.

Trophic disturbances manifest themselves in many ways, depending in part on the different body types involved, the length of time
these "septum-washers" have been impaired, the sensitivity of the specific tissues protected and nourished by the fascias, and the presence
or absence of other disease or traumatic conditions. The degree of
disability may vary, but there is a sense of both a general problem as
well as a specific one. True, all disease and traumatic conditions involve trophic disturbances, but often in whiplash injuries, there are
minimal changes in the beginning that accumulate their effects through
the following days, weeks, months and years, until the results can be
expressed in the words of Dr. Still: "Cause and effect are perpetual.
Cause may not be as large in the beginning in some cases as in others,
but time adds to the effect until the effect overbalances cause, and the
end is death. Death is the end or the sum total of effects."[2]

Thus trophic changes and their effects can manifest in any cellular,
visceral, or musculoskeletal system of the body in our whiplash case
because the patient has been exposed to a total pattern of potential
disability. The pattern localizes in specific areas with the passage of
time for the maintenance of specific symptoms, but both the specific

areas and the "silent" areas are involved.

The cheerful side of this picture is that these trophic changes have a high degree of reversibility towards the normal, when the total picture is taken into consideration and the patient is treated as a whole to restore the fascial pumps of the body. There have been many a case that I did not feel would make a good response, which in fact returned to a physiological capacity far beyond my own and the patient's expectations. The body has potentials far beyond our comprehension if we give it a chance.

Chronicity

This aspect of whiplash injuries can be summed up quickly. From the moment of impact until something is done to really diagnose and correct all the multiple factors involved in the whiplash syndrome, our patient is going to suffer from one or more phases of his whiplash injury. I have seen and have diagnosed cases in which this syndrome is still contributing to a share of their disabilities 40 years after their automobile accidents. I have made the diagnosis on the grounds of the physical findings of a whiplash injury and later elicited a history to go with the findings. They came in with other complaints, but these had not responded either to other doctors' treatments or to my own. Reexamination of the underlying disturbed mechanisms of the body revealed an old whiplash mechanism, standing like a reef in the channel, over which and around which the patient had to maintain his health pattern.

To briefly review the basic whiplash syndrome findings, there is a generalized limitation of function of the shoulders, neck and upper extremities; a generalized limitation of the craniosacral membranous articular mechanism; a locked sacrum at the level of the second sacral segment, the respiratory axis of the sacrum; a generalized feeling of limitation of the soft tissues of the body and the fascial pumps, with specific restricted areas in the regions of the patient's complaints; a sense of fatigue throughout all the tissues of the body; a sense of feeling as if the whole patient is involved in a total change towards dysfunction; and specific changes in each case depending on body type and individual characteristics.

I have learned to feel the functioning or dysfunctioning of these patients' anatomicophysiological mechanisms, not merely the degree of mobility or motility of the lesioned areas. Every structure in the body goes through rhythmic change during the respiratory cycle. All midline structures flex during inhalation and extend during exhalation. All bilateral structures externally rotate during inhalation and internally rotate during exhalation. The motion is minimal but perceptible to the touch, if you train yourself to feel for the functioning of the tissues. Limitations of these factors aid in diagnosis. Generalized limitation means a whole person is involved in a total dysfunction to a varying degree. Localized dysfunction means specific details must be examined to explain the limitation.

The term chronicity often has a negative connotation when used to describe a patient. In using the term, I am referring only to the length of time the patients are burdened with the whiplash injury. These people are not just "chronic pain patients;" they never have been, nor will they be. These disabilities are effects that can be diagnosed and treated, and thanks to the potential reversibility of pathology, a high percentage of them manifest a considerable degree of restoration to more normal functioning. That automatically takes them out of the "chronic psychosomatic," negative classification. I say this because it has been as much or more my surprise to find these people getting well as it was the patient's relief to find himself recovering from long-standing complaints. I have had my failures, primarily due to inadequate diagnostic skill as well as too short a time in which to invoke the necessary corrective changes. It takes time to crank up the motor in some of these long-standing static fascial pumps, but when they finally come to life, restoration to some new level of health is axiomatic.

1. A.T. Still, *Philosophy of Osteopathy*, pp. 164-5 and pp. 167-8.
2. A.T. Still, *Autobiography*, p. 202.

WHIPLASH

This article is the result of having extensively edited and merged three papers on the subject of whiplash. One, entitled "Whiplash Injuries," was originally published in the 1958 Yearbook and reprinted in the 1964 Yearbook of the Academy of Applied Osteopathy (currently named the American Academy of Osteopathy). The other two papers, dated March 1970 and December 1970, were written for American Academy of Osteopathy seminars on whiplash.

Normal Anatomical And Physiological Mechanisms

THE TERM "WHIPLASH" REFERS to a type of energy to which a patient is subjected, often in the form of rapid acceleration or rapid deceleration or a combination of both. In approaching a patient with a whiplash injury, we must first determine what would be the normal for the patient as a whole. How did they function anatomically, physiologically, psychologically and emotionally before they were hurt.

What is health? It is all parts functioning in harmonious interrelationship. All systems are "go" and are free to adapt to the ever-changing environment of the individual's life. Everything is working together, and the patient is not conscious of any part because his nervous system is not reporting to him that anything is wrong. He accepts wellness as a natural component of his daily living. He has freedom to live without conscious thought of any limitation of function in any of his systems. He can walk, stand, sit, work, play, eat, sleep, dream, and do all the things he needs to do with a sense of moving in his environment according to his needs and desires. He is a living, *whole* man or woman in tune with the universe, both internally in his homeostatic balances and externally with his environment.

His pattern of health is individually right for him, and it is this pattern for this one individual that should be evaluated by the physician in determining the baseline of health for diagnostic and treatment purposes. The health present in a man or woman in their sixties is obviously different from a man or woman in their twenties. The physical characteristics of a body system that is long and slender are different from one that is short and stocky. The impacts of past illnesses and injuries that have occurred during a lifetime and to which the patient has made adequate recovery and compensation are all a part of the total pattern of the health for that individual. All of these factors are a part of the baseline evaluation.

Let us consider the various systems of the body in more detail. The connective tissue system is a framework of multiple layers, bands, and intricately designed mechanisms with millions and trillions of spaces for the inclusion of the working cells of the body. It is a living system which has tone quality that expresses health or disturbances of health to the palpatory hands of the physician who is examining it. Within it is the musculoskeletal system.

The skeletal system can be compared to a living, intricately patterned mobile, including the shapes and contours of the individual bones of the foot to the 22 bones that comprise the cranial mechanism. Each bone articulates with its neighboring bone or bones so that the total skeletal mechanism is one of efficiency in man's walkabout on earth. All of them are in motion from the top of the head to the bottom of the feet throughout life. The muscular systems of the body, together with the connective tissue fascias that unite them to the skeletal system, form a framework of coordinated locomotion for the use of the individual. There are other muscular systems in the body that serve to maintain the internal functioning of life—the cardiovascular, costorespiratory, gastrointestinal and urogenital systems. Again, these musculoskeletal systems have a living tone quality that is palpable to the physician's diagnostic and therapeutic hands and can be evaluated as part of the baseline of health for the individual. There are many other soft tissue systems in the body, including all the viscera. The central and peripheral nervous system and the autonomic nervous system are included in the soft tissues of the body and are the vast communication network for total body functioning.

Each one of these systems is complex in its organization and has normal values for functioning that are a part of the armamentarium of every physician's diagnostic insight. There is a biorhythmicity of function that is organically interrelated to functioning patterns for all hours of the day and night for all systems of the body, and this information is a part of every physician's training.

It is interesting to consider all the fluids that make up the normal physiology of a patient's health pattern. These include the cerebrospinal fluid, blood, lymph, interstitial and serous fluids. All of them interchange in body physiology with each other and with all the living cells which they surround and bathe. There is tone quality and quantity in function that is palpable to the physician in his evaluation of the patient's baseline of health, through his examination of many of these fluid systems.

Finally, there is the psycho-mental-emotional-mind and Mind of the patient, which shares in importance with the total health of the patient as much as does the physical health of his body physiology. How does this patient view his health level of functioning? What is his stability factor as to his emotional make-up? Is he basically a nervous type, sensitive to every little change that takes place in his environment, or is he more phlegmatic in his approach to his health and his needs? How does he react to the stresses of life: Does his musculoskeletal system have that constant feeling of tension that we find in so many of our patients today? Does he react through other systems of the body with palpitations or gastrointestinal symptoms? These and many other factors may be a normal part of this patient's health pattern and would have to be considered *normal* in his baseline evaluation—for this is how he functions. His or her reaction to the situation that has created this whiplash type of strain is a factor in each case.

The general structural analysis of the total body has been discussed. To this analysis should be added this detail. Examine the patient for the type of scoliotic tension patterns that may be present. The described normal curvatures of the spinal mechanism are rarely seen, as most individuals have some lateral scoliosis or anteroposterior variations.

Many people will have a flat area in the upper or mid-thoracic spinal areas, with a flexion curve above and below the site of the anteroposterior flattening. The crossover areas for various types of scoliotic tension patterns are particularly vulnerable to the strains of the whiplash type of injury.

In terms of physiological dynamics, structure and function are intra- and interchangeable in their functioning relationships. We have discussed, briefly, the structural aspects. The physiological capacity to function within the human body can be broadly divided into two main categories. One is the voluntary use of the body in everyday activities. In health, this is a largely unconscious use of all the resources of the body for the multitudinous actions of daily life, from getting up in the morning, doing our daily work or play, and going to bed to sleep the night through to get ready for the next day. The musculoskeletal system, digestive system, respiratory system, cardiovascular system, and all other systems are doing their jobs easily and competently.

There is another functioning complex taking place within the body. This, too, is essential to the total health of the whole man. It is the primary respiratory mechanism, which is broken down into five parts: the inherent motility of the brain and spinal cord, the fluctuation of the cerebrospinal fluid, the mobility of the intracranial and intraspinal membranes, the articular mobility of the cranial bones, and the involuntary mobility of the sacrum between the ilia. All five units work together in a harmonious, rhythmical pattern of total functioning and cannot be separated one from another in their inherent capacity to function within the total body physiology from the head to the feet. This simple, rhythmic movement (which is alternating flexion/external rotation and extension/internal rotation) takes place in the total mechanisms of the body, no matter what other patterns structural analysis may reveal: the scoliotic curvatures, the different types of body build, and all other data.

It is a small movement and not easily perceptible to the untrained palpatory sense of the physician, but it is there and can be found when the physician gears his sense of touch down to its level of functioning motion. Its importance lies both in the fact that it is an essential part of normal physiology and that this rhythmic movement contributes to maintaining the normal health of the individual. This is the individual, then, that is going to be subjected to a whiplash type of strain.

Pathologic Anatomical And Physiological Mechanisms

Whiplash Energies Plus Body Physiology

The whiplash type of injury can occur in many forms, but here we will focus on the automobile accident. The automobile-induced whiplash involves far more than the cervical area; the total body physiology from the soles of the feet to the top of the head is subjected to the whiplash energies and all of the body physiology is influenced by the accident. In order to better understand the forces involved in whiplash energies, let me quote from an article:

When an auto comes to a crash halt, a second collision occurs inside the car milliseconds later. Inertial force propels the occupant forward with an impact equal to the deceleration rate times his own weight. Instrument readings in simulated accidents sometimes attain 200 G at peak deceleration, or an impact of 200 times the weight of the occupant. If the motorist weighs 150 pounds, he strikes with an effective weight of 15 tons. Unless restrained, motorists in a front-end collision are projected violently upward and forward. If not diverted by intervening factors, they are hurled in a straight course toward the point of collision.

Two important points need emphasizing: The patient is suddenly a mass of body physiology weighing up to 15 tons *in motion*, and it is a *unidirectional* energy directed toward the point of collision.

During the accident, there's a force field within body physiology, unidirectional in character. In theory, this increment of energy from 150 pounds to 15 tons is dissipated during the time of the accident. By the end, the patient again weighs 150 pounds, and the energy field projected towards the point of collision no longer exists. Ideally, afterwards, it is totally dissipated. However, in practice, this force field within the body physiology can still be present in the patient; it is still unidirectional towards the point of collision; it is continuing to influence body physiological functioning for weeks, months, and years after the accident; and it can be found by palpation by the physician within the body physiology of the patient. The total fascial connective tissue framework, together with the fluids of all the cells of the body, has been subjected to this force, which creates a chronic state of less efficiency for all structures invested by the fascia. Since fascia envelops practically all somatic structures within the body, this can be a contributing factor to preventing total restoration to health.

Many cases will totally dissipate the whiplash energy field during or soon after the accident, and only the acute, traumatic injuries and decompensated, body physiological mechanisms will require treatment to restore health. However, there is also a definite percentage of cases in which it does not dissipate, and it becomes an added factor in body physiological functioning in the patient's health pattern. It becomes a part of body physiology for the patient to handle in his body's effort to heal itself.

Finding the presence in the patient of the force field in its unidirectional action is easier in the case of a recent automobile accident. As the weeks, months, and years go by after an accident, it gradually becomes less demonstrable. I have found it present in some cases as late as 35 years after the accident. It is not necessary to find it, but it is necessary to understand the potential presence of it in fascial functioning in body physiology. Its presence is a clinical entity, observable by palpation, and it does contribute to persistent fascial dysfunction.

Technique for Determining the Presence of a Non-dissipated Whiplash Energy Field: In the case of a patient who has been in a front-end collision, the patient lies on their back on the examination table. The physician is seated at the head of the table and slides his hands under the patient so as to make contact with the thoracic area. The weight of the patient is sufficient to make a good contact for the physician's hands; however, the hands do not lie inertly under the patient. The physician projects his sense of touch through his hands so as to gain a total impression of the whole body, then, specifically, tries to sense through to the anterior chest wall. Continuing to project his sense of touch, the physician should close his eyes and sense the presence or absence of a unidirectional vector of force passing anteriorly throughout the whole body. Closing the eyes is not necessary, but it serves to gain a better palpatory sense of touch for this phenomenon. If such a vector of force is present, it will show itself through the body physiology of the patient towards the ceiling within a minute or so.

In the case of a patient who has been in a rear-end collision, have the patient lie face down on the table. The hands slide under the patient on the anterior chest wall, and the sense of touch is projected towards the posterior chest wall. In a case of side collision, the patient can be on their back or face down, and the force field will demonstrate itself going through the body laterally to one side or the other, depending on the point of collision.

Mechanisms of Injury

An understanding of the pathological effects that occur to the individual in the whiplash injury begins with a careful history of the positioning of the patient in the automobile at the time of the accident. Since this is an accident and the patient is being subjected to a unidirectional force field passing *through* his body physiology, the following considerations should be taken into account.

If the patient is in an upright position looking forward, his normal flexion-extension mechanisms will bear the brunt of the force in front- and rear-end collisions and his sidebending mechanisms in side collisions. If his head is turned to one side or the other, or if he is partially turned in the seat, fascial planes throughout his body physiology will be subjected to additional torsional effects.

If he is the driver of the automobile and his foot is on the brake or accelerator, the force field will have a more direct application through the fixed limb of the patient into his body physiology. Even in minor accidents, this can be a component in the damage to body physiology. If the patient is lying down in the back seat of the car, many different factors are introduced into the effect taking place at the time of the accident. Children may be in any type of positioning at the time of the accident if unrestrained.

The rear-end collision produces a hyperextension of the cervical area and the rest of the spine, with associated injuries to anterior and posterior structures. It places traction upon the anterior longitudinal ligament and compressive forces upon the posterior structures. It is possible to find cervical muscle tearing and fractures of the spinous process, laminae, articular elements or odontoid process of the axis. Rotation of the head at the time of the accident produces torsional effects and may cause greater damage to one side than the other. The vertebral arteries may be affected. Front-end collisions cause forceful hyperflexion of the neck and spine, again with multiple anterior and posterior structures being potentially injured. Side collisions often produce a complex pattern of movement and injury.

During the automobile accident, there is the additional factor of a unidirectional force field of hundreds of pounds of inertia going through the body physiology towards the point of collision. These vectors in the force field do not follow the normal planes of motion of the ligamentous articular mechanisms of the midline structures in body physiology (flexion, extension, and sidebending with rotation). They intercept the planes of motion of the midline structures at angles of momentum contrary to the normal motion. Therefore, the hyperflexion, hyperextension, and hypersidebending rotation within body physiology are taking place against strong resistance. The vectors of force from the accident towards the point of collision subject the total, fascial connective tissue, ligamentous articular mechanisms of all the body physiology to unphysiological forces.

The effects of an auto accident upon body physiology begin with shock to the entire body cellular physiology from the soles of the feet to the top of the head. It is a common story in major and minor accidents that the patient gets out of his car, if he is able to do so, and states that he is not hurt. The shock wave has passed through his body physiology rapidly to create the pathology he will feel later, but the initial experience is one of a numbed sensorium in the central nervous communication system. This shock begins to wear off within a few hours, and his pathology can express itself as symptoms. This tissue shock can last for days before final resolution, and I have seen cases in which tissue shock was still present three months after the accident.

Injuries to the brain are common from direct blows to the head. There is also forceful hyperextension of the neck in rear-end collisions, causing a sudden drag on the base of the skull through all the muscles and ligaments fastened to the base of the cranial mechanism. Injury to the brain and to the brain stem may be the result of pressure gradients created by pressure buildup or by shearing forces and mass movement of the intracranial contents. The entire dura mater, arachnoid, and pia mater layers around the brain and spinal cord are involved—from inside the cranial cavity, along the course of the spinal canal, out the dural sleeves that accompany each spinal nerve through the intervertebral foramina, and down to their attachment within the sacral canal and the coccyx. Emotional reactions which occur sometimes after rapid acceleration and deceleration injuries indicate that brain damage is more common and extensive than generally recognized.

Injuries of the lower back are frequent, involving the muscles, ligaments, and loss of functional motion for the lumbar spine and of the sacrum between the ilia. The seat belt is a protective device that serves its purpose well, but it also provides a fulcrum restricting the movement of the pelvis against which the inertial forces may produce many strain patterns.

Other sites of damage particular to the individual are the crossover areas of the various scoliotic patterns of the spinal curvatures. These may be in either the lateral scoliotic patterns or in the anteroposterior scoliotic patterns. The compensatory normal functioning of these areas is seriously disturbed, not only in the time of the acute phase but also during the entire chronic phase, which may be a matter of weeks, months, and years.

Ligamentous articular strains will be present from the upper cervical areas through to the pelvis and in the appendicular areas. But do not look for mere osseous immobility. Most of the strain patterns are soft tissue in nature, and careful evaluation and corrective measures to bring them back to normal functioning will permit normal mobilization of osseous elements. The fascias of all the organ systems will be involved, and membranous articular strains will be found in the craniosacral mechanisms.

Physiologically, any ligamentous articular or membranous articular area must be an automatic, shifting, suspension fulcrum in order to fulfill its capacity to express health. In daily use, it must be able to shift into any position and return to a floating neutral position again for subsequent action. In the whiplash injury, every ligamentous articular area in the thoracic and cervical regions involved becomes limited in this physiological capacity. The segments involved become relatively fixed fulcrums, unable to perform their natural functions until the strained ligaments have healed. This loss of automaticity as a fulcrum mechanism is even more important when it involves the membranous articular mechanism with its resultant venous drainage and cerebrospinal fluid fluctuation disturbances.

The forceful movements of the body, and the forces to which it is subjected, create the potential for microtrauma to all the fascias of the body. The somatic cellular elements within the fascias and enveloped by the fascias with their fluid contents are equally involved. This microtrauma will lead to minute patterns of fascial fibrosis and leave sleeves of increased tensity in fascial planes affecting the future functioning of the somatic structures within the fascia. This includes muscles, nerves, blood supply to and from various tissues, and lymphatic drainage. There is disruption of compensated homeostatic mechanisms. Scoliotic tension patterns from within the basilar areas of the skull through the spine to the sacrum develop and become facilitated focal points of decompensated body physiology. Also, patterns of previous disabilities that the patient may have had earlier in life and from which he has developed adequate compensation break down and decompensate. I refer to these disruptions as "awakened tigers."

In this context, "tigers" describes the old injuries, old illnesses, and old patterns of physiologic disturbance to which people have compensated. They have been feeling fine for many years or months and have not had any serious difficulty with these problems. But these problems can come back to life when a person has been in an automobile accident. Many times when a patient comes to you, they will be complaining, not about the fact that they've been in an automobile accident but about the fact that this problem, which they had many years ago and which was under control, now is causing them trouble again. They have tried the treatments that worked before, but the problem does not subside. If you will check into the history of that patient, you will often discover that they had an automobile accident a few weeks, a few months, or sometimes even a year before this awakened tiger came back to annoy them. It is not the awakened tiger that is the problem. The whiplash injury, with all its effects on the primary respiratory mechanism, has disturbed this tiger, and the tiger has come back to life and is tearing at this patient and causing their symptomatology. The answer to the problem is to find out if they have been in an accident they did not remember, or in which they feel they were not hurt, and treat that. Then the awakened tiger will go back to sleep.

Craniosacral Mechanism

The craniosacral components of injury in whiplash cases deserve a more detailed understanding. For it is these changes in the primary respiratory mechanism, particularly the sacrum, that serve as the maintaining factors in the difficult cases that fail to respond to the usual methods of treatment applied to the cervical and thoracic areas. Often there are no symptoms reported in the cranial or sacral area, so treatment remains focused on the areas of complaint in the neck and upper back.

The ligaments involved in whiplash injuries as they relate to the spine and rib cage are the anterior and posterior longitudinal ligaments, interspinous and intertransverse ligaments, radiate ligaments between the body of the vertebrae and the neck of the ribs, and the capsular ligaments. With a whiplash affecting the relationship of the occiput and atlas, occipitoatlantal and atlantoaxial ligaments also become involved. A deeper analysis of the anatomic structures reveals even more extensive involvement. The anterior longitudinal ligament fastens firmly to the anterior surfaces of the bodies of the vertebrae from the second thoracic through the second sacral segment. Superiorly, a portion of the anterior longitudinal ligament lies anterior to the bodies of the cervical vertebrae and fastens to the basiocciput. It is connected with the tendinous expansion of the prevertebral muscles in the cervical area and with the crura of the diaphragm in the lumbar region. The posterior longitudinal ligament extends from the occipital bone above to the coccyx below. The last well-marked expansion of this ligament inferiorly is situated between the first two segments of the sacrum. Thus, ligamentous articular strains occur in the thoracic and cervical areas and, through the extension of these ligaments, to the occiput and the sacrum.

Membranous articular strains and stress can also occur in and around the occipital area. The Sutherland fulcrum, which is the joining of the tentorium cerebelli and the falx cerebri, becomes limited in its capacity to function freely in full physiological excursion. With the production of membranous strains within the cranial mechanism, disturbances of cerebrospinal fluid fluctuation also occur. This in turn prevents an adequate transmutation of nerve vitality to the central nervous system, a major factor needed in the healing of the injured nerves caused by the whiplash injury. Drainage from the venous sinuses of the skull also becomes more difficult and is another contributing factor to central nervous system pathology.

The cranial lesions accompanying whiplash injuries include membranous restrictions of the Sutherland fulcrum and the lining membrane of the cranial bowl, occipitoatlantal lesions (unilateral or bilateral), temporal bone lesions, modified forms of the occipitomas-toid lesion, and others. Disturbances of the fluctuation of the cere-brospinal fluid always accompany lesions of the primary respiratory mechanism and are always present in these cases.

This modified form of the occipitomastoid lesion is an interesting one. Instead of it being produced by a blow upon the occiput driving it inward, as is the usual form of lesion, this restriction is produced by the sudden pull of the whiplash force acting like the suction cup of a plumber's plunger upon the base of the occiput through the deep cervical fascia. Its crippling, clinical effect may or may not be as severe as the usual occipitomastoid lesion, depending upon its specific impact upon the venous sinuses and tentorium cerebelli within the cranium.

The reciprocal tension membrane is frequently restricted in its normal mobility. This includes the dura that lines the skull, the falx cerebri, the tentorium cerebelli, and the spinal dura that surrounds the spinal cord and accompanies each spinal nerve as it leaves the spinal canal through each intervertebral foramina. Because the Sutherland fulcrum becomes restricted in its total pattern of normal functioning and the two halves of the tentorium cerebelli fasten to the petrous ridges of the temporal bones, these lesions can affect any of the nine cranial nerves that pass through the dura around each temporal bone. This can produce many bizarre patterns of symptoma-tology. Also, each sleeve of dura around each spinal nerve can be restrictive in its influence, much like the restriction of dura that causes tic douloureux in the fifth cranial nerve within the cranium. The dynamic of this mechanism is to interfere with the free fluctuation of cerebrospinal fluid, which is so important to the normal metabolism of neural functioning. I have observed this phenomenon in hundreds of whiplash cases. I feel it is a dynamic factor in explaining the many entrapment neuropathies that we find in acute and chronic disabilities in post-whiplash cases.

The Role of the Sacrum

The sacral portion of the primary respiratory mechanism is almost always involved. With the extension of the anterior and posterior longitudinal ligaments through the second sacral segment, the sacrum shares in the whiplash injury. Even more important than the pull of the spinal ligaments is the pull of the dura upon the sacrum, particularly at the second sacral level. This occurs not only from direct sacral effects of the whiplash but also from the membranous articular strains produced in the area of the occiput, which automatically affect the caudal connection of the dura at the sacral area. Any limitation of the Sutherland fulcrum is reflected inferiorly in limited functional capacity at the sacrum, particularly at that most important anterior convergent, posterior divergent spot on the second sacral segment so vital to good physiological functioning of the primary respiratory mechanism.

The direct effects upon the sacrum from the trauma of the whiplash injury occur at the moment of impact. As the patient is initially thrown backwards, forwards, or sideways, depending on the direction of the impact, the sacrum is forcibly lifted towards the head and, during the recoil, just as forcibly driven back into the pelvis. During this short but violent journey, ligamentous and membranous strain occurs at the sacroiliac and sacrolumbar articulations. The lesions may be bilateral or unilateral.

Associated with this injury is an important fascial drag upon all the fascia fastening to the entire pelvic rim—bilaterally from iliac crest to iliac crest and anteriorly-posteriorly from the fifth lumbar to the pubic rami. The pelvis is normally a floating base for body physiological motion, for the extremities below and for areas up to the shoulders and basiocciput. After this jamming takes place, it becomes a fixed base of limited functioning for body physiological activity. All physiological activities of the cervical and thoracic areas, and upper extremities, are working against a resistance from the fixed pelvic base. Thus, pathological stresses in these regions are maintained in their pathological state of poor efficiency, and the sacral jamming, with a loss of its involuntary flexion-extension motion, becomes a major contributing factor in the breakdown of compensatory homeostatic mechanisms and of scoliotic tension pattern decompensations.

Because the sacrum has been forcibly lifted from its pelvic seat and forcibly reseated into a combined ligamentous and membranous articular pattern of strain, there is direct loss of its capacity to act as an automatic, shifting, suspension fulcrum. The sacrum has become fixed in its pelvic bed at the level of the second sacral segment. The larger, L-shaped areas of the sacroiliac are not usually too deeply involved. The upper thoracic and cervical areas, having lost a floating fulcrum 18 to 24 inches away at the sacrum, find it necessary to compensate for this loss by becoming even more whip-like in their action. Ligaments and tissues that are already under stress in healing are forced to work even harder to maintain dynamic, spinal functioning.

An analogy can be made by seeing the difference between a tree and a stick driven into the ground. The tree is able to bend with the breezes and shows no stress because its root structures give and take in adequate compensation. A stick driven into the ground can be bent backward and forward, but the resistance is much greater because of the portion that has been driven into the soil. It does not have the elasticity of the normal root structure of the tree. Similarly, the sacrum that has become fixed by the whiplash injury is offering resistance to every motion of the thoracic and cervical areas.

The sacrum normally flexes and extends involuntarily between the ilia (during extension of the cranial base, the sacral base drops and moves anteriorly, while the coccygeal end moves posteriorly; then in flexion it does the opposite). A free sacral mechanism permits freedom for function superiorly for the trunk and cervical areas. If the sacral mechanism is tied down in its free mobility and works with the ilia as a unit, it is a fixed fulcrum creating resistance of mobility for the trunk and cervical areas. Restoration of sacral function and mobility is necessary in almost 100% of all auto accident cases.

Examining the Sacrum: Diagnosing this lack of movement in the sacrum is difficult because an area of little or no involuntary motion is harder to find than one of obvious displacement. One of the ways to diagnose this problem is to have the patient supine and to slip the hand under the sacrum. Let the palm of the hand mold with the sacrum so as to be able to read its mobility and motility, the inherent motions of the patient's respiration, and inherent ligamentous and membranous tonal qualities. A sense of restriction may be immediately felt, and the age of the injury can be assessed. By this is meant that if the whiplash injury is only a few weeks old, the sacral fixation feels that it is of relatively short duration. On the other hand, if it is an injury of several months or years of age, the tone quality of the sacrum gives that impression. Of course, whiplash is not the only injury that produces this restriction, but a careful history and the associated findings in the thoracic and cervical areas will serve to differentiate the pattern under examination.

Having secured a molded sense of the sacral capacity, bridge the anterior superior spines of the ilia with the forearm and hand of the free arm. Contact them lightly for accurate reading of the potential motion of the ilia as the next step is carried out. Then have the patient dorsiflex and extend the feet, rhythmically, slowly enough to feel motion in the pelvic area. With acute or chronic restriction of the sacrum at the second sacral segment, the relatively independent motion of the sacrum and ilia is lost. Normally, with all the pelvic articulations working physiologically, individual motion of the pelvic articulations can be felt through the palpating hands and arm. In a bilaterally jammed sacrum between the ilia, the whole pelvis moves as one unit instead of many individual units. During flexion and extension of the feet, you feel one piece at the pelvis instead of individual motion between the two ilia, sacrum, and fifth lumbar. In a unilaterally jammed sacrum, one side of the pelvis moves with individual motion between the ilia and sacrum and the other is a one-unit motion between the jammed sacrum and ilia of that side.

It is interesting to note that when the sacral jamming has taken place, the presence of this problem can be inferred through palpation from above in the cervical and thoracic areas of the spine. If the physician is holding those areas gently for diagnostic information, he will sense that he is at the end of a lever in motion with the quiet pattern of motion of physiological functioning and respiration of the patient. It feels as though this motion is operating from a fixed base at the pelvis, which, in fact, is true. Normally, with a floating pelvic mechanism, one does not feel the end of a lever type of motion in the cervical and thoracic areas. There is only the local movement of cervical and thoracic functioning. If such a lever type of movement is palpable in the cervical and/or thoracic areas, check the pelvis for a jammed sacral mechanism.

Treatment In The Chronic Whiplash Case

THE KEY WORDS FOR a therapeutic program are physiological function. This applies to both diagnosis and treatment because all treatment programs are continually monitored diagnostic analysis from the initial visit through to the final discharge. It takes diagnosis to determine what is or should be the health pattern of normal physiological function for the patient; it takes diagnosis to determine the pathological anatomicophysiological functioning present at the time of the first and subsequent visits; and it takes diagnosis to determine the efficacy of a treatment program during the course of the case to know when physiological function within the patient has returned to health. Chronic whiplash cases offer many complexities in a treatment program for the reason that physiological function is disturbed in so many diverse patterns, and these cases require a great deal of diagnostic thought and modifications of treatment to fit the individual patterns presented by each case. It is sometimes difficult to recognize a chronic case as post-whiplash because the potential patterns of disabilities involve the whole person and have developed through the years in subtle dysfunctioning, and the focus of the individual complaints may involve any given system or combination of systems within the body. Most often, the patient does not relate his presenting complaints to his old, frequently forgotten whiplash experience.

An example of this was seen in a woman in her mid-fifties, stockily built, strong in physique, and relatively phlegmatic in disposition. Her complaint was chronic chest pain for six years. She had several medical evaluations, but the tests were always negative, and she had been told she should see a psychiatrist. My physical examination revealed the presence of a locked sacrum between the ilia; a characteristic, deep, resistant type of spinal tension; an immobile chest pattern of functioning; and a cervical area that gave me the impression that all the dural sleeves in that area were chronically on tension. This tension extended into the cranial cavity, involving the rest of the reciprocal tension membrane. When questioned, she reported a severe auto accident 14 years before. After the initial injuries had healed, the incident was forgotten. But we know that the fluid pumps of vital functioning through the months and years were not doing their job 10 to 14 times a minute. Microfibrosis was slowly developing in restricted tissues through the months and years. This was an accumulative pattern of pathological physiological functioning that resulted in the chronic complaint of chest pains. Treatment to restore correct functioning in the mechanisms corrected the chest pains, and her health pattern should be better ten years from now than it is at present.

The case history that follows is taken from a lecture
Dr. Becker gave in the 1970's.

ANOTHER CASE THAT ILLUSTRATES the trophic influence of this alternating primary respiratory mechanism-in-action is a patient who had been in a major automobile accident about 30 years before he came to see me. His complaints were of chronic neck and upper back pain. He had a sacrum that was a solid cement block; it had lost its tone quality; it didn't even feel like bone. Also, the muscles of his upper thorax had a glass-like quality to them, like you see in Parkinson's syndrome. Here was evidence of a trophic influence being blocked; he was not getting the trophic influence of the rhythmic balanced interchange between the fluids of the body and his living mechanism. The sacrum was absolutely fixed between the two ilia, and it did not move forward, backwards, upside down, or otherwise, independent of the ilia. The normal rocking motion was not being fed up through the muscles and ligaments from the pelvis. There was just no motion there—it was locked. All the involved muscles were getting withered, the "withering fields."

We began treatments on a once a week basis, and all I did was sit with my hands underneath that sacrum and work within, trying to allow for anything that would come out of the total mechanism. Anything at all that would have any influence on that sacrum, we just wanted it to happen. I put enough compression on an already compressed sacrum to let the sacrum know I was there and told it to wake up. For a time, nothing happened. Then three months later, all of a sudden it dawned on me that it was beginning to act like a piece of very hard wood instead of like stone. In another three months, it hinted that there almost was some motion in that sacrum. Finally, at the end of nine months, he came for a treatment, and that sacrum was really alive; it was functioning as an involuntary mechanism. Sometime during that previous week, with the cumulative effects of nine months of treatment, the sacrum had come alive and was in full, vigorous functioning. At that point, I fired him, since that was the sole purpose of treating him in the first place.

Five years later, he came back, and the tone quality and everything else in the upper thorax was completely normal—there was no glass-like feeling, it was in perfect shape. I see him on occasion socially, and 20 years later, he's just as strong and healthy as you've ever seen. Would he have been that healthy if he'd stayed locked up with that sacrum. No way.

There are literally hundreds of patients who present themselves with cervical and upper backaches and who have forgotten they were in an auto accident. Physical evidence for the lingering effects of a whiplash injury will be found when sought by the physician. The case that is slow to respond to the physician's usual care should be re-examined with this thought in mind.

The first goal of the physician is to secure health for the patient; the second goal is to secure corrective changes in existing pathology in order that health may be restored. In other words, determine the normal for the individual and devote your efforts to bringing that picture into functioning capacity. Do it clinically with each office visit.

Here are a few general comments to be made about a treatment program. The essential difference between allopathic care and osteopathic care is that the allopath understands most of the pathology present but is able only to give supportive care, which includes all types of physiotherapy, exercises, etcetera. The osteopathic physician understands the pathological picture much more clearly because he takes into consideration all the normal factors of physiology and pathology discussed earlier. Then he has the ability to diagnose the lesion complexes present and give physiological corrective treatment that will allow the body to normalize its lesion patterns.

Physiotherapy for deeply involved whiplash cases is not the answer in a therapeutic program for correction. The milder cases may respond, but it is highly likely they would have responded without any care. Mere manipulative mobilization of osseous elements and physiotherapy is also not enough to correct all post-whiplash cases. Deeply involved cases require specific diagnosis and specific treatment to restore health. The lesions of the whiplash case are primarily soft tissue lesion pathology in the ligaments, in the fascias, in the membranous dura mater, in the muscles, and in the central and autonomic nervous systems. Think physiologically and deeply into each individual case and devise techniques that will permit physiological functioning to reassert itself without blind force from without, and the osseous elements will automatically resume their functioning relationship with each other.

It is not necessary to give symptom relief in the case before you today. Seek the physiological cause for the patient's complaints, secure corrective action and the symptom relief will follow naturally.

Many times, in fact most times, a treatment will make the patient feel worse for a few hours or a day or two. It should. You have given physiological orders to sick tissues to make a change, and they respond, not react, by complaining about going to work to create the corrective changes you will find have taken place the next time you see the case.

Very few cases will stay with you until you can completely restore the normal pattern of function they had before the whiplash injury, but practically all of them can be brought back to a well-balanced, compensated, symptom-free state of good function for their daily life. Irreversible pathological areas cannot be restored, but don't be too hasty in making up your mind that some of the problems you see are irreversible. You may be surprised at your results, if you follow through adequately.

Your goal is to seek health within the patient and bring it into active, physiological functioning again. Anyone can find abnormal functioning, including the patient. He hurts. I specifically use the physiological forces within the patient by changing latent, dormant, or quiescent physiological energies within the patient into active or kinetic physiological energies that literally cause the body to treat itself at each office visit. I physiologically plan what is needed for that particular visit and make the patient's body physiologically participate in creating its own treatment program. In treating patients, think physiological function in order to meet the ever-changing patterns presented to you, and you will have rendered the osteopathic service that will heal.

Treatment for chronic whiplash will now be discussed under four headings:

1. Dissipation of unidirectional, unphysiologic whiplash energy fields through the total body physiology of the patient;

2. Restoration of involuntary flexion and extension mobility of

the sacrum between the ilia and release of pelvic fascial drags;
3. Correction of specific ligamentous articular strains associated with the auto accident;
4. Reconstruction and restoration of compensatory myofascial scoliotic tension functioning to "easy" normal for the individual.

1. Dissipation of unidirectional, unphysiologic whiplash energy fields: The presence of this force field can be found by diagnosis as described at length in "X....Whiplash Injury" and "Force Factors With Body Physiology." Briefly, the patient is lying on his back on the table. The physician's hands are slipped under the thoracic area, and the weight of the patient is on the physician's hands. The physician projects his sense of touch so as to sense through the body towards the whole anterior surface of the body. He quietly waits for about a minute or two until he feels as though he can attain this sensation.

He finds a point of balance for the whole of the patient, from the posterior side next to his hands towards the anterior surface of the body. He sits there quietly at that point of balance until he senses that a change has taken place within all the body physiology he is capable of feeling. This usually occurs within approximately five minutes and represents the amount of dissipation that can take place for that one treatment session. The physician is initiating the body physiology to release its nondissipated energy field, and this process will continue between office visits.

The next office visit will reveal a modification of the pattern of nondissipated energy field in comparison to the last visit. The technique is repeated with each visit until the physician is satisfied that body physiology has released the unidirectional, unphysiologic whiplash energy field. After the physician has gained experience with this, in many cases he will actually feel the energy field "come to life," so to speak, as he finds the point of balance, and he will feel a change take place within that energy field as it releases itself in body physiology.

The key to this technique is the projection of the sense of touch through the hands under the thoracic area. This does *not* mean pushing firmly up into the body physiology of the patient. The weight of the patient on the hands is firm enough contact. It does mean trying to project a sense of touch *through* to the anterior surface of the body while the hands lie quietly alert under the thoracic area.

2. *Restoration* of involuntary flexion and extension mobility of the sacrum between the ilia and release of pelvic fascial drags: To summarize the technique for diagnosis of sacral jamming given earlier in this article, the one hand is under the sacrum, and the other forearm and hand are bridged across the anterior pelvis. Then, when the feet are flexed and extended, the pelvis is felt to move as one unit if the sacrum has been jammed into the pelvis in its involuntary flexion-extension mobility.

One technique for release of this jamming is to continue to have the patient flex and extend the feet rhythmically as the motive force for release. The physician, with the hand under the sacrum, projects his sense of touch towards a balance point of function similar to that of projecting a sense of touch for dissipation of whiplash energy forces. In other words, the physician works to transform the inertia of a sacrum lying on his hand into a sacrum that can move during the flexion-extension cycle of the moving feet. The arm and hand across the anterior superior spines of the two ilia are simultaneously cooperating by increasing the pressure on each anterior superior spine gently, so as to anteriorly approximate the two ilia and posteriorly pry them apart, allowing the sacrum room in which to unjam itself. Further assistance by the patient can be obtained by having the patient take a deep breath while he is working his feet and the physician is securing his point of balance. Have him hold the breath to the limit and expel it. Repeat two or three times.

This rhythmic flexion and extension of the feet and opening of the pelvic bowl by the physician is continued until the physician can feel any initiating change of release at the pelvic girdle that is permissible for that one treatment session. It is not necessary to get a total release. The total time for this technique need not be more than five minutes at any given treatment session. Body physiology will work on the problem until the next visit and through subsequent visits until a total release can and does take place.

Again, the key to a better palpatory sense of touch for the physician for both diagnosis and treatment is for the physician to project his sense of touch from the hand under the sacrum towards the contacts on the iliac crests and to project the sense of touch from the arm and hand on top towards the hand under the sacrum. In this manner, the physician gains the maximum insight into what is happening in the pelvic girdle, while the patient adds his cooperation by moving his feet and/or holding his breath.

Correction of the diagnosed strain is one of careful consideration of all the factors present within the injured ligamentous and membranous articular processes. It should be of utmost gentleness, trying to allow the physiological processes within to manifest their own unerring powers to release the strain, with the hand under the sacrum merely guiding and analyzing the process. Thrust and other forceful techniques are too severe for this type of problem. Many of these patients have experienced the use of these techniques for the problem before, and the restrictions are still present. A gentler approach is more effective because it does not add to the trauma by introducing an external force. Any release secured is compatible with the patient's total capacity to utilize the newly gained freedom physiologically for healing and function. Remember that the purpose here is to resecure normal fulcrum function and not merely to force a change of position within the given area.

This type of stress pattern, as with all stress patterns, manifests as loss of freedom of voluntary motion and loss of involuntary motions inherent within the second sacral segment as part of the body's homeostatic function. Remember, then, that it is important to restore the voluntary use of the second sacral segment, and it is equally important to restore the automatic-shifting-suspension-fulcrum activity of the second sacral segment to its full homeostatic capacity for function. It may perhaps be thought that if one is corrected, the other is corrected automatically. This is not true. With persistence of either problem, the patient's distress pattern will recur. With a total correction of both phases, there is very little chance for recurrence.

After correction of the sacrum has been attempted and as much released as is advisable for the patient's problem at that particular treatment, the test for motion can be rechecked. If some motion has been regained for this area, there will be an immediate change in the motion perceived between the bridged ilia and sacrum. It is well to make haste slowly in these cases and to let the newly acquired, more efficient automatic fulcrum manifest its healing impacts upon the injured thoracic and cervical areas.

3. Correction of specific ligamentous articular strains associated with the auto accident: The patient has been thrust violently against some object in the car. Even in minor accidents, there is considerable forceful action in the contacts made upon the body against the parts of the seat belt or automobile. Add to this the unidirectional, unphysiologic whiplash energy fields. As a result, there is microtrauma to all the fascias of the body and to the somatic cells enveloped by those fascias. Ligamentous articular strains are produced, especially in those areas of the spine that make direct contact against specific parts of the automobile and as a result of the rapid, whiplike action of the head and cervical area in its action pattern of motion during the first moments of the accident.

The physician may use any of the osteopathic techniques in which he has perfected his skills to make a diagnosis and to give treatment for these specific ligamentous articular lesions. He should keep in mind the following points: These lesions may be found from the cranium through the spine down to and including the sacrum, the rib cage, and the appendicular areas; they are traumatic in origin, with a lot of energy involved in their production, and thus they have an organic connotation rather than just being functional in character; the deeper layers of fascia on a cross section through the entire body at the level of the lesioned area are involved as well as the deeper layers of fascial planes superiorly and inferiorly to the lesion.

It has been my clinical experience that using the dissipating techniques for the relief of general myofascial strains and the unlocking of the jammed sacrum, if either or both factors are present in the case, does a great deal to promote the release of the soft tissue strains associated with the specific lesion pathology. I use these techniques prior to my specific corrections of the lesion in question. The osteopathic techniques used for the correction of these specific lesions should include an awareness of the depth of tissues involved rather than just focusing on securing mobility in a specific facet syndrome. Try to sense a corrective change taking place through all the cross section of soft tissues for the specific lesion area as well as for the facets as the technique is applied.

4. Reconstruction and restoration of compensatory myofascial scoliotic tension functioning to "easy" normal for the individual: Microtrauma to fascial planes throughout the body and the production of specific lesion pathology have contributed to the breakdown of well-compensated scoliotic functioning from the sphenobasilar synchondrosis above to the sacrum below. This decompensation will not be voiced by patients in the presenting complaints when the patients come in for care in chronic whiplash cases, but it can be found by careful palpatory diagnosis by the physician in his examination of the patients. Well-compensated scoliosis is a part of normal health for the patient and the decompensations should be corrected.

The corrective steps proceed as follows: release of unidirectional unphysiological myofascial drags; release of the jammed sacral mechanism; correction of specific ligamentous articular lesions. Usually the corrections of these three factors will permit the body physiology of the patient to restore its own compensation of the scoliotic tension patterns, but there are some cases that require additional help. This is done by evaluating the pattern that should be present in the patient and gently exaggerating the rotated spinal bodies above and below the crossover areas of the scoliosis to the point of balance for the whole cross section of the body at that area. Hold for a few moments while body physiology secures its own myofascial release. Do this at each crossover pattern of scoliosis. Repeat this at each treatment session until you are satisfied that recompensation is assured for the patient.

In summary, four factors have been given as being present in chronic whiplash automobile accident cases: the presence of unidirectional, unphysiologic energy fields; the loss of involuntary flexion and extension of the sacrum between the ilia; the presence of specific ligamentous articular lesions; and decompensations of scoliotic tension patterns. Diagnosis and treatment programs for the patient do not have to include all four of them at every office visit, but the presence of them should be evaluated and worked on as indicated by whichever is dominant and needs attention for that particular day. The body physiology of the patient is constantly trying to automatically release these strained patterns back to normal health. It is up to the physician to assist that body physiology in those areas of dysfunction indicated by his diagnostic insight and treatment skills, in cooperation with the body physiology of the patient.

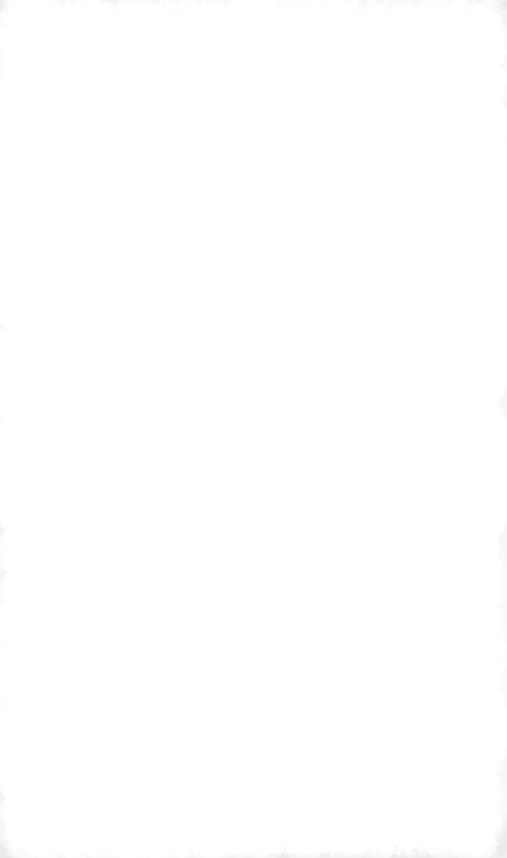

Clinical

Considerations

APPROACHING CLINICAL PROBLEMS
This material is excerpted from a paper dated January 1958.

BEFORE A DISCUSSION OF any clinical topic is broached, I think it is wise to lay down a big picture before it gets clouded by too many details. The cranial concept is a portion of a broader concept–the osteopathic concept as envisioned by Dr. Andrew T. Still. Dr. William G. Sutherland insisted that his work be credited to that started by Dr. Still. It was never meant to be a separate study apart from the general science of osteopathy.

Throughout the writings of Dr. Sutherland, one can see his broad understanding of the cranial concept and its relationship to osteopathy in general. From these writings, further conclusions can be reached: His was a total concept in its construction, and the tools of it were the cranial-sacral, anatomical-physiological mechanisms, the inherent living quality of its capacity for self-sustained functioning, and the role of the operator to elicit knowledge of its mechanisms for diagnosis and treatment. This type of reasoning necessitates at least some degree of insight before any of its parts may be lifted out of context and defined or discussed. The same is true for the writings of Dr. Still.

It is important when dealing with the works of men like Drs. Still and Sutherland that one think in terms of the whole person. The physiological processes that constitute the normal and the dysfunctions in those processes that constitute disease are merely part of the total picture. These individual portions should always be thought of as part of a total pattern and their place evaluated on that basis. Drs. Still and Sutherland wrote their works with that totality in mind. They did not separate the person from his physiological processes or his disease processes. They kept the whole person in the forepart of their minds as they worked with the physiological or disease process that they were studying. The total patient was the reference point for their reasoning, and the processes under observation for diagnosis and treatment were the tools with which they worked.

In all clinical problems, it is important to think in terms of a whole person or whole cranial mechanism that is suffering the disability and to visualize this disability in terms of the total process, rather than just the local one under consideration. It makes for more cohesive thinking and for a more complete diagnosis and thorough treatment.

CLINICAL OBSERVATIONS
This is an edited transcription of a lecture given in 1976 at a Sutherland
Cranial Teaching Foundation basic course in Milwaukee, Wisconsin.

I would like to bring out a few things that I have observed in my practice.

Hypertension: It is interesting that in most cases of essential hypertension, you will find the tentorium cerebelli seems to be pushed down and spread out; it's relatively flattened and does not want to dome up. I've treated a number of them. That reciprocal tension membrane has to be retrained to function normally; this is done slowly, over time—how many years does it take to develop that essential hypertension? But you can gradually teach that reciprocal tension membrane to do its job of domeing rhythmically, and the essential hypertension will be brought under control with less drugs than it would ordinarily take.

Dyslexia: You're going to run into dyslexic children once in awhile. The parents often come to you, not because the child has dyslexia but because of something else, and in passing, they report the dyslexia to you. As a supplemental treatment, it is possible to help them. As a clinical finding in practically all dyslexic children, there is an intraosseous lesion of the temporal bone in which the petrous portion is twisted into an internal-rotation type of strain, whereas the squama is more or less like it's supposed to be. In checking these kids, this temporal bone almost feels as if it were an occipitomastoid type of strain, with a traumatic tensity on that tentorium that says that this is not correct. But it is an intraosseous lesion of the right temporal bone usually, sometimes the left, depending upon the child. Through molding techniques and directing the cerebrospinal fluid tide down along the petrous connections, the articulations down along the occipitomastoid suture, and at the junction with the squama, things can change. Gradually mold that temporal bone back towards the capacity for function—once a week for awhile, then every other week, and then once a month. Things change slowly. If you give a child this treatment now, let's say this is June, then not the September of this school year but the September of the next year, that child will be showing marked improvement and will continue to modify his dyslexia.

Parkinson's Disease: I've had good results in three cases of Parkinson's syndrome by putting them on crutches. Make them walk on crutches for a solid year, and they will treat themselves. It springs the upper dorsals and ribs where the sympathetics come from. What happens in Parkinson's? They get bound down tighter and tighter and tighter in the thorax and choke off the autonomic nerve supply that controls the blood supply to the brain. Parkinson's is a chronic, degenerative, central nervous system disturbance, and these individuals are years preparing themselves to express symptoms. That's why it takes at least a year—every step they're on their feet—of walking on crutches adjusted to reach up into the axilla to gradually spring that thing loose. Eventually, they will correct some of their problem and keep it under control through this self-treatment at home. You don't need to treat them. Dr. Still, the founder of osteopathy, said he never saw a man that had to walk on crutches that ever had a case of shaking palsy. That's where I stole the idea from.

Multiple Sclerosis: I have four cases of multiple sclerosis that insist that I work on them every other week, and I'm perfectly glad to do so because I feel that it encourages remission and helps prevent exacerbation in this up-and-down condition, though I'm not planning on making an organic change in their multiple sclerosis.

Sternum: The sternum is supposed to recede during inhalation and come out during exhalation, the same as the bregma and glabella recede during flexion and extend during extension or exhalation. The sternum is supposed to do the same thing, but when you hold your posture with your chest back, you're locking it up. Letting things relax allows this movement to happen.

Rheumatoid Arthritis: CV4 is a fantastic treatment for rheumatoid arthritis. Utilized on a once a week basis for six months to a year, depending upon the severity of the case, you can wash out the stasis of the connective tissues of the body and give those people a symptom-free pattern for function. It builds up their vital capacity to be alive and feel well, and it takes once a week for six months to a year to achieve the results you want. This is a supplement to their medical program or anything else you want to do.

Brachial Neuropathy with Locked Sacrum: I mentioned elsewhere that in whiplash injuries, make sure the sacrum floats along with the rest of the mechanism. I only bother to reiterate this because there are usually no complaints coming from the sacrum. Almost invariably, you have to go shopping for it. They're not going to say they're hurting down there, they'll say they're hurting up higher somewhere.

This concept was illustrated in a non-whiplash case of a young man with bilateral brachial neuropathies that he had experienced for 15 months. When I took ahold of his neck and shoulders to find out why he had a brachial neuropathy, I felt as if I was at the far end of a lever because no matter what I was doing at this end, as I was sitting quietly, I was being moved around. Well, if I'm at the end of a lever that is moving, obviously there must be some fulcrum point somewhere that is relatively still. So I went down to check the sacrum, and, yes, it was completely locked in its respiratory function. On further questioning, I got the pertinent history. The guy was a sports car enthusiast, and he weighed 150 pounds. One day, he picked up his car engine himself to put it into the car and locked his sacrum.

The first two times he was in the office, I was trying to figure out what the score was. The third time, I found the sacrum and released it. The fourth time, the sacrum was free, and the fifth time, there was no brachial neuropathy, period. Now that was the end of that case. Because his sacrum was fixed and locked, up in the shoulder girdle he was doing everything against resistance. Your pelvis is supposed to give when you move your arms. With the loss of this micromovement, every time he moved, he had to move both the ilia and the sacrum, and there was a constant tension on his brachial nerves. When the sacrum released so there was free movement, there was no tension on the fascias around the brachial plexus. This is the same situation that maintains the chronic whiplash case.

Vault Compression: It is possible to get a tremendous, traumatic compression of the entire vault by its getting jammed down into whatever cranial base they may have. You go through the windshield of a car, or you get tossed off of a horse in a rodeo accident and come down on the top of your head, and what happens? The total vault is compressed down into a marked external rotation position and jammed into a cranial base that may be a flexion or extension base, a torsion or sidebending-rotation base, or whatever base it is, and there it sits. One fellow I've seen had this condition for seven years standing; he had a long, narrow base with this big, wide top. He did not have headaches for seven years, he had head pain. Gradually, as we were able to get a reduction of this mechanism back towards the normal, his whole head became long and narrow again and felt free. Now what has been accomplished there? Not only are we changing the position and the function of that cranial vault, we're also dissipating the forces it took to allow this to happen in the first place.

Mild Occipitomastoid Lesions: Occipitomastoid lesions are common, and most of them are minor. The more severe ones are going to present with enough reactions and clinical symptoms to indicate you'd better go looking for them. But the milder ones are not going to tell you so clearly that they are there. Here is a clue. If there is an occipitomastoid lesion present, the occiput is jammed up inside the temporal bone, and even when modest, the lesion limits some of the function of this joint. Well, that temporal bone influences the sphenoid and the fascias on the base of that skull, affecting their normal flexion and extension mechanism. So what is the effect of their limited functioning on the fascias on that half of the body? They are relatively immobile. So what are you going to get from the history of a patient in this situation? You're going to get a patient who says, "All my problems have always been on the right side; I've never had any trouble with the left." Look for a mild occipitomastoid lesion in these people.

The Balance of Energy: This type of approach tends to dissipate unwanted energy and also permits wanted energy to again flow into a patient who is at a very low ebb. When a patient comes in, I register in my own mind that patient's voltage. A patient who has any degree of health at all should be 110 volts of alternating current—they just feel alive. (I'm not too much interested in the rate of the cranial rhythmic impulse, the CRI—how much does it move per minute—I am mainly interested in the quality of it.) But a patient may only have 50 volts for some reason or other, and they may have been that way for a long while. Then as you work with them, you are revitalizing that field of energy that is their life force upwards towards the normal 110 volts.

You can also drain off the excess energy if it is an overload for them. I'll give you a clinical example. A man came into the office for a treatment, and I read his mechanism as having basically 110 volts. It was a relatively normal mechanism in some ways, but there was a sense of it being a suspended 110 volts, a suspended mechanism that says, "I would like to work, but I'm not too sure that it's a good idea at this particular moment." As I was doing whatever I was for that treatment, probably a CV4, I was in contact with the fluid drive and the reciprocal tension membrane, and all of a sudden, there was a change or shift within it, and he began to cry. Then he told me he had just finished building a new swimming pool and had opened it up the day before; the neighbor's child had come over and drowned in it. So what he had was a total shock and a totally locked mechanism, and with the treatment, he drained off this emotional load and came back to function again. The energy that was locking him up went back to wherever it came from. Where energy comes from, we care not, but we know the mechanism can tune into it and either build it up or dissipate it as needed. It requires a certain amount of care and caution in working with these emotional strains in patients.

So you can read the pattern in people. In patients you have treated over time, when you are looking to pick up the pattern that you're ordinarily accustomed to finding in them, you can find little areas of overload or underload that perhaps could use a little drainage or a little recharge. So you have many uses for what you've learned this week—far more than you can realize at this time.

Timing a Lesion: You can learn to sense the time a problem has been in existence. People ask me, "How do you know this guy's had this problem ten years?" There's nothing to it. When I find some old, chronic ligamentous articular or membranous articular strain, I ask the patient, "When did you have an accident in this particular area?" They might answer, "Ten years ago." Well, that's what a ten-year-old strain feels like. It's simple. As you do this over and over again, you begin to recognize what is a ten-year-old strain. Keep it simple.

VISCERAL CONSIDERATIONS:
CARDIAC AND GENITOURINARY
This is an edited transcription of a recorded conversation between
Dr. Rollin Becker and his son, Donald Becker, M.D., in 1967.

BEFORE ANSWERING YOUR QUESTIONS about your cases with cardiac and urinary tract problems, I would like to interject a few comments about osteopathic technique in general. There is a tendency in discussing osteopathic technique to think of it in terms of osseous relationships only. The osteopathic physician has a tendency to say he fixed the fifth lumbar, corrected a third dorsal, manipulated a fourth cervical, or moved the sixth rib on the left side. In other words, he describes the osteopathic lesion in terms of osseous relationships when, as a matter of fact, this is not what he's doing at all. He is giving it a title according to the general area in which he is operating. But I have never yet seen a skeleton walk into my office to get an osteopathic treatment.

When you look at the complexity of the myofascial, ligamentous, articular, total mechanism of the body, you get a different picture. Get an anatomy text and look at a cross section of the body at the level of a thoracic vertebra. You see the musculature surrounding it, the lungs internally, the nerve supply, the blood supply, etcetera. Now when you place your hands upon a tissue, you are feeling all that mass of tissue—muscles, ligaments, nerve supply, venous drainage, arterial supply, lymphatics, the whole works—and as you read it through your perceptive touch, you are getting a coordinated pattern of functioning and dysfunctioning of the entire mechanism and not of the osseous relationship alone.

Getting motion into the osseous relationship is not the primary purpose of osteopathic treatment. The primary purpose of diagnosis and treatment osteopathically is to secure function in the total mechanism at that particular segment you are working on, not merely to mobilize or create motion in an osseous relationship. The total area is involved in terms of dysfunction. If you have a strain pattern, normalizing the function of that area to function as it was designed to do in that particular patient according to their physiologic need is the purpose of diagnosis and treatment.

I give you this brief analysis because your next two questions on specific pathologies, cardiac and urinary tract, both require a broader viewpoint than the mere osseous relationships described for the typical osteopathic lesion. We are dealing here with the capacity for organ functioning, and we've got to think in terms of functioning anatomy and physiology as it applies to that organ, and its capacity to be sick and its capacity to get well.

The Heart

In dealing with cardiac pathology—myocardial infarction, coronary insufficiency, chronic congestive failure—we have to think in terms of the nerve supply, the blood supply, and the functioning of the total cardiac mechanism as it lives and breathes literally within a functioning thoracic cage. The cardiac area rides on the top of the diaphragm and is being rocked up and down rhythmically with the motion of the diaphragm. It receives its basic nerve supply from the autonomic nerve plexuses in the upper thoracic areas.

These lie on the heads of the ribs, up and down the thoracic chain, and give off branches that go up into the cervical area, into the cardiac ganglion, and then descend down to the heart for the sympathetic division. The parasympathetic division comes from the vagus nerve in the basilar area of the skull through the jugular foramen. If we're going to do anything for these patients, we're going to have to think of the normal anatomy and physiology that helps control the functioning of that cardiac mechanism, and that is very briefly the anatomy and physiology of the central control over the cardiac mechanism.

I'm treating a young medical pediatrician for a low back problem, and I had him listen to the tape you sent me, and he was very much interested in how I was going to answer the problem I am discussing with you right now, this cardiac situation. So I gave him the same story that I just got through giving you, and he was asking me why all cardiac cases have strains in these areas anyway (which is what I find). Well, it's not due to the fact that they've had a cardiac problem that you have stress and strain and problems with tension in the upper thoracic area—that probably has little or nothing to do with it. You can't differentiate and be so specific as to say: Because you've got these strains in this particular area, this is the cause for heart problems.

Instead I answered him by saying that everyone has a scoliosis, some degree of lateral curvature, mild and always functional, and never severe enough to demand attention or even to look at very carefully. But the standard scoliotic curve that occurs in most individuals is going to have crossover areas where the bodies of the vertebra are shifting to the right or left to create the scoliosis they have. With this scoliosis, the usual pattern is to find a lot of tension at either end of the spine in the upper cervicals and at the pelvis. Additionally, there usually are two main crossover areas of tension: one in the lower thoracic and upper lumbar and another as the curve crosses over at the upper thoracic.

This means that vertebral bodies that have swung to the right are having a struggle in cooperating with the ones that are swinging to the left in the upper thoracic area and vice versa. And very frequently, we do not find the patient has only a simple scoliosis such as I have described, but they may also have multiple variations of scoliotic tension patterns. They may have a flat upper thoracic area and a prominent lumbar spine. We may find they have a little dipsy-doodle area of about four or five segments of the upper thoracics that are relatively anterior in that position instead of the posterior, gentle roundness we're supposed to find in normal spinal mechanics.

So there can be any kind or combination of postural strain patterns that have existed all the patient's life. And often the crossover is in the general area that is supplying the heart with autonomic functioning. This means that the rib, the musculature, the ligaments and so forth associated with that upper thoracic area are also slightly embarrassed in their functioning. All this is a contributing pattern to potential maintenance of cardiac pathology.

Now let's get down to the diaphragm. Good, normal diaphragmatic action is very important in the functioning of the cardiac areas as well as for the kidneys, which we are going to discuss in a few minutes. Think of the cardiac area and the diaphragm in this respect: The left crura of the diaphragm is supplying musculature for the right side of the diaphragm; the right crura of the diaphragm is leading up to and forming part of the musculature of the left diaphragm. So if we can do something to release the tone or the tensity of the crura in the upper lumbar area on each side, we are going to have a tendency to normalize the diaphragmatic freedom of motion.

Figure five in the "Diagnostic Touch" series (see Chapter Five) is the general application I use to get to this crura of the diaphragm. The figure is entitled "Upper Lumbar and Psoas Muscle," but what I am doing is sliding my fingertips just underneath the twelfth rib pointing towards the lumbar vertebra. The crura of the diaphragm, as well as the psoas muscle, lies anterior to and on the sides of the body of the vertebra, so you have to think deep into this thing. You get your fingertips underneath and close to the head of the twelfth rib and just beneath the twelfth rib in this general area. Then think deep and into and through to the crura of the diaphragm, and bring your fingers slightly laterally, following the course of the twelfth rib. Think deep until you can sense or feel a change taking place up anteriorly in the crura on that particular side. If you are working on the right side, you are going to be releasing the right crura and affecting the left diaphragm. Get around under the left side, and you're going to be working on the crura of the left side and affecting the diaphragm on the right. So this takes care of releasing the crura of the diaphragm on each side of the lumbar area.

You then can get your hands underneath the upper thoracic area, as shown in "Diagnostic Touch" figures seven and eight (see Chapter

Five), and you try to feel the functioning of the upper thoracic area, the normalization–the releasing of the tension in the upper thoracic area as well as in the upper rib cage on each side. By taking care of the upper thoracic area and securing the functioning of the vertebra as well as the ribs and associated muscles and all the works, you are releasing the origin of the cardiac plexus, which travels up to the cervical area (which is generally fairly mobile in that area) and then goes down to the heart. The parasympathetic innervation travels by way of the basilar area of the skull, and some gentle attention to the temporal and occipital area is in order to see to it that the functioning between the temporal bone and occiput is sufficient to help the vagus nerve do its job.

Another point of interest in cardiac cases–I have seen it several times and you perhaps can learn to sense it also–is that when a patient has had a myocardial infarction, this represents an implosion, if you want to call it that, within the chest. The infarction comes on suddenly, it hits like a ton of bricks, and the patient is shocked. In these cases, I find a general shock throughout the total thorax, as if there had been an implosion of a bomb that went off within the chest. For this, I place one hand under the thoracic area, with the patient on their back, and the other hand is on top over the midchest and cardiac area. Then I just sit there for a little while to allow the shock effect to resolve itself as an energy field back toward the place from whence it came, the environment around it. I usually spend a very short time on this–two to three minutes at the most–each time that I am working with those other specific areas that control cardiac functioning.

These cardiac cases are not situations that suddenly come out of a clear blue sky, having had a healthy heart, so practically all these problems are relatively chronic cases. The tensions in the thoracic area, rib cage, and crura of the diaphragm are long-standing, tense areas that are going to take a series of treatments to respond. You might see them weekly or twice a week, whatever you decide, and usually within a month, you will see an appreciable difference in this type of case. In your patient with congestive heart failure, you could produce results within a month or six weeks, and it's noticeable to the patient. They're a lot more comfortable, and it will be a good supplement to the digitalis they're taking.

Also, you're not only correcting diaphragmatic function for the cardiac mechanism when you release the crura and lower ribs, you are also restoring the capacity of the liver to move up and down freely, as it was designed to do, and you are releasing the tension in and around the lung trees. So you are affecting the total capacity of the heart, the lungs, the liver, and the renal area to prevent the congestive failure that follows cardiac cases. I think if you try this for a period of five or six weeks on two or three cases, you will find that there will be more to discuss when you get some experience with it.

The Genitourinary System

Let's move into the other problem you brought up in our discussion: a young female, with recurrent urinary tract infections, where concerns for future kidney problems make her a candidate for the use of suppressive antibiotics. We have to consider the basic anatomy controlling these areas. There are pelvic splanchnic nerves supplying the parasympathetics and carrying with them some of the sympathetic flow. The lower thoracic and upper two lumbar splanchnic nerves supply the sympathetic nerve supply to the kidneys and suprarenal structures as well as the sympathetic flow to the bladder and pelvic organs.

We also have something else to consider. From the standpoint of the movement of these kidneys, they move up and down with respiration and move with every body movement of the patient. They ride on the surface of the crura of the diaphragm and the psoas major muscle on either side of the lumbar spine. The uterus and bladder sit on top of the pelvic diaphragm.

There are several diaphragms in the body, if you stop to analyze it. There is the pelvic diaphragm, which goes across the middle of the pelvis; the thoracic diaphragm, separating the thorax and the abdomen; and a cranial diaphragm, which is the tentorium cerebelli bilaterally, separating the cerebral hemispheres from the cerebellar content underneath. All three diaphragms descend during inhalation and ascend during exhalation—you know this to be true for the thoracic diaphragm, and it is equally true for the pelvic and cranial diaphragms.

The pelvic diaphragm gets bound down in a lot of these problems that you're discussing, especially in young females; it gets crowded downward so that it doesn't move up and down rhythmically. The pelvic diaphragm can be held down on one side or bilaterally, as a result of having given birth to children or from gynecologic surgery, which acts as a deterrent to free functioning of the pelvic diaphragm. In this case, the bladder, vagina, and other organs are all being interfered with in their fascial envelopes in a mild sort of way—they're not getting the motion they should during the respiratory cycle.

Therefore, because healthy tissues throw off germ infections of all kinds, our treatment goals are to restore the nerve supply controlling the blood supply to these organs and also to create the motion that should be available to these areas. The treatment to release the pelvic diaphragm is relatively simple. In 1949, Dr. Howard Lippincott wrote an article on some of the techniques of William G. Sutherland.[1] One of the techniques he describes is the so-called pelvic lift. It is an approach to lifting the pelvic contents, which include the pelvic diaphragm, and freeing up the fascial connections in and around the organs of the pelvis.

To do this, the patient is turned on their side, and you position your fingers so that two or three fingers are placed on the medial side of the ischium in the ischiorectal fossa. You allow the palmar surface of the fingers to follow upwards on the inner side of the tuberosity of the ischium, lifting the pelvic fascias towards the head during the exhalation of the patient. As the patient takes a big breath, you'll feel these tissues come down against your fingers; then as the patient exhales, you can very gently feel your fingers working their way cephalad, up along the inner rim of the tuberosity. At the end of each exhalation, you hold that position gently—you don't try to crowd it—and as the patient inhales, you just don't let it come down; and during the next exhalation period, you follow it up another step. After the patient has inhaled and exhaled four or five or six or seven times, all of a sudden, it just feels as if your fingers kind of give. I mean by that they just feel as if they flow upwards into the pelvis with little resistance. Have the patient turn over on the other side and repeat on the opposite side.

It is also good to check the relative functioning of the various diaphragms. While your hand is in position contacting the pelvic diaphragm, you can take the other hand and put it up on the side of the lower rib cage and see if the pelvic diaphragm on that side is rising and descending in cooperation and at the same time that the thoracic diaphragm is going up and down. I have seen some cases after pelvic surgery, or after the birth of a baby, in which the pelvic diaphragm would actually be descending while the thoracic diaphragm would be ascending—there can be some confusion of function down in this area. The idea is to get that pelvic diaphragm to rise and descend during normal inhalation and exhalation.

There is another thing that can be done in bladder problems. If you look at figure number two in the "Diagnostic Touch" series (see Chapter Five), you'll see that one hand is placed underneath the sacrum, and in the very next picture, number three, you'll notice that the fingers of the opposite hand are slid under the fifth lumbar from the side. In bladder problems, there's always a strain or a tension in the area between the fifth lumbar and the sacrum. There's a tissue tension in and around and all through the fifth lumbar and sacral area. Interestingly enough, by releasing the tension (with the one hand under the sacrum and the opposite hand under the spinous process of the fifth lumbar to see what's going on)—by working in that area for a little while until you can begin to feel function restored to it in terms of its ability to do what it wants to—you're going to have a lot of control over bladder irritability.

When your grandmother was visiting us several years ago, she had enough bladder incontinence that she was wearing pads. She was here for six weeks, and I gave her daily treatments doing no more than what I just got through describing to you, and at the end of that time, she didn't have to wear anything, and she was perfectly comfortable for two to three hours at a time. After she left, she eventually went back to the same degree of bladder incontinence, but, of course, it was a long-standing, chronic problem, and she needed ongoing treatment. But the idea is to get into that area for bladder irritability and get some correction for the fifth lumbar and sacral mechanism.

In these genitourinary problems, we also go up to and free the crura of the diaphragm on each side as described for the cardiac case. This does two things: It releases the tension in the psoas muscle and the crura of the diaphragm both, and it is a stimulatory influence upon the autonomic nerve supply to the kidneys and the pelvis. While you are under the sacrum and fifth lumbar, you are automatically tending to tone up the nerves there, the pelvic parasympathetic nerve supply.

I believe these simple maneuvers—the so-called pelvic lift or pelvic diaphragm release, the fifth lumbar and sacral mechanism release, and the psoas-crura release for the floating action of the kidneys as well as the autonomic nerve supply—will contribute towards normalizing or giving some help in these chronic bladder cases. Check out the pelvic diaphragm and lumbosacral area rather carefully in these people, and work to get a very definite release in the two areas. See if it doesn't make a difference in symptomatology and their need for suppressive medication; give me a little report on it later on.

1. Howard Lippincott, "The Osteopathic Technique of Wm. G. Sutherland, D.O.," 1949 *Yearbook* of the Academy of Applied Osteopathy. Reprinted in *Teachings in the Science of Osteopathy*, pp. 233-284.

KNEE INJURIES

This is an edited transcription of a recorded conversation between
Dr. Rollin Becker and his son, Donald Becker, M.D., in 1967.

YOU ASKED ABOUT KNEE injuries, about a 16-year-old boy who was going to have a cartilage removed. In my book, if and when they actually tear ligaments or cartilage and disturb the relationship, then it probably is necessary to operate and take out that particular cartilage. However, there's another layer of the problem that also needs to be checked, and this is what I wanted to give you some detail on.

The same strain or stress it took to produce the knee injury is also going to be reflected into the acetabular area. This creates a functional change in the acetabular area as follows: Everyone has an acetabulum that wants to rotate more fully into either internal or external rotation, depending on their pelvic pattern. In my particular case, I have a right acetabulum that likes to rotate externally, and the left acetabulum likes to rotate internally. That's the configuration in my pelvic functioning.

Now, in these cases where they have torn a knee up pretty badly so as to create problems down in that area, it is possible to create a strain in the acetabular area so that it goes against the normal pattern of functioning for that pelvis. In my case, since I have an external rotation pattern in my right hip, if I were to have a knee injury that forced the acetabular mechanism into an internal rotation strain, that would be contrary to the balance between the pelvis and upper ends of the femur.

To assess this, I cup my hands behind the knees of the seated patient, resting my own elbows on my knees, and I simply rotate the acetabulum in each leg to find out in what direction it would like to rotate (see figure 24 in the chapter, "Diagnostic Touch"). I check the good leg, and I find out whether it wants to go into internal rotation or external rotation. Then, I check the leg in which the strain has occurred at the knee and find out if it prefers to go into the opposite pattern because normally in each patient, one side will be in external rotation and the other side, internal rotation.

Then, if I do find, let's say, an internal rotation pattern strain, I deliberately take it in towards that pattern of strain, utilizing the same approach as viewed in figure 24, until I feel the release in and at the level of the pelvis. I will then find that the pattern has reversed itself back to fit the normalcy for that particular patient. This correction of the acetabular strains in the relatively mild knee cases, or the ones that have not had extensive ligamentous tear patterns, will promote healing to take place in the knee by the readjustment of the long leverages of the hamstring and anterior thigh muscles. The knee problem can then go ahead and make a more adequate correction in its own right, as long as it does not have to operate from a partial strain in the acetabular area. So all cases of knee injuries should have the acetabular area checked to establish the normal pattern that is right for that particular individual's pelvis and to correct any internal or external rotation strains that might be present there.

SINUS PROBLEMS

This is an edited transcription of a recorded conversation between
Dr. Rollin Becker and his son, Donald Becker, M.D., in 1962.

STOP TO THINK FOR a minute: Where do sinus problems begin? What sinuses are involved? Every individual is going to have his own private set of sinus problems.

The sinuses to consider include the ethmoid sinuses, which are multiple, small, air cells within the ethmoid bone. Then there are the maxillary sinuses in each of the maxillary bones and the frontal sinuses, which can be a single large sinus in each of the frontal bones. (I use the plural because at birth there are two frontal bones, and throughout life, even though they unite, they act independently in the respiratory mechanism.) There is also a sphenoid sinus back in the sphenoid bone.

All these sinuses are composed of air cells within bony cavities that interchange air rhythmically during the primary respiratory movement. But what guides the respiratory movement? We find that each of the sinuses has a "plumber's friend," a mechanism similar to the stick with a rubber cup on the end used to pump out toilets. There is a plumber's friend which literally pumps each of the sinuses involved within the cranial cavity. The plumber's friend for the maxillary sinus is the zygomatic bone; for the sphenoid sinus, it is the vomer. The plumber's friend for the frontal bones can be thought of as the ethmoid bone—the perpendicular plate of the ethmoid, which, with the crista galli, is rocking up and down during respiratory movements of the cranial base. The plumber's friend for the ethmoid sinuses is that same rhythmic motion of the crista galli, moving up and down (actually posteriorly and anteriorly).

We have talked about the zygomatic bone, the vomer, and the perpendicular plate of the ethmoid. But where do they get their motions from? We have to reach deeper and deeper into the cranial mechanism to understand sinus problems. Fastening to the crista galli of the ethmoid bone is the anterior end of the falx cerebri, which curves backward, going back to the junction with the tentorium cerebelli. The tentorium cerebelli has a strong attachment to the junction with the falx cerebri and also fastens to the right and left petrous ridges of the temporal bones. Dr. Sutherland called these the three sickles: the left tentorium, the right tentorium, and the falx cerebri. So actually, when we are dealing with sinus problems, we're dealing with membranous articular strains involving the falx cerebri or the tentorium cerebelli.

The tentorium cerebelli attaches to the petrous portion of the temporal bones, and the temporal bones fasten into the zygomatic bones. Restrictions of the right temporal bone in its full respiratory movement would restrict the motions of the zygomatic bone on the right, in turn, restricting the up-and-down, pumping action of the plumber's friend involving the right maxillary sinus.

Restrictions involving the falx cerebri physiologically interfere with the normal motility and mobility of its anterior attachments to the crista galli of the ethmoid bone and to the sphenoid bone. The sphenoid is responsible for practically all the normal mobility of the fourteen facial bones. Most of the bones that comprise the face have a direct connection with the sphenoid bone or a clear, indirect connection with the motility of the sphenoid bone. So whatever happens to the sphenoid is going to have direct influence over all the facial bones.

During the normal respiratory cycle, when the sphenobasilar synchondrosis moves into flexion, the sphenoid rises at its posterior connection with the occiput, the anterior end of the sphenoid dips slightly, the posterior end of the ethmoid dips with it, while the anterior end rises. Immediately beneath the perpendicular plate of the ethmoid is the vomer. The rocking motion of the sphenoid and ethmoid creates a motion within the vomer; as the sphenoid nosedives, the movement of the vomer affects the sphenoid sinus acting through the rostrum. In addition, the lateral side of each frontal bone is carried laterally by the large, angular, frontosphenoidal articulations. They're carried laterally during inhalation and inwardly during exhalation. Due to the expansibility of the bone itself, the various ethmoid sinuses are also expanding laterally in inhalation and inwardly during exhalation. So the ethmoid and frontal sinuses have their back-and-fro motion during inhalation and exhalation, which acts as a pump to permit normal sinus drainage.

Given all this, in the diagnosis and treatment of sinus problems, we're not too concerned about the sinus itself. That's the end organ that's doing the complaining; it is bound into inactivity and is showing the disturbance deep within its mucous walls as a congested phase. The sinus condition is the end result of the problem. The bug that settled into that sinus is also in all the other sinuses that are not disturbed. But that particular sinus has become restricted. Perhaps there was a little blow on the forehead, more or less freezing the free action of the frontal bones, not allowing them to move freely during inhalation and exhalation; so the plumber's friend is involved. When we restrict the plumber's friend, that allows stasis within that sinus, and any bug within it gets a fertile field in which to set up a sinus irritation. If the maxillary sinus gets an infection in it, almost invariably you can go back to the temporal or zygomatic bone on the same side, and you'll find there is a loss of the normal mobility which is working on that maxillary sinus.

Another aspect we haven't touched upon is the little palatine bones. These small bones can have big effects. We once spent three solid days with Dr. Sutherland just studying the palatine bone. The palatine affects the area around the sphenopalatine ganglion, which receives and sends out orders through the autonomic nerves to all the sinuses and a lot of other important structures of the facial mechanism.

To recapitulate, sinus problems are not necessarily due to a specific infection in a given sinus at any given time. Each sinus within the facial mechanism depends for its normal functioning upon a plumber's friend, which in turn is dependent upon a normal mechanism deep within the cranial mechanism. It can seem to be difficult to visualize this cranial and facial mechanism as one unit. Yet it isn't difficult when you get to thinking about it. There is a sphenobasilar synchondrosis rising and falling during inhalation and exhalation and three sickles—the falx cerebri, right tentorium, and left tentorium—moving forward and expanding during inhalation and narrowing during exhalation. The membranes are controlling the movements of the temporal and sphenoid bones, which in turn are controlling the movements of the 14 facial bones, which in turn are controlling the rhythmic, to-and-fro movements of the various sinus mechanisms.

In chronic cases, as the cranial mechanism is restored to normal functioning, there can be a delay in the resolution of all the associated symptoms. Chronic congested cells only know how to make too much mucous. More healthy cells at the basement level of development work their way to the maturity of surface cellular structure and only form as much mucous as is physiologically needed. In severe cases, this can take three months.

DELAY FIX FOR cHRonic Sinusitis

DENTAL MEMBRANOUS ARTICULAR STRAINS
This paper was dated September 1, 1984.

DENTAL MEMBRANOUS ARTICULAR STRAINS are a frequent source of problems found in facial mechanics. In one unusual case I treated, a dental device could have led to total disability and death. A man, age 62 years, had a dental device made of metal that fit into the roof of his mouth. The device was kept firmly in place by prongs anchored to the posterior maxillary teeth. It extended forward to include the hard palate of the maxillary bones. He wore it continuously, taking it out only for cleaning.

Within six months after getting the device, he developed grand mal seizures and other symptoms of disability. This continued for about three months before he sought osteopathic care; his condition was gradually worsening as time passed. My initial examination revealed that, with the device in his mouth, his total anatomicophysiological involuntary mechanisms were locked, with extension of his midline structures and internal rotation of his bilateral structures. This included all the body's fascias and related tissues, not just the craniosacral mechanism. There was no palpable involuntary mobility towards the flexion-external rotation pattern of physiological motion.

With the device removed, treatment was administered to initiate a restoration of the involuntary flexion of midline structures and external rotation of bilateral structures towards its rhythmic cycle of function. In about 30 minutes, a palpable effort on the mechanism's part toward an involuntary flexion phase was faintly present, and the treatment was finished for that day. The patient was told to return in two days and not to use the dental device.

He returned in two days with palpable evidence of a more healthful, alternate involuntary mobility throughout the body and fascia, including the craniosacral mechanism, not with the strength as found in health, but at least, it was present. To test the effects of the device, he was requested to replace it in his mouth while his involuntary mobile mechanisms were monitored through palpation at the sacrum. The response was immediate. His involuntary craniosacral mechanism and fascial tissues went into an extension-internal rotation pattern, completely occluding any rhythmic involuntary flexion-external rotation phase of functioning. The time involved for this transition was 30 seconds to one minute. The device was removed and evidence of the return of alternate involuntary movement towards the 8-to-10-times-per-minute, rhythmic health cycle could be palpated. He was told to cease using the dental device.

With supportive treatment at irregular intervals (because he lived out of town) over a period of several months, his grand mal seizures and other disabilities gradually were alleviated. The question arises: What would have been the outcome of his health pattern if he had continued to use this device? When he was asked this question, his answer was, "Death." His answer is physiologically correct. When a body dies, its mechanisms go into extension and internal rotation.

This extreme and unusual case as well as the lesser traumatic problems to be described later demonstrate the need to know and understand what is health in facial, involuntary, anatomicophysiological mobility and function. The face is the anterior portion of the craniosacral mechanism and is on the forepart of the neurocranium. The craniosacral mechanism includes the articular mechanisms of the sphenoid, occiput, temporals, frontal(s), and parietals; the to-and-fro mobility of the reciprocal tension membrane; the coiling and uncoiling motility of the central nervous system; the fluctuation of the cerebrospinal fluid; and the involuntary mobility of the sacrum between the ilia.

The face is composed of 15 bones. These are the ethmoid, two zygomatics, two maxillae, two palatines, vomer, two nasals, two lacrimals, two inferior conchae, and the mandible. Technically the ethmoid belongs to the cranial base, but it is considered here. There are 79 articulations in the face and 43 articulations in the neurocranium.

The involuntary mobility mechanisms of the face are controlled by the sphenoid with exception of the mandible, which is controlled by the occiput and temporals. The sphenoid is part of the main drive shaft in the cranial base, and it directly articulates with eight facial bones and, through these eight, influences all the others. It is this mobility of the sphenoidal-facial unit of function, in reciprocal integrated mobility with the occipital-temporal-mandibular unit of function, that determines the quality of life for the face and its mucous membranes, sinuses, muscles and ligaments, trigeminal and sphenopalatine ganglia, orbital and nasopharyngeal cavities and their contents, and venous and lymphatic function.

Further understanding as to what is health in the face is to know that body physiology as a whole expresses life in motion through both voluntary and involuntary mobility, while the craniosacral mechanism is basically expressed through involuntary mobility. Nevertheless, body physiology is one unit of integrated activity–that which is voluntary movement becomes part of the activity of the involuntary craniosacral mechanism, and involuntary activity of the craniosacral mechanism is palpable throughout the total body, whether the voluntary movement is at rest or in use.

What is this simple rhythm of life in the involuntary activity of the craniosacral mechanism? It is a vital 8-to-10-times-per-minute cycle fluctuation of the cerebrospinal fluid, flexion of all midline structures and external rotation of all bilateral structures alternating with extension and internal rotation. It is present and palpable throughout life, bathing and moving every cell of the body rhythmically. The relative health of the face and its 79 articulations is dependent upon this vital interchange.

A case in point is the man who came into the office with a complaint of chronic maxillary and sphenoidal sinusitis over a period of ten years. Functionally, each sinus has a plunger-like mechanism, which pumps its individual sinus and keeps it aerated. The zygomatics are the pumps for the maxillary sinuses, and the vomer is the pump for the sphenoid sinus. In his case, they were not doing their job, and the mucous membranes were in a state of stasis. Corrective treatment to restore basic involuntary mobility for the zygomatics and vomer allowed the mucous membranes of the sinuses to heal from their bottom layer to the surface in three months, and the patient was in health for that area.

Considering the complexity of the facial mechanisms, there are multiple ways in which dental membranous articular strains can be found to be interfering with the inherent, basic involuntary mobility of the face. I spoke to a dentist about this problem, and he offered the following list of procedures, which show a potential for traumatic results: improperly applied occlusal equilibration techniques, mass crowning of teeth, incorrect use of splints for the temporomandibular joint problems, and traumatic extraction of teeth that have variations in their root system, to name a few. To prevent as much trauma as possible in the extraction of teeth, he dissects the tooth to be pulled so as to pull each root in its plane of motion rather than pulling the whole tooth and injuring the jaw bone. This discussion should not imply that the use of all dental devices is harmful—the majority of them are beneficial in their applications for specific needs.

Another type of dental membranous articular strain following a tooth extraction involves the temporal, sphenoid, maxilla, and mandible. The findings on the side of strain are: The temporal bone with its petrous portion is in internal rotation; the pterygoid process of the sphenoid is upward and lateral; the maxillary is downward, and the mandible is in malalignment at its articulation. The mechanics of this strain can begin with the dental chair, if there is a V-shaped headrest. The patient's occiput rests upon the V-shaped headrest so as to cause compression upon the mastoid portion of the temporals immediately anterior to the lambdoidal suture. With the occiput and temporals relatively immobilized, the dentist applies inward side-leverage downward on the opposite side, causing tension upon the sphenomandibular ligament and swinging the pterygoid process on the lesion side upward and laterally.

Editor's note: The V-shaped headrest is rarely found in dental offices anymore, but traumatic strains can still develop.

The results of this type of trauma, involving the unit of the occiput, temporal, mandible, maxilla, and sphenoid, can affect the trigeminal and sphenopalatine ganglia and lead to symptoms of facial neuralgia or tic douloureux. The increased tensity of the reciprocal tension membrane within the neurocranium on the lesion side plays an important role in the maintenance of this lesion complex during the months and years the patient may carry this strain. A woman with this type of strain developed a severe tic douloureux 11 years ago, after the extraction of a tooth. She has been under corrective treatment for four years and is slowly progressing towards health for this sick fifth cranial nerve. The more modern, relatively flat headrests on dental chairs and the elevator type of dental tools for the extraction of teeth have lessened the potential for this type of strain.

Most dental membranous articular strains are not diagnosed or treated at the time of their production but are found weeks, months, or years later by skilled palpatory diagnosis of the mobility patterns of the structures involved, which demonstrate a loss of the innate basic involuntary mobility. If one understands the mechanics of this multiple facial articular functioning, one can read the areas of health and compare those with the areas of strain. Following a treatment, one can reevaluate the health and stress areas to determine the quality of the treatment results.

The important factor to consider in palpatory diagnosis and treatment is not just the correction of lesion mechanics; it is the restoration of membranous articular health and the return of the basic rhythm of involuntary mobility. This restoration is what gave the man with the dental device an opportunity to head in the direction of health again. This restoration also returned mobility of the plunger-like pumps, the zygomatics and vomer, in the case of chronic sinusitis. This seeking of health for facial functioning applies equally for all dental membranous articular strains.

THE EYE
Practical Application of the Cranial Concept to the Common Refractive and Muscular Disturbances of the Eye
This paper was dated January 1958.

THE CRANIAL CONCEPT HAS tremendous possibilities to offer in the field of the common refractive and muscular disturbances of the eye. The limiting factors for aid in these cases are those of the degree of organic disability in the disease processes and the operator's understanding and skill as a technician in the cranial concept. The more complete his knowledge of the cranial mechanism, the more opportunity he will see to reverse the pathological processes under observation.

Eye Muscle Disturbances

The muscular disturbances of the eye are generally due to neurological disturbances in the structures that innervate the involved muscles. A partial outline would include: extrinsic eye muscle palsy, palsy of associated eye movements or gaze palsy, convergence-divergence disturbances, and intrinsic eye muscle palsy. To this may be added disturbances of the seventh cranial nerve, with palpebral fissure disturbances, and fifth cranial nerve disturbances as they affect the orbit.

Extrinsic eye muscle palsies affect the various patterns of movement within the eye. Strabismus, or convergence-divergence disturbance, is a deviation of the eye, which the patient cannot overcome. The visual axes assume a position relative to each other different from the normal. The various forms of strabismus are spoken of as tropias, their direction being indicated by the appropriate prefix, such as esotropia or exotropia.

The term "palsy" refers to both paralysis and paresis and may involve cranial nerves III, IV, VI, or a combination thereof. There will be different clinical findings depending on which part of which nerve is primarily involved. Possible locations of pathology and disturbance include nuclear, medial and dorsal longitudinal fasciculi, root, basal, cavernous, fissure, apex, neuritic, and to this, for purposes of discussion in the cranial concept, will be added the calcarine fissure. The etiology of eye muscle palsy can be from an array of disease or physiological disturbances. These include brain injury, tumors, central nervous system infections or neurologic diseases, vascular problems, and congenital palsies. There can also be diseases of the nerves themselves, such as polyneuritis and other systemic disease conditions. To this list may be added the anatomical-physiological factors known to the cranial concept. A complete and thorough knowledge of the anatomy and physiology of the cranium and orbit will add greatly to the insight into the majority of these disease processes, as well as adding many factors for more complete diagnosis and potential treatment.

For example, disturbance in the area of the calcarine fissure would imply that there is lesion potential in the area of the tentorium cerebelli and the Sutherland fulcrum. Dr. Sutherland used to refer to this fact in his discussion of visual field disturbances. A boy who had the difficulty of perceiving two different-sized images had the physical finding of a flattened occiput on one side in the interparietal area. Treatment to this area, which necessarily would be directed to freeing the Sutherland fulcrum and tentorium cerebelli as well as molding the disturbed occiput, resulted in remarkable improvement in his visual pattern.

In nuclear disturbances of the III, IV, or VI cranial nerves, potential pathology in the context of the cranial concept would be in the area of the fourth ventricle and the brain stem. These could include trauma to the base of the skull, occipitomastoid lesion, occipitoatlantal lesions, cervical or upper thoracic lesions, disturbances of the fourth ventricle and its cerebrospinal fluid content, and restrictions of the Sutherland fulcrum.

As the nerves are followed forward toward the orbit, the next area to consider is the brain stem and midbrain. Here the cranial concept suggests a number of potential pathological factors: sphenobasilar synchondrosis compression, traumatic torsion or sidebending-rotation patterns, vertical or lateral strain patterns, condylar parts compression, the petrous portion of the temporals in any of its diverse patterns, and dental traumatic patterns. The tentorium cerebelli and the Sutherland fulcrum are again in the picture. It will be remembered that these cranial nerves slip into the cavernous sinus through folds of the dura mater near the posterior clinoid processes. In this way, disturbances in the pull on the dura in this area can contribute to eye nerve palsies.

The next area is the cavernous sinus and the area of the optic chiasm. Here, potential primary lesions will be found in the sphenoid bone and its relationships. The sphenoid is one of the most important osseous structures to consider in eye pathology. It articulates with all the bones of the cranium and five of the face—the two zygomatics, the two palatines and the vomer. Its lesion potentials are as numerous as its articular maze. The sphenoid is also involved in all the strains of the sphenobasilar synchondrosis.

In considering the cavernous sinus, remember that it is part of the membranous system that aids in the venous drainage of the eye. Diseases affecting membranes—such as encephalitis, meningitis, and toxic states—can have serious effects resulting in eye disturbances. The tone quality of the meningeal membranes must be perfect to insure good venous drainage from the skull and the orbits. The tone quality of the membranes after encephalitis, meningitis, or toxic states may be likened to that of wet cardboard or several folds of damp Kleenex. It is dull, flat, and has lost its capacity for reciprocal tension. It is almost impossible to secure lesion reduction within the cranial structures with this serious loss of tone of the reciprocal tension membranes. If a correction is made while the patient is on the table, his getting up to leave the room is all that is necessary to cause a reoccurrence of his entire lesion pattern. Much work is needed here to restore the normal tone quality before any attempt is made to correct osseous cranial patterns. For several visits, the use of cerebrospinal fluid mechanics, such as the compression of the fourth ventricle and the alternating lateral fluctuation techniques, seems to offer the possibility of the quickest recovery of the tone quality of the membranes in these disease conditions.

The author has had some rather dramatic results in correcting eye palsies following meningitis or encephalitis by restoring the tone quality of the membranes to bring them back to their normal reciprocal tension action. However, achieving these dramatic results took time. It takes time to restore this vital function. The more quickly these pathologies can be treated following illness, the shorter the time that a patient must suffer from disabilities.

This is another area where the Sutherland fulcrum is involved. The Sutherland fulcrum contains the straight sinus, which provides the venous drainage for the great cerebral vein of Galen, which drains the areas associated with the medial and dorsal longitudinal fascicular types of eye nerve palsy. Any loss of tone quality within the dura mater of the cranium is going to reflect itself into the Sutherland fulcrum and in turn be reflected by the Sutherland fulcrum in its functional capacities in relation to the dura mater of the cranium. This effect extends to include the sacrum through the dural sheath. The presence of any whiplash injury, recent or old, will add its patterns of disabilities to the functioning of the Sutherland fulcrum. Eye symptoms are common after whiplash injuries. It is important to recall that the sacral fixations at the second sacral segment following a whiplash injury may be the maintaining factor for the entire syndrome.

The Sutherland fulcrum serves as a focusing agent for the reciprocal tension membranes. Its full physiological functioning is essential for normal cranial or orbital mechanics. Through the falx cerebri, it influences the parietals, ethmoid, and sphenoid areas; through the tentorium cerebelli, it reaches the temporals, occiput, and parietals. The reciprocal tension membrane is continuous with the lining dura mater of the entire skull and the sheath following the spinal cord and cauda equina to the sacrum. Like any lever, the Sutherland fulcrum acts over a still point where the falx adjoins the tentorium. It is an

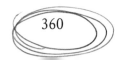

automatic, shifting, suspension fulcrum whose still point can be read by the skilled hands of the cranial technician. The operator can initiate the potency in this still point for the skillful reduction of reciprocal tension membrane strains. He can determine and influence cranial and orbital functioning, if he understands this lever principle with its automatic-shifting-suspension-fulcrum capacities.

The cranial nerves traveling to the eye then pass into the superior orbital fissures of the sphenoid, the apex, and the orbit itself. The eye muscles take their origins from the annulus tendon of Zinn (common annular tendon). This is oval on cross section and encloses the optic foramen and part of the medial end of the superior orbital fissure. It is divided into two parts: the lower tendon of Lockwood, which is attached to the inferior root of the lesser wing of the sphenoid and gives origin to part of the medial and lateral rectus muscles and all of the inferior rectus muscle; and the upper tendon of Lockwood, which is attached to the body of the sphenoid and gives origin to part of the medial and lateral rectus muscles and all of the superior rectus muscle.

Developmental Anatomy of the Sphenoid: Because of the importance that the epiphyseal units of the sphenoid can play in eye muscle palsies as well as in refractive errors of the eyes, it is well to review the development of the sphenoid and the times that the various epiphyseal units become a part of the matured sphenoid bone.

Up to about the eighth month of fetal life, the sphenoid bone consists of two distinct parts: a posterior or post-sphenoid part, which comprises the pituitary fossa, the greater wings, and the pterygoid processes; and an anterior or pre-sphenoid part, to which the anterior part of the body and the lesser wings belong. It develops from 14 centers: 8 for the post-sphenoid and 6 for the pre-sphenoid.

In the posterior sphenoid division, the first nuclei to appear are those for the greater wings. They make their appearance between the foramen rotundum and foramen ovale about the eighth week, and from them the external pterygoid plates are also formed. Soon after, the nuclei for the posterior part of the body appear, one on either side of the sella turcica, and become blended together about the middle of fetal life. About the fourth month the remaining four centers appear, those for the internal pterygoid plates being ossified in membrane and becoming joined to the external pterygoid plate about the sixth month. The centers for the lingulae speedily become joined to the rest of the bone.

In the pre-sphenoid division, the first nuclei to appear are those for the lesser wings. They make their appearance about the ninth week, at the outer borders of the optic foramina. Shortly after, a second pair of nuclei appear on the inner side of the foramina and become united, forming the front part of the body of the bone. The remaining two centers for the sphenoidal turbinated bones (conchae) do not make their appearance until the end of the third year.

The pre-sphenoid is united to the body of the post-sphenoid about the eighth fetal month. Thus, at birth the bones consist of three pieces— the body in the center and on each side the great wings with the pterygoid processes. The lesser wings become joined to the body at about the time of birth. By the first year after birth, the greater wings and body are united. From the tenth to the twelfth year, the membranous vault bones are partially united to the sphenoid, their junction being complete by the twentieth year. Lastly, the sphenoid joins with the occiput from the eighteenth to the twenty-fifth year.

The following muscles have their attachment to the sphenoid bone: the temporalis, external pterygoids, internal pterygoids, superior constrictor, tensor palatini, levator palpebrae, superior oblique oculi, superior recti, medial recti, inferior recti, and lateral recti.

Knowing this detailed information is important when one wants to correct the distortions that may occur at birth in patients with orbital muscle palsies. The time to get to these problems is as soon after birth as is reasonably possible to get the maximum correction for the bent-twig patterns that appear. Since the lesser wings along with the optic foramen are the origin for most of the muscles controlling the eyeball and since they fuse about the time of birth, it behooves the cranial technician to get an early start on these problems. If there is disturbance in this area, it may be only one portion of the disturbances affecting the cranial base and mechanism. The whole picture must be unfolded as completely as possible for permanent benefit. These osseous lesions are also intricately tied in with the total reciprocal tension membrane pattern because there are no sutural articulations in the skull at birth. One has until almost the end of the first year after birth to correct the disturbances associated with the great wings of the sphenoid before these parts become part of the permanent bone structure of the sphenoid and less responsive to change.

The orbit is composed of seven bones: the sphenoid with its lesser and greater wings, ethmoid, lacrimal, maxillary, zygomatic, frontal, and the little orbital plate of the palatine. It is the free and easy, normal articular relationship between these units that makes for normal orbital functioning and contributes to normal eyeball functioning. A disturbance in any of these units can be a contributing factor to orbital and eyeball pathology.

There are 12 muscles within the orbit: the six extraocular muscles and the ciliaris, dilator pupillae, sphincter pupillae, orbicularis, orbitalis, and levator palpebrae. The six extraocular muscles are the ones concerned in eye muscle palsy. All have their origin around the optic foramen except for the inferior oblique, which originates from the medial side of the orbital plate of the maxilla. The superior oblique takes its origin from the optic foramen and passes through a trochlea, a pulley-like arrangement, on the medial side of the orbital surface of the frontal bone. All six muscles have their insertion into the sclera of the eyeball near its forward pole. The oculomotor nerve supplies the inferior oblique, inferior rectus, medial rectus, and superior rectus as well as the levator palpebrae muscle and the sphincter pupillae. The trochlear nerve supplies the superior oblique, and the abducens supplies the lateral rectus.

Given this anatomy, bent twig patterns or trauma to the lesser wings of the sphenoid can affect the majority of the muscles of the eyeball; trauma to the frontal bone can affect the action of the superior oblique muscle; and trauma to the maxilla can affect the inferior oblique muscle. Trauma is rarely confined to one osseous unit, and usually its effects will be transmitted to all the osseous units of the orbit. Practically every child who is brought for diagnosis with a serious cranial distortion will exhibit some type of eye muscle palsy or refractive problem.

A traumatic pattern resulting from injury to any part of the membranous vault creates a potential for eye muscle pathology, either through injury to the nerve tracts or to disturbances of the eye muscles themselves. Blows to the vertex have their contrecoup effect upon the condylar parts, occipitomastoid areas, sphenobasilar synchondrosis, or directed forward toward the optic chiasm and the orbit. Blows upon the posterior part of the skull commonly produce symptoms of double or blurred vision. Traumatic occipitomastoid lesions have a direct effect on visual disturbances to the same side through venous sinus drainage impairment and contrecoup effects to the vision of the opposite side.

Next, a few words will be added concerning intrinsic eye muscle palsy. These muscles include the ciliaris, dilator pupillae, and sphincter pupillae. The ciliaris affects the shape of the lens in visual accommodation. Its nerve supply is the short ciliary nerves via the ciliary ganglion. These nerves have their origin from three sources. The sensory division comes from the nasociliary nerve, which is part of the ophthalmic division of cranial nerve V and supplies the intraocular structures. The parasympathetic fibers come from the inferior division of cranial nerve III and supplies the sphincter pupillae. The sympathetic division is derived from the superior cervical ganglion and is distributed to the dilator pupillae, ciliary muscle, and blood vessels of the eye. The superior cervical ganglion receives its fibers from the upper thoracic sympathetic ganglia. Thus, it is important to normalize

the cervical and thoracic areas of the spine as well as the cranial structures, if the patient is to receive the total benefit of treatment. The
second thoracic area is an important segmental stress area in eye pathologies.

Eye pathology described

Refractive Errors of the Eye

The refractive errors of the eye most commonly seen are myopia,
hyperopia, presbyopia, and astigmatism. In myopia, or nearsighted-
ness, the rays of light are focused in front of the retina, while in hyperopia, or farsightedness, they focus in back of the retina. In presbyopia, there is impairment, associated with aging, from the
diminution in the power of accommodation due to a loss of elasticity
of the crystalline lens, causing the near point of distinct vision to be
removed farther from the eye. Finally, in astigmatism, the ray of light
is not sharply focused upon the retina due to defective curvature of
the refractive surfaces of the eye. These problems can occur singly in
a patient or can be seen in combination. These phenomena are not
fixed; they do not remain the same year in and year out.

The very fact that there is a shifting character in these changes in
the refractively disturbed eye is a clue to the potential for modification of these patterns. If they were fixed patterns, the potential for
modifying them would be considerably lessened. The eyeball, with its
intrinsic refractive surfaces, is a liquid mass in a sclerous envelope
and subject to the forces that surround it in its orbital home. It responds readily to any environmental change, and the intraocular
change is reflected as a refractive pattern.

Each of the refractive error patterns—the myopias, hyperopias, and
astigmatisms—can be broken down into various classifications and
descriptions. The ones that might be of greatest interest at this point
are the axial myopia and axial hyperopia. In axial myopia, there is an
elongation of the axis of the eyeball. Might it not be due to an extension pattern of the skull with an elongated orbit affecting the shape of
the eyeball so that the rays of light would fall in front of the retina?
And in the axial hyperopia, might it not be due to a flexion pattern of

the skull foreshortening the orbit and the eyeball so that the rays of light would tend to focus in back of the retina? Or in a marked torsion pattern, one eye might show the hyperopia disturbance and the other a myopia condition. The same possibility might occur in a marked sidebending-rotation pattern, although to a lesser degree.

The astigmatic patterns are much more numerous in their variation than are the others. There are several refractive surfaces within the eye, and the name of the astigmatism will vary according to the type of refractive medium involved. The cornea, the lens, and the vitreous humor all play their roles in these disturbances. Here, again, the fluid mass of the eye in its sclerous envelope is responding to environmental changes of the orbital cavity. Specific pathologies in relation to various diseases of these mediums are major contributing factors to astigmatism. Any pattern other than the normal functioning orbital cavity will potentially show the patterns of some type of astigmatism. In treating astigmatism, it is well to try to discover some form of unphysiologic abnormality within the orbital cavity or some form of trauma that has so changed the physiologic capacity as to create the situation for astigmatic disturbances.

In this discussion, I have tried to cover the broad field of these disturbances in a manner that would give the operator an opportunity to make a diagnosis and form the foundation for a treatment program. When one is using the cranial concept in the analysis of eye muscle palsy or refractive error, a thorough knowledge of the anatomy and physiology of the skull and orbit is as valuable a tool for diagnosis and treatment as is the knowledge of the specifically named disease and its symptomatology, perhaps even more so. The same contributing factors in two individuals might well manifest as different, specifically named pathologies because of the difference in their anatomicophysiological makeups. With anatomical and physiological knowledge, the operator is in a position to determine more accurately the site of beginning or existing pathology and is in a better position to prescribe a treatment program for that case.

The cranial concept offers the operator an opportunity to develop an understanding of the pathology present with far greater insight than the mere review of the end products of the pathology as manifested by the symptomatology and the gross pathological picture. With the knowledge of the cranial concept, the operator is able to read the functioning picture of the pathological status of the disorder. It is to his advantage to try to read into the skull, orbital cavity, cervical and thoracic areas—to form as complete an analysis of all the factors present as is possible. And the sacrum should be added to this picture if a whiplash injury was ever a part of the patient's history. Try to bring together a picture which will serve as a total concept of why this patient exhibits this pattern of disability that has brought him to the office. If there is a traumatic pattern that contributed to his disability, it is absolutely essential to take into account the elements of such force as it took to produce the trauma, the direction it came from, the quantity and quality of its action, and the degree to which this force is still an operative factor in the traumatic pattern under observation. It is a physiological fact that one can apparently correct the cranial distortions, the malalignments of the orbital units, and the individual anatomical disturbances and still not eliminate the reoccurrence of the patient's disability. What has been left out of the picture? Correction of these disturbed anatomical units can take place to the operator's satisfaction while the patient is in the office, but if the total picture is to be understood, the force that brought that picture into manifestation and is still acting as a focus for the pattern must be recognized. When that patient resumes his active, day-to-day living, this added focus of force will remold the newly corrected, anatomical picture back into a modification of the original pathological phenomena. The force and its focus have become a physiological unit along with the anatomical units, and this unit seeks to establish the only reciprocal tension balance it knows—that of the anatomical-physiological pattern plus the force.

It is imperative to understand this focus of force and resolve it so that the normal anatomical-physiological patterns of the patient's body can reestablish their full, functional capacity. The operator can learn to read these force fields within the patient's problem with a fairly high degree of skill. He can then direct the resolution of them by creating as complete an anatomical-physiological picture of the total pattern as is possible to make at the time of diagnosis. Thus, the normal factors of the inherent living body will have the chance to resolve the force factors that have been added to the picture, and the normal factors will again gain the ascendancy in the patient's body and correct the pathologies present. The eventual recovery rate will be greatly increased by this procedure.

The osteopathic and cranial concept offers more than mere palliative relief. It is a total understanding of the patient and his problem that presents a challenge in every case that comes to us for diagnosis and treatment.

BIBLIOGRAPHY

* Still, Andrew Taylor. *Autobiography of Andrew T. Still.* 1905. Reprint, American Academy of Osteopathy, 1981.

* _____. *Osteopathy: Research and Practice.* 1910. Reprint, Seattle: Eastland Press, 1992.

* _____. *Philosophy of Osteopathy.* 1899. Reprint, American Academy of Osteopathy, 1977.

≈ Sutherland, William Garner. *Contributions of Thought: Collected Writings of William Garner Sutherland, D.O.* Edited by Adah Strand Sutherland and Anne L. Wales. Sutherland Cranial Teaching Foundation, Inc. 1967.

≈ _____. *Teachings in the Science of Osteopathy.* Edited by Anne L. Wales. Sutherland Cranial Teaching Foundation, Inc., 1990.

† _____. *The Cranial Bowl.* 1939. Reprint, The Cranial Academy, 1994.

Books available from:

* The American Academy of Osteopathy, 3500 DePauw Blvd., Indianapolis, Indiana 46268. Phone: (317) 879-1881.

≈ The Sutherland Cranial Teaching Foundation, Inc., 4116 Hartwood Dr., Fort Worth, Texas 76109. Phone: (817) 735-2498.

† The Cranial Academy, 8606 Allisonville Rd., Indianapolis, Indiana 46250. Phone: (317) 594-0411.

ABOUT THE SUTHERLAND CRANIAL TEACHING
FOUNDATION, INC.

THE SUTHERLAND CRANIAL TEACHING FOUNDATION, INC. is a not-for-profit organization which was established in 1953 by Dr. Sutherland and senior members of his teaching faculty. Dr. Sutherland conceived of the foundation as a way of providing a continuity for his teaching.

Dr. Sutherland was the first president of the foundation, serving until the time of his death in 1954. The presidents who followed him were Howard Lippincott, D.O., Rollin E. Becker, D.O., John H. Harakal, D.O., and Michael P. Burruano, D.O. In 2006, Melicien Tettambel D.O. became the sixth president of the organization.

The charter of the Sutherland Cranial Teaching Foundation calls for the organization to dedicate itself to purely educational activities. It specifically states its objective as using its resources to establish the principles of osteopathy in the cranial field as conceived and developed by William Garner Sutherland, to disseminate a general knowledge of these principles and the therapeutic indication for this approach to treatment, to encourage and assist physicians in osteopathy, and to stimulate continued study and greater proficiency on the part of those practicing osteopathy in the cranial field.

In its endeavor to carry out these objectives the Sutherland Cranial Teaching Foundation supports research, produces publications, and offers both basic and continuing studies courses. As a not-for-profit educational foundation it accepts charitable contribution to support its work of perpetuating and disseminating the teachings in the science of osteopathy as expanded by William Garner Sutherland, D.O. The current address of the SCTF is 4116 Hartwood Dr., Fort Worth, Texas 76109.

ABOUT THE EDITOR

RACHEL E. BROOKS, M.D. met Dr. Rollin Becker in 1975, just before she entered the University of Michigan Medical School. That first meeting with Dr. Becker inspired her to pursue the study and practice of osteopathy. She remained in contact with Dr. Becker through medical school, graduated in 1979, and in 1980 took her first formal course in osteopathy in the cranial field with the Sutherland Cranial Teaching Foundation.

After completing a residency in physical medicine and rehabilitation, she moved to Massachusetts in 1982 and began her private practice in osteopathy the following year. In 1986, she first taught with the Sutherland Cranial Teaching Foundation (SCTF) and served as a member of its board of trustees from 1988 through 2004. Over the years she has taught a variety of courses and worked on numerous publication projects. Her first editorial project was assisting Anne Wales, D.O. in the editing of *Teachings of the Science of Osteopathy*. Since then she has worked on a number of editing projects for the SCTF and her own Stillness Press, LLC.

Dr. Becker provided the initial inspiration for Dr. Brooks, profoundly influenced her approach to osteopathy, and continues to inspire her work. Dr. Brooks currently is in private practice in Portland, Oregon.

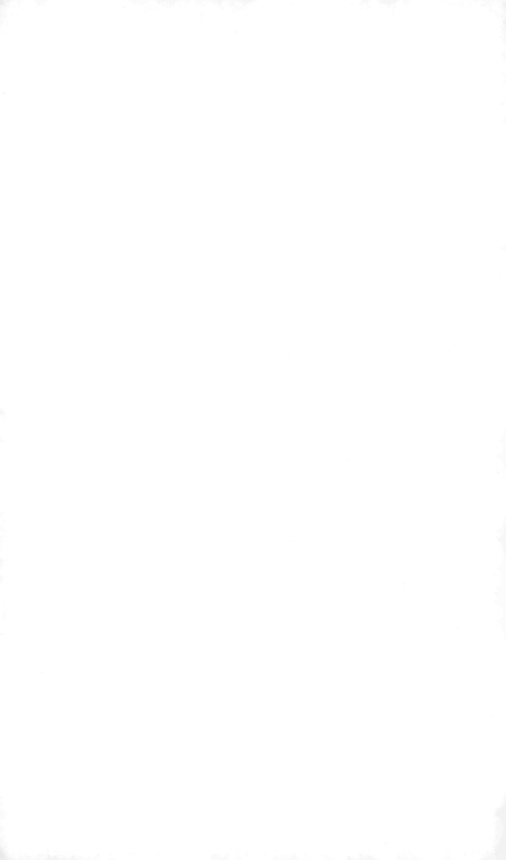

INDEX

Bold type indicates chapter heading or subsection.